MEDICAL ASTROLOGY
IN ACTION

The Transits of Health

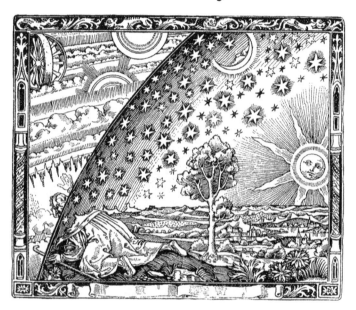

JUDITH HILL

Sequel to:
Medical Astrology:
A Guide to Planetary Pathology

Foreword by Matthew Wood

MEDICAL ASTROLOGY IN ACTION
The Transits of Health
Sequel to: *Medical Astrology:*
A Guide to Planetary Pathology

by Judith Hill

Edited by Mark Polit
Design, Layout, Cover:
Dawn King Fine Design

STELLIUM
P R E S S

Published in 2019 by Stellium Press
Portland, Oregon
Copyright © 2019 by Judith Hill
JudithHillAstrology.com

ISBN: 1-883376-75-0
ISBN: 978-1-883376-75-8

Medical Disclaimer:
The following information is intended for general informational purposes only, and does not constitute medical diagnosis, opinion, or advice. Individuals should always seek their physician's approval before considering any suggestions made in this book. Any application of the information set forth in the following pages is at the reader's discretion, and is his or her sole responsibility.

Revised Edition 2019
Illustrations are by Judith Hill unless otherwise specified.
Cover Illustration: "Flammarion Man" by unknown artist.
Facing page: Depiction of the god Mercury with flute & caduceus,
by German engraver Hans Burgkmair.

DEDICATION

For wise physicians, skilled astrologers
and great herbalists.

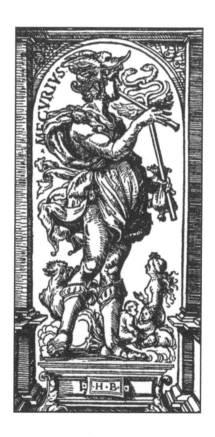

ACKNOWLEDGMENTS

Gratitude is due my dear friend of decades, and research colleague Mark Polit for his patient editing direction, wisdom and support. And, to Dawn King, my guardian angel, for her immeasurable assistance in the design, typesetting, editing, and timely completion of this project.

Salutations are due to three remarkable friends of profound influence to my life and work, who departed Earth during this book's formation: the great maverick physicist Buryl Payne, Ph.D.; the remarkable publisher Robert M. Briggs; and my beloved friend and fellow harmonica player, that old Texas cowboy turned vegetarian, Will Thompson.

CONTENTS

FOREWORD

There are very few books in print, in the astrological field on the subject of medicine, that detail the distinctive physical and medical influences of *transiting* planets and Lunar Nodes upon the human body as reflected in the natal chart. In one stroke, in this historic tome, Judith Hill has remedied that situation.

Here, from the pen of one of the most experienced medical astrologers in modern times is a book that makes the subject easy-to-understand. Basically, the planets are the "energies" (hot, cold, damp, dry, tense, relaxed), the signs are the zones and major organs, and the angles and aspects bring out the curative or adverse health effects observable from the chart. In addition, Judith has added sections on timing of disease-onset and what times are best for operations and medical procedures.

As if this were not enough, our author is deeply acquainted with the properties of medicinal herbs, gemstones, and other therapeutic tools. I don't mean this in the abstract: Judith has proven their properties in practice, not in theory only. As a professional herbalist, I attest to her acumen in the field.

Medical astrology, pragmatically grounded in the body, rather than in the more subjective psychological or social worlds, brings clarity to the whole endeavor of astrology. Hence, it is a subject all serious astrologers should become familiar with. Here's their chance.

It is quite possible that astrology was invented in large part for the purpose of medical evaluation. From the original Greek texts, the late Robert Schmidt effectively showed that the originator of astrology was the Greek mathematician, priest, lawgiver, and medical doctor, Eudoxus of Cnidos, a contemporary of Plato and Aristotle. Schmidt's material is not yet published, and may never be (he did not receive the support of the astrological world), so this valuable contribution to astrological history and the understanding of our science, will probably remain no more than a rumor.

In the ancient world, the use of the chart of decumbiture (the moment the patient went to bed or asked for help) was the standard method of medical astrology. Today, both the decumbiture and natal chart are used. The latter is particularly popular, and is the approach used here.

The present work is based on Renaissance medical astrology, which evolved since ancient times and is also different in some details from modern practice. Yet, it is the same system, shining through, from Eudoxus to the present: signs, planets, aspects, houses. Astrology is such a wide ranging field that the individual needs to choose their approach, including whether they want to be Greek, Ptolemaic, Arabic, Jewish, Byzantine, Medieval, Renaissance, or Modern, any of which was available in many varieties. Judith is virtually "an incarnation" of Renaissance astrology, when the medical element of the art was at a peak. She carries this heritage gift down to the present, in a form totally suited to the Modern astrologer. All is here, in abundant detail, proven by a lifetime of experience.

– Matthew Wood, MSc *(Herbal Medicine),*
American Herbalists Guild
The Matthew Wood Institute of Herbalism

INTRODUCTION

At birth, the current dance of cosmic light is mysteriously embedded into the mental, emotional and physical fabric of our beings. The natal chart is truly a "permanent planetary resonance imprint." In most cases, this imprint is fixed for life. Following our first life-breath, the planets continue about their cyclic trajectories around and around. We call their motions "transits."

The Need for This Book

In reference to one's lifework, my father (who taught me astrology) advised, "find a hole and fill it." His advice prompted the writing of this book.

As an herbalist, I've lamented the limited use of real physical energetics in modern astrology. Classical, Medieval, Renaissance and Jyotish physicians all understand planetary influences as primary tools for assessing health, diagnosing illness, and prescribing treatment. In their view, how could one understand a disease without first discerning the excesses and deficiencies of planetary light and temperature? Hopefully, this book will help revitalize this useful approach.

Renaissance doctors accepted diseases of astralic origin as one of at least thirteen recognized etiologies. With the assistance of astrological charts, physicians determined if the cause of a disease was food (ingested poison), constipation, air, accident, psycho-emotional causes (grief, broken heart, or shock), astrology, fairy revenge, elves (and "elfshot"), inherited conditions, witchcraft, worms, possession; or simply "of God." The fun part is that astrological charts were used to diagnose the other twelve etiologies!

I'm always bemused at the enthusiasm with which Western healers accept and adopt Traditional Chinese Medicine (TCM) and India's Ayurveda, seemingly blind to their own similar and equally venerable ancient medical system. The culpability lies with the

Western scientists and "new" physicians of the late seventeenth and eighteenth centuries, who set about to crush and besmirch their own medical heritage in a kind of frenzied collective suicide.

Their goals at the time were many, and certainly not all bad. These included stamping out superstition, replacing unsanitary and unproven medical practices with scientific methods, and improving knowledge of the body. But they were also seeking to crush the competition, make money, and last, but not least, suppress female healers. This last trend began full-scale centuries before, when in 1421 physician Gilbert Kymer and colleagues petitioned Parliament to ban all women physicians.

The Foundation of Western Medical Astrology

Astrology springs from the ancient fountain of "energetic analysis," common to most preindustrial peoples. Individual forms arise from the great sea of universal matter, and then return to it. We are all composed of the same "universal stuff," but, then, what exactly makes an individual? To deduce this, we must first discern the light and vibrational patterns behind these temporarily individual forms.

Each individual person, herb, or stone expresses an emphasis of some energetic patterns at the expense others. It's like baking—no cake is ever quite the same! And neither are any two snowflakes. It is obvious that the universal forces habitually and constantly create individuals. For people, the horoscope offers an unparalleled portrait of individual energetics, symbolized.

Medical astrology analyzes the pattern of health and disease. Ancient physicians were as preoccupied with the patterns behind individual bodies as are today's physicians with the body itself. Energetically, a sparrow is obviously different from a watermelon!

The ancient Greeks described four types of universal matter, or *Elements*, based on their densities: Fire, Earth, Air and Water. Each element was further defined by rates of matter in motion, known as the three astrological *Modes*: Cardinal, Fixed and Mutable. Modern healers may be familiar with a comparable system of modes known as the *Ayurvedic doshas*. The Greeks also recognized that each planet had distinct characteristics, including temperature, color, level of moisture, and speed.

Planetary individuality is indeed a delicate affair, full of descriptive nuance! Yes, Mars is "hot and dry," but he is so much more. His qualities and influence vary during his travels through the twelve zodiac signs, as each imparts its own natural character to their lusty guest.

Of course, the signs themselves are hybrids of Element, Mode, and planetary influence! The avid student soon begins to comprehend these subtleties, and to understand how they impact health. And, as testified by their own formal statements, physicians who discern the astral energetics behind disease manifestation are physicians, indeed: H. L. Cornell, William Davidson, Joseph Blagrave!

In this system, excess and deficiency of elemental, modal, sign, and planetary energies create the natal health portrait. Transiting planets acting to disturb this underlying pattern are observed to cause disease. This book hopes to elucidate this process in a useful manner.

Medical Astrology in Action provides a practical guide to the characteristics of transiting planets and their demonstrable physical effects. This knowledge allows an immediate insight into energetic excesses and deficiencies, their bodily seat, and how to cure them. Antipathetic and sympathetic herbs are one effective method favored by early and Renaissance physicians. There are many other useful methods. The insights of medical astrology are uniquely suited for use in almost every branch of the medical arts, including surgical timing, as amply detailed in this book.

We use microscopes, MRIs, and X-rays to see what isn't visible to our naked eyes. The natal chart and current transits comprise an "astroscope" that allows the healer to view the astral frequencies behind disease in all their full glory.

It is essential that this profoundly useful art and science of medical astrology is not lost to future generations. Thankfully, there now arises a collective yearning in Western medicine for its ignored predecessor and estranged spouse: the "old knowledge."

Let's recall the renowned words of the great herbalist-astrologer Nicholas Culpepper:

"A physician without astrology is like a pudding without fat."

Uses of Medical Astrology

This book is designed to give information on how medical transits work, how specific alignments translate into physical maladies, when that may happen, and the weight of probability of its occurrence. This information is critical for both astrologers and physicians in addressing most medical questions.

This knowledge is equally useful for the medical evaluation of natal charts. Medical astrologers would pay homage at the grave of Dr. William M. Davidson if they only knew where it was. Here are his own words:

"Almost every disease has its 'pseudos.' More than that, there are many diseases which have very different types, and to differentiate these types is imperative if you are going to be successful in practice.

"You can tell in the twinkling of an eye if you use astrology; to the doctor, it gives great insight. The quickness, the speed of it is unbelievable; it's like reading a piece of music. After all, that's what a horoscope is: it's a music of the soul projected into the body."

As discussed in *Chapter 1: Essentials*, the descriptions of health influences of the current planetary transits can also be applied to the aspects between exclusively natal planets in the birth horoscope! Also, many of the maladies discussed are specific to natal aspects. Therefore, the information in this book can be used for the following purposes related to the nativity itself.

This is all information of inestimable value for health practitioners, for use in: disease preemption, case evaluation, surgical timing, and remediation. My hope is that this work will support a new generation of astrologers, herbalists and cosmically aware physicians by providing a foundation to further advance this venerable field.

Practical Uses

- Forewarn of an approaching crisis, allowing for preventative measures. Forewarned is forearmed!
- Determine etiology. Reveal the specifics of a malady's seat and nature. This is especially valuable for the solving of medical mysteries.
- Suggest to the medical practitioner methods of preemption or treatment.
- Select remedies appropriate to the internal energetics of the case; e.g. "Should a warm or cold expectorant be used?"
- Select times for herbal harvest, decoction and administration, supercharging the effectiveness of herbal medicines. *(See Chapter 7: The Moon, The Herbalist's Companion).*
- Indicate the direction of disease in time. Will it worsen or soon improve? How long will it last without intervention?
- Identify mortal danger.
- Select safe dates for surgery. Note this complex procedure is described in more detail in the companion book: *Medical Astrology, A Guide to Planetary Pathology.*
- Fertility timing for pregnancy.
- Ascertaining the strength and type of the patient's vital force and personal idiosyncrasies.
- Delineating the patient's disease tendencies and the weakest (and strongest) organs and bodily systems.
- Identifying the life periods that may bring natal weaknesses to fruition.

Other uses of medical astrology that are not directly addressed in this present book include:

- Distinguish "physical" from purely psychological causation.
- Determine "natural" from "supernatural" etiology.
- Match patients and surgeons.
- Match patients and physicians.
- Donor selection assistance for fertility purposes.

TRANSIT AND NATAL APPLICATIONS

Chapter 1
ESSENTIALS

The foremost intention of this book is to present the planets and elements as the ancients did, as distinctive cosmic energies, vibrations, temperatures, speeds and colors. Building on this foundation, this book incorporates knowledge developed over two millennia by practitioners, as well as my own experience over the short span of one lifetime. By adhering to this method, we hope to revitalize the original understanding and uses of medical astrology.

Planetary and elemental energies are traditionally envisioned as *hot, cold, moist, or dry*. Later traditions added *fast, slow; and tense, relaxed*. We can also add the intermediate qualities, *warm, cool and neutral*, those normalizing Venusian qualities so often neglected by both ancient and modern writers. In the ancient viewpoint, *health problems occur when energetic balances shift into the red zone*.

Descriptions are provided herein for the potential health effects of major aspects, as delivered from transiting planets to the planets in the natal chart. Allow me to highlight that *most planetary transits, most of the time, do not manifest as physical symptoms or disease processes!* However, when they do, you will see apparent in the birth chart the planetary and elemental imbalances suggestive and/or causative of the physical manifestation.

As discussed below, these descriptions are equally useful for the medical study of exclusively natal charts. Key rulerships, elements, dignities, temperatures and colors are listed in each chapter on the planets, the two Lunar Nodes, and the Lights.

Unique to this book, we provide many notes on possible herbal remedies specific to many of the health transits listed. For many of the transits of health, information on surgical timing and other medical treatments are given specific to those aspects. And finally,

Field Notes from my own casework have been sprinkled throughout. These constitute helpful and sometimes entertaining examples to better comprehend medical astrology in action.

When Do Natal Planets Manifest Pathology? It's Complicated.

Natal chart placements and chart inter-aspects are imprinted on each of us for a lifetime. *This does not mean we express them physically, or ever will. Neither does it suggest that if we do express our planets physically that this will endure for life, or cannot be overcome.*

Our physical health, stamina, maladies, and longevity depend on the interactions of the natal chart, transits, our lifestyle decisions, environmental toxins, thoughts, the company we keep, DNA, and the mitigations we take to either improve our wellbeing or ward off disease. The wise practitioner never assumes that natal planetary positions will manifest as health maladies and doesn't frighten their client with definitive disease predictions!

As astrologers, we strive to give our clients actionable information so that they become more aware of their physical strengths and weaknesses, and understand timing, so they may take preventive or mitigating measures. Thus, the natal chart of outwardly healthy individuals is best used for preemption. Forewarned is forearmed!

In truth, most natal planets do NOT express themselves as health maladies. For this reason, readers are reminded throughout this book that the maladies listed are only potential health outcomes, or "**health potentials.**" Also, for most maladies to manifest, the natal chart, or "nativity," must be **predisposed** to the ailment in the first place. The Great Rule: "Plums Cannot Grow From Pear Trees."

We can assess if the nativity is predisposed to manifest a malady by looking for multiple testimonies, including extreme aspects, multiple difficult aspects, debility, malefic placement, temperature extremes, and house placement. The natal planets tenanting the natal 6th, 8th, and 12th signs as counted from the Ascendant (the ascending sign as "1") are more likely to express health issues. Likewise, a natal planet strongly afflicted anywhere in the chart by another planet out of these malefic houses is more prone to physical complaints. A strongly afflicted planet in any of the twelve houses bears the potential of health manifestations at some point in the life. These considerations are central to determining if a planet may express physically. Thus, they are discussed in more detail in *Chapter 5: The Planet in Trouble.*

To summarize, the vast majority of transits pass by each day without a noticeable physical manifestation other than a rise or fall of energy, a mysteriously dribbling nose, or stubbed toe. Nevertheless, in the path of living, most people will experience significant medical issues, and when this happens the transits almost always show us why.

Medical Astrology and the Medical Professional

This book is designed to be of benefit to all astrologers, whether or not they are licensed or certified in a medical field. However, most astrologers are not licensed medical practitioners. Nor do they have the knowledge of the body and disease, nor of treatment methods such as medicines and herbs, that treating professionals should have.

For the non-health-practitioner, the possible physical manifestation of transits provides a greater scope of astrological information, keeping in mind that astrologers, per se, may not be licensed in their given nation to provide medical opinion or advice.

This book is written because of the tremendous wealth of knowledge that medical astrology can provide. We see this as a complement to the tremendous wealth of knowledge that medical professions have developed.

For this reason, we provide admonishments throughout this book. For example, **surgery dates must be coordinated with the responsible physician.** The astrologer may assess that a given surgery date is dangerous; but the responsible physician must be consulted to see if the surgery can be postponed. This must be a decision between the patient and the doctor. And if the wisdom of deferring to medical expertise is not convincing, perhaps the legal liability for medical advice gone wrong would be.

Similarly, this book provides many suggestions for herbal remedies for specific planetary conditions. However, we emphasize that this information, while useful for lay people, is intended for professional herbalists. And we admonish throughout to not self-treat.

For the medical practitioner who is conversant with astrology, this book overflows with invaluable prompts. Alternatively, the health professional who knows little or nothing about astrology should find easier fare in the layman's text *Medical Astrology for Health Practitioners*, and from there graduate to *Medical Astrology: A Guide to Planetary Pathology*.

The Most Significant Planetary Precursors of Disease
Saturn, Mars, The Lunar Nodes, Quincunxes, and Lights

The study of physical maladies inevitably leads the skilled astrologer to acknowledge the outsized influence of the malefic planets, malefic houses, the quincunx, the Lunar Nodes, and of course, the Lights. Therefore, this book seeks to mirror their importance in the way it is organized.

To acknowledge their importance, and draw the readers attention, the Lunar Nodes, are placed front and center in the chapters on the planets. So often in astrological literature, the nodes are placed last in the list of planets. While not intended, their placement makes them seem almost an afterthought. The Lunar Nodes wield great power in both natal and transit astrology, and medical astrology is no exception.

Eclipses always occur near the Nodes. Their distinctive health influences through the twelve signs are detailed in the book *Eclipse and You*. The transiting Nodes always carry along, and transmit, the positive and negative implications of "their" recent eclipses.

By no means is it suggested here that the unlisted planets cannot produce powerful medical influences. *Au contraire*. Mercury, Venus, Jupiter, Neptune Pluto, all produce a litany of specific diseases and concerns.

Quincunxes are little understood, in part because they are so difficult to understand! This has led to a paucity of literature on their effects, especially with respect to health! Yet, the quincunx is the preeminent medical aspect. We have therefore devoted a separate chapter on understanding the quincunx, as well as given detailed information in each of the planet chapters.

It is no surprise that the malefic planets, especially Mars and Saturn, can have serious impacts on the native's health. These are discussed in detail in their respective chapters. The malefic houses are discussed in various planet chapters. However, the influence of these houses is so pervasive that the astrologer must be able to apply this knowledge when called upon. *It is important to understand the definition of the malefic house in medical astrology.* Therefore, a section of this chapter, below, is dedicated to this.

Finally, the Sun and the Moon are the "lights" of the nativity. They are the centers of the health horoscope, along with the Ascendant. While the Sun and Moon are informally called "planets," they are of course not planets. The Sun is the star of our Solar system around which the planets rotate. The Sun gives light and life to the Earth and illumines with its rays all the planets and their many moons. It is summed up so beautifully in the ancient Vedas:

> *Oh, Golden Sun in the blue sky*
> *Impeller of all that lives.*

The Moon is a "moon" that rotates around our own planet. *Since the Lights are not planets, it should be no surprise that their meaning and use in medical astrology are different than the planets.* Their respective chapters explain how.

Malefic Houses
Definition for Physical Effects

As discussed throughout this book, planets in the malefic 6th, 8th, and 12th *angles to the Ascendant sign* are highly inclined to produce physical symptoms.

When considering physical effects of the planets, and the bodily regions affected, the traditional "Whole Sign" house system is the system preferred by this author for defining malefic houses.

In this system, **the sign of the Ascendant is the first house, the sign after the ascending sign (counting counter-clockwise) is the second house, and so forth.**

Disease vulnerability of bodily regions is based, in part, on a deficiency of vital force current available to the sign governing those body regions. This deficiency of vital force is angularly based. Traditionally, the zodiac signs located at the natal 6th, 8th, and 12th angles from the ascending sign comprise the "malefic" houses.

The signs positioned at angles 150°and 210° to the ascending degree, are associated with the health-perplexing *quincunx* aspect. These angles receive, and likewise send, less vital current to and from of the Ascendant. Similarly, the 12th sign from the Ascendant is considered as *inconjunct* the ascending sign, with significant mental and physical health implications. For an explication of the quincunx aspect and the related *inconjunct,* please see *Chapter 4: Quincunx!*

This author finds in her experience, that for the medical applications of astrology, best results are achieved with the Whole Sign house system. However, if you prefer an alternate system, there is no argument, but only this caveat: While the topic of house systems is an ongoing rich and productive discussion in the astrology community, no one should overlook the physical deficiencies noted for signs that are angularly placed 6, 8, and 12 signs from the Ascendant. Do so at your client's peril!

A thorough discussion of why malefic angles (houses) produce health problems and what can be done about this, can be found in my book *Astrology & Your Vital Force, Healing with Cosmic Rays and DNA Resonance.*

Natal Versus Transit Planets
Embedded Versus Temporary Influences

This book is written largely from the standpoint of the impact of *planets in motion* upon the planets embedded in the natal or birth chart. This decision was made because it is the best way to actively understand planetary energetics—both in current time but also when permanently embedded in the natal pattern.

When studying the planets in motion, the astrologer keeps in mind how transiting planets affect the natal chart. Visualize the transiting planet as a celestial postman delivering a "right now" package of energetic influence **to** the natal planets and houses. The transiting planet is the *active principal*. The natal planets act as recipients and symbolize various *potentials*.

Now visualize a garden full of seeds. The planets of our natal chart symbolize seeds of character and karma, all due to hatch under the right kind of planetary weather. The transiting planets inform us when the right type of weather approaches to "hatch the seed" symbolized by the natal planet. Sometimes a natal planet represents a latent health issue!

The reader can use the transit details provided in this book in two ways: 1) transiting planets as influencing the natal chart or birth horoscope; and, 2) natal chart aspects between natal planets. These are explored below, along with a brief discussion of how to use this book for exploring collective health aspects.

Natal Aspects: The planets are in constant motion through the signs of the ecliptic as seen from the Earth. In devising the natal or birth chart of a person, we note the positions of the transiting planets at the time of birth by sign, degree, element, and house. These natal chart placements and chart inter-aspects provide each of us with *a permanent planetary resonance imprint*. Astrologers know that most people retain this birth resonance throughout life.

According to Hindu tradition, the planets influence us through subtle cosmic light vibrations of various colors. The inestimable Dr. William Davidson explained:

"The reason the planets indicate health condition is because flowing into the body are invisible radio-like frequencies, which control and build and maintain all the tissues, and those frequencies are conditioned by the planetary forces in operation at the first moment of breath, in other words, the cosmos is impressed upon you, the moment you take

your first breath. Because you breath a cosmic ether as well as air: the scientist doesn't believe that there is any such thing as a cosmic ether. I prefer to believe the people who can see and who have studied it. And so the ether has a sum total of your vibration, as when you take the cap off a camera lens, the surroundings are impressed on the place; so the reason the planets indicate health is because they indicate the frequencies radiating at that moment."

Davidson's Medical Lectures, Dr. William Davidson, edited by Vivia Jayne, 1979, Published by the Astrological Bureau.

The planetary positions in the birth chart are known as the "natal planets." Their interactions are known as "natal aspects," which are, of course, distinct from "transit aspects." Despite the difference in terminology, **the interactive aspects of the natal chart are in fact, *transits frozen in time!***

Because the natal chart is effectively transits-made-permanent, the interpretations provided in this book for planetary transits can also be used to interpret *exclusively* natal planetary positions and aspects. However, the viewpoint is quite different, as explained in the following.

Aspects by Transit:

We refer to a current-time transit as an "aspect to the natal chart," or more directly put, a "transit." Like storms, health transits are temporary affairs, but may leave behind a long wake. Transits are the cosmic weather that hatches the seeds of karma lying dormant in the natal chart. These seeds bear all kinds of fruit, including the occasional health malady. A brief transit is capable of sprouting chronic health problems of long duration that are suggested in the original natal pattern at birth. *However, if health problems could not be preempted or prevented, why consider medical astrology?*

Collective Transits:

The public responds to transits en masse, and sometimes this is reflected in health trends. Transiting planets and the transiting Sun and Moon constantly interact with each other in complex cycles influencing all life on Earth collectively. These influences are collectively important, although not as useful to the astrologer for targeting individual outcomes. For example, today is Thanksgiving in America smack dab on the full Moon in Gemini. This makes *collective* travel a nightmare, but not for those who stay home!

Physicians may wonder why their office suddenly fills up with knee cases, or five patients call with migraines in one day. Astrology is very good at predicting public health trends! Some examples of health manifestations on a grand scale are given below:

• **Infection/Accidents/Inflammation: Mars**
The body regions ruled by the zodiac sign that Mars transits through will correspond with an increase in accidents, inflammation, flus, muscle strains and infection! For example, when Mars passes through Aquarius, ankle injuries will be in vogue, because Aquarius rules the ankle. *(See Chapter 12, section: "Mars Through the Signs.")* Mars usually spends at least six weeks per sign, although it varies considerably.

• **Chronicity (chronic disease): Saturn**
The body regions ruled by the zodiac sign that Saturn is passing through will experience an increase in chronic problems, and bone and structural issues. For example, when Saturn passes through Scorpio, constipation and colon complaints increase, because Scorpio rules the colon. *(See Chapter 14, section: "Saturn Through the Signs.")* Saturn remains in a sign approximately two and a half years.

• **Collective Fatigue: South Lunar Node**
The body regions ruled by the zodiac sign that the South Lunar Node is passing through will correspond with an increase in failure within that bodily region, or mysterious viruses. For example, when the South Node transits Cancer, there will be an uptick in cases of malnourishment due to poor appetite, because Cancer rules the stomach. *(See Chapter 9, section: "South Lunar Node Through the Signs.")* The South Lunar Node remains in a sign approximately one and a half years.

• Mass Public Health Events: Eclipses

Eclipses strongly impact public health by indicating the body systems most under stress during the year and a half that a specific "eclipse system" reigns. Think of these as you would a long weather system! It behooves the wise physician to know if it is currently "the eclipse season of the heart" or "the eclipse season of the pancreas", and so forth. The medical implications of eclipses by sign (body zone), with calendar, can be accessed in my book *Eclipses and You.*

Dwarf Planets, Astroids and Comets

Except for Pluto, which has long been studied, these minor or very distant bodies are not included in this work. The reasons are many, but not least because they have been recently discovered, and little research has been conducted on their physical effects, if any. When it comes to advising clients on their health, I prefer to rely on well established effects.

The newly discovered asteroids, dwarf planets, and cometoids (e.g. Chiron is a cometoid), have provided a great deal of excitement, discussion and exploration in the astrological community. This book is not the place for these discussions. However, as research astrologers may consider these bodies for potential physical effects, some issues are worth bearing in mind.

Do we really want to continue the recent tradition of pre-deciding a planet's influence based exclusively on its mythological namesake? Or, do we follow the older model of carefully documenting transit influences for decades, then meeting together at council and finding what traits follow through.

We also need to understand the relative impact of these new bodies, including some that roam far flung from the ecliptic plane. For instance, even if we establish that Chiron, (a tiny ice comet) is everything his mythological namesake suggests, should he be regarded in chart readings as Jupiter's equal?

These and many other questions must be carefully considered before our charts are deluged with an ever-growing number of tiny bodies of unknown or predetermined meaning that are immediately relegated the respect of the gas giants.

Note on Gender Semantics

A new thrust has appeared in our field to remove gender pronouns from astrological signs and planets. Proponents would prefer that the planets, Sun, and Moon not be described as "he/him" or "she/her," but rather, as either genderless or non-binary. There are some sound reasons for this request. Conversely, some schools of astrology assert that the planets and Lights are in fact, sentient beings with real gender. However, as space is limited, I'll leave that discussion to others and another time.

Gendered or not, in medical astrology, some planets do govern the physical gender parts, sex hormones, gender roles, and gender specific maladies. For instance, Luna governs the menses. In adherence to known rulerships, and because they work, the author retains these traditional medical assignments.

At the time of publication, proponents of the genderless approach have not yet adequately sorted the issues in terms of stylistic elegance. Therefore, reader of this book will encounter planets mentioned in the classical style as "he" or "she," in part because this is far warmer than "it."

Readers who prefer that no gender pronouns be applied to planets, are invited to substitute "it" (or any other term) for he or she where you personally feel needful. However, when quoting text, please retain my original wording, or first contact me for permission to reword sections. There are some important reasons for this request.

Mind, Will, and Transits

Planetary transits comprise a sort of subtle "astral weather," not dissimilar to our better understood terrestrial weather. The skilled astrologer describes the planetary weather in the same manner that your local meteorologist provides a useful daily weather report (albeit, the astrologer views a far greater scope of time).

In relation to the planetary influences, the owner of the horoscope, or "native" can be likened to a farmer. The vegetable farmer cannot halt the weather, but she can design ways to utilize it for greatest advantage. Conversely, the wise farmer knows when to act to protect her crops!

Most people have some latitude of choice in how best to utilize the astral weather in manifold ways. In respective of health (the topic of our book), one can choose to ignore, utilize, deliberately channel, direct, neutralize, antidote, deflect, absorb, or enhance any specific transit influence.

For centuries, astrologers have designed manifold ways to do just that: herbs, stones, metals, chants, deliberate activities, exercise, cautions, music, prayer, scents, etc. Most essentially, the deliberate use of entrained thought can nullify, antidote or enhance any planetary transit (C. C. Zain). There are many books that discuss transit and natal chart remediations *(see Bibliography)*, including my own *Astrology & Your Vital Force: Healing with Cosmic Rays and DNA Resonance.*

True, there are both terrestrial and astral hurricanes that influence whole populations, overwhelming individuals. We also have the hand of "karma," playing out in individual lives. However, most of us have a substantial control over the development of our character and health. Similar to the terrestrial weather, the planetary rays hatch what we ourselves have planted in our own gardens!

One must never allow fear and worry over past, present or future transits to govern one's life, because the planetary influences are "just the weather." The seasoned astrologer knows that astral weather is very real, and should be duly noted, and worked with. However, our will power must reign supreme over the vagaries of both astral and earthly weather, and not the other way around! It is intended for us to reign as the kings and queens of our moods, minds and mortal bodily castles. This discipline is one of the true goals of astrological training.

When asked: *"Is it proper for us to study the effects of the planets upon our lives, in order to understand our tendencies and inclinations better, as they are influenced by the planets?"* the great twentieth century medical psychic and prophet, Edgar Cayce could not have stated a better response:

"When studied aright, (it is) very, very, very much worth while. Then how studied aright? By studying the influence (of the planets) in the light of knowledge already obtained by mortal man. Give out more of that knowledge—giving the understanding that the will must ever be the guiding factor to lead man on, ever upward." (3744, A-35)

Astrological Herbalism

In medical astrology, the first level for the herbalist in prescribing herbal remedies is the knowledge of planetary energetics. Each planet has its own influence. For instance, the transit South Node is profoundly weakening, Mars is heating, and Saturn is cooling.

To see how this is especially useful in practice, let us take for our example a case of bronchitis occurring as transit Mars conjoins natal Mercury. Then, let's compare this against a second case of bronchitis coincident with Saturn's transit conjunction of natal Mercury. In the first case we have the arrival of heat and inflammation (Mars), while in the latter case, the entrance of cold and dry (Saturn). Mars stimulates, whereas Saturn represses!

Obviously, the cooling, demulcent respiratory herbs work best for allaying Mars, whereas the warming expectorants perform for Saturn's chilling conjunction. This substantial difference in treatment, for the same malady, is essential knowledge. And, yes, these principles would likewise hold if you observe these same aspects in the natal chart; for example, natal Mars conjuncting natal Mercury.

The second level of assessment brings in the specific nature of elements and signs. These always temper the innate quality of the planets. In our example, the question is now: *What sign is natal Mercury in? In what sign and element is transit Mars, or Saturn?* This is why I've devoted sections in this book to the planets through all twelve signs and four elements. You will find these sections reiterate similar material in previous works, although these present form a more distinctly energetic approach, (hot, cold, etc.).

Mars' action is hot and dry, but more or less so, depending on his transit or natal sign. In Water signs he boils the water, becoming "hot and wet." He is at his most inflammatory in Fire signs and parching dry in Earth. Conversely, Saturn is innately cold and dry, but warmer in the Fire signs and less drying in Water (instead, trapping moisture, creating stagnation and torpor). These distinctions are essential for subtle diagnosis and effective herbal selections. This is one reason why added commentary entitled *Herbal Notes* are included for each chapter on the Lights, Nodes and Planets.

Chapter 7, The Moon: The Herbalist's Companion provides direction for the harvest, preparation, and administration of herbs, to be potentized in the traditional manner. More material of relevant assistance can be found in *Astrology & Your Vital Force.* Additional material, tailored just for the non-astrologer herbalist, is available in: *Medical Astrology for Health Practitioners.*

Armed with the knowledge herein, plus a copy of Matthew Wood's *Earthwise Herbal Repertory,* you have a complete system of astrological-herbal medicine, shorn of the confusions typical of medieval planet-herbal lists. These lists abound. You may have seen one of many extant Renaissance-era catalogs of herbs listed collectively under "their" planet headings. However, there is a real problem here in the matter of practical usefulness.

To elucidate this mess, I'll use Mars again, for our example. Herbs are assigned to Mars, sometimes, by color (red for Mars), season of flowering (Aries or Scorpio), physical attributes (thorns), organ affinity (muscles), symbolic associations (looks like a phallus), mineral content (iron), or actual properties (stimulant).

Are we really supposed to "just pick one" for any deduced Mars complaint? I doubt this, considering that Blagrave, Culpepper, and others were master herbalists, as intimately involved with their herbs as they were their patient's symptoms.

First, physical, emotional and mental symptoms were noted, and the horoscope consulted, not necessarily in that order. Then, specific herbs were selected appropriate to the individual case.

Herbal Notes are largely relegated to the sections in each

chapter that is devoted to planetary conjunctions. In most cases, these tips can be utilized for fellow sections on squares, oppositions and quincunxes, should symptoms agree.

The admonition, "Do not self-treat" follows all herbal sections for obvious reasons. The information in this book is designed for educative purposes, and not for literal use by unlicensed medical practitioners.

In recognition of the conscious individualities of herbs, it was decided to capitalize herbal references.

The field of Astrological Herbalism is vast and endless. Herbal examples are included so herbalists can see the method of selecting specific herbs according to planetary energetics.

Reiterations

The reader may notice that the sections of planetary chapters providing descriptions of planets by sign, and also the material of *Chapter 2: Zodiacal Human* are partial reiterations from my previous work *Medical Astrology: A Guide to Planetary Pathology*. These were necessary to include again for the greater convenience and comprehension of the reader. These form a small percentage of the material herein.

However, the approach of these reiterated sections is distinctly new, crafted to distinctly explicate *planetary energetics*, and those health effects in current action *(as transits)*, as they play out within the natal chart, or what I like to call the "permanent planetary resonance imprint."

Additional Texts

Foremost pioneer of astrology-based nutrition, Eileen Nauman, DHM, provides an excellent section on the health and nutritional implications of natal hard aspects in her breakthrough tome *Medical Astrology*. Herbalists are well advised to obtain a copy of Matthew Wood's *Earthwise Herbal Repertory* for more complete herbal options listed by body system and organ affinity plus their distinct uses. My own book *Medical Astrology: A Guide to Planetary Pathology* fleshes out the surgical and other sections in this present text, whereas *Astrology & Your Vital Force* provides further and exhaustive detail on extant remediation techniques for planetary-based health problems. The book *Eclipses and You, (Hill)* provides details on the medical impacts of eclipses through all twelve signs.

Maintaining Prudence

Planetary aspects do not always manifest as health concerns or benefits.

Applicable to both natal and transit charts, the partial lists of expressed symptoms in each section apply only to predisposed nativities. These conditions are obviously uncommon and require multiple testimonies beyond the presence of any one celestial body.

Manifestation of symptoms may be enhanced by lifestyle choices, and taking preemptive measures can reduce, remove or prevent potential issues from manifesting.

This material is published for informational purposes only. It is not intended to be a substitute for professional medical advice and should not be relied on as health or personal advice.

Planetary and Sign Symbols	
Planets	*Signs*
Sun ☉	Aries ♈
Moon ☽	Taurus ♉
Mercury ☿	Gemini ♊
Venus ♀	Cancer ♋
Mars ♂	Leo ♌
Jupiter ♃	Virgo ♍
Saturn ♄	Libra ♎
Uranus ♅	Scorpio ♏
Neptune ♆	Sagittarius ♐
Pluto ♇	Capricorn ♑
North Lunar Node ☊	Aquarius ♒
South Lunar Node ☋	Pisces ♓
Pars Fortuna ⊗	

Chapter 2
ZODIACAL HUMAN
SIGN-BODY CORRELATION

For the reader's convenience and necessity, this section is reiterated from my other texts on this subject. Great benefit goes to any astrologer who memorizes these traditional sign-body correlations, so useful in many branches of our field. It is essential to note that some body parts are co-ruled by two signs, and often share rulership with a specific planet as well.

In a general way, the signs govern the bodily regions whereas the planets rule the internal organs, but this is far from consistent. Medical astrology is an evolving science. Many bodily parts and functions have not yet been assigned to planetary and sign rulership, e.g. brain hemispheres and blood constituents. Additionally, the signs are subdivided into thirty degrees, each governing very precise body parts.

Zodiacal Degrees: The twelve signs can be subdivided into thirty tiny subsections, each of 1°. A list of the specific body parts assigned to these degrees, entitled *Anatomishe Entsprechungen der Tierkreisgrade,* was created by the iconic Elsbeth and Reinhold Ebertin, and translated into English by Mary L. Vohryzek as "Anatomical Correspondences to Zodiacal Degrees." While woefully incomplete (where is the clitoris?), this seminal article remains the best available and bears out tolerably well in practice, sometimes precisely.

A list of specific maladies associated with the zodiacal degrees, as compounded from the collected findings of many authors (including my own) is available in *Medical Astrology: A Guide to Planetary Pathology*, section: "Degrees, Fine Tuning the Signs."

Body Zones: The use of numbered "Body Zones," in lieu of traditional zodiac sign names, is my own device. *(See Figures 1 and 2 at the end of this chapter.)* This was created to assist the medically inclined non-astrologer to understand *(and use)* the system with less prejudice. It is hardly possible to list all body organs here. For individual vessels, vertebrae, and muscles, please refer to Dr. H. L. Cornell's *Encyclopedia of Medical Astrology.*

Aries – Body Zone 1: Crown of the head: cranium, forehead, eyes, motor centers of brain, upper jaw and teeth, some head nerves. Adrenal glands (shared with Libra and Mars), the mandible (with Taurus).

Taurus – Body Zone 2: Lower head, lower teeth and jaw, ears, tongue (shared with Venus and Mercury), vocal chords (shared with Venus and Mercury), Adam's apple, salivary glands, thyroid (shared with Uranus, Venus, and Mercury), neck, cervical nerves and vertebrae, neck muscles, gullet, throat, upper esophagus, swallowing reflex, epiglottis, jugular vein, carotid arteries, and atlas and axis bones. Taurus may have some influence sensory, taste and hearing centers of the brain. Taurus and Scorpio share the tonsils.

Gemini – Body Zone 3: Bronchial tubes, upper lungs, inspiration (as opposed to expiration), shoulders, clavicle, scapula, arms, radius and ulna, hands, bodily capillaries, speech centers of brain, peripheral afferent nerves, and coordination tubes of the body in general.

Cancer – Body Zone 4: Lower lung, breast, stomach, lower esophagus, uterus (when pregnant), meninges and pleura, thoracic duct, rib cage, sternum; scapula (shared with Gemini), elbow, armpit, pancreas (shared with Virgo), diaphragm; this sign exerts influence over temperature regulation, the hypothalamus and thalamus; posterior pituitary, gums, the umbilicus *(Hill)* although Cornell says Virgo. The solar plexus *(Hill)* co-ruled with Virgo *(Cornell).*

Some authors allot all hollow bodily cavities to Cancer, including the eyes sockets and cheeks. This author is not in full agreement. Cancer and Pisces both hold a significant rulership over the lymphatic fluid and nodes. Cancer may have some influence over the temperature sensing function of the hypothalamus (the body's thermostat). Davidson says that Cancer rules the bone marrow, whereas Cornell says Jupiter and Venus; and Jyotish tradition gives it to Mars!

Leo – Body Zone 5: Heart, aorta, dorsal vertebrae, general spinal alignment, spinal sheaths. Gallbladder (shared with Capricorn, Saturn, and Mars). Governs the longissimus, latissimus dorsi, transversalis, heart muscles. The forearms and wrists (shared with Gemini).

Virgo – Body Zone 6: Upper intestinal organs; liver (shared with Jupiter with influence from Leo and Cancer), pancreas and spleen (shared with Cancer), upper intestine and ascending colon (shared with Scorpio); immune system (shared with Pisces), automatic nervous system, and sympathetic nerves; portal vein (shared with Aquarius). The fingers (shared with Gemini and Mercury).

Libra – Body Zone 7: Kidneys, ovaries, lumbar spine; buttocks (shared with Sagittarius) sense of balance, acid-alkaline balance, salt and fluid balance; adrenal glands (shared with Mars and Aries). Cornell places the buttocks themselves (but not the hips) under Libra, although these are usually assigned to Sagittarius *(Nauman)*, with influence from Scorpio (the sacrum and anus is under Scorpio, and the coccyx under Scorpio and Sagittarius).

Scorpio – Body Zone 8: Excretory system (shared with Mars), nose, bladder and bladder sphincter, cervix, neck of uterus, (with Cancer and the Moon, this sign greatly influences the uterus) genitals, urethra, colon, rectum, anus, sweat glands, sacrum, brim of pelvis.

Sagittarius – Body Zone 9: Hips, thighs, femurs, arterial circulation (with Jupiter); lower spinal nerves, buttocks (shared with Libra and Scorpio). This sign has a significant influence on the coordination processes of the central nervous system and on the motor nerves and voluntary muscular system (shared with Mars and Aries). Sagittarius and Scorpio both influence the sacrum and coccyx.

Capricorn – Body Zone 10: Knees, patella; the skin, ligaments, tendons, and cuticles of the body in general. This sign has a significant influence (with Saturn) over the entire skeletal system, joints and bones.

Aquarius – Body Zone 11: Ankles, shins, venous circulation (shared with Venus); the oxygenation of the blood (shared with Gemini); general quality of blood, and the little known electrical system of the body. Some authors cite the rods and cones of the eye as under the dominion of this sign.

Cornell gives "the pyramidal tract of the spinal cord" to this sign. This sign, with Sagittarius, greatly influences the spinal nerves, (whereas Leo governs the spinal sheaths).

Pisces – Body Zone 12: Feet and toes; lymphatic system (with Cancer), parasympathetic nervous system, sleep, supernatural etiologies, and the extracellular matrix, and cellular hydration. Pisces influences the cecum and duodenum (shared with Virgo). Pisces influences the lymphatic matrix.

The two illustrations *(Figures 1 & 2)* more clearly depict the 12 Body Zones than do Renaissance models. The first drawing shows the anterior view. The organs located within these zones share rulership with various planets.

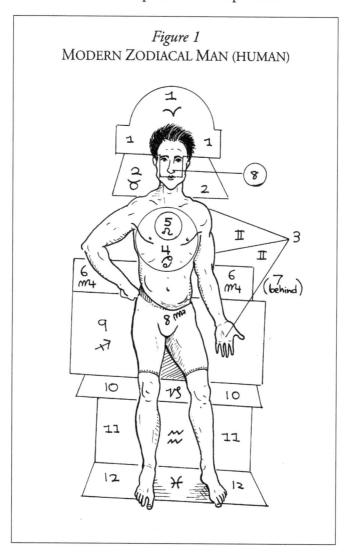

Figure 1
MODERN ZODIACAL MAN (HUMAN)

Lateral view, exposing the Leo and Libra regions not visible in the old frontal views. The organs located within these zones share rulership with various planets.

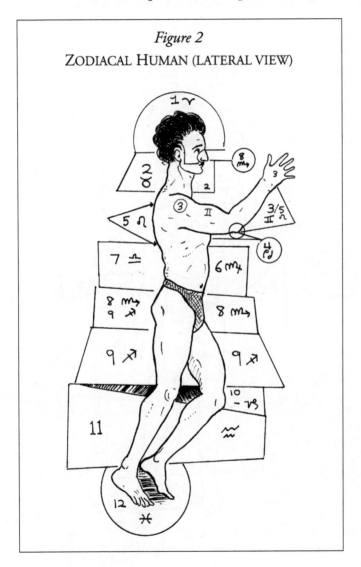

Figure 2

ZODIACAL HUMAN (LATERAL VIEW)

Figure 3
HOMO SIGNORUM – THE MAN OF SIGNS

From Johann Regiomantus' *Kalendarius Teutsch*, printed by Johann Sittich, Augsburg, 1512.

Also known as "Zodiacal Man," similar images were displayed in Renaissance surgeon's offices for guidance in the selection of safe surgery dates. The use of the Moon's transits through its four phases and the twelve signs was essential knowledge for the selection of safe surgery dates.

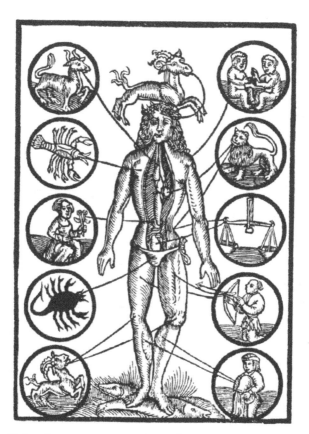

Klarhayt der zeit beſſert alle Laßtag

Chapter 3
ASPECT MECHANICS
PHYSICAL INFLUENCES

Why Transits Work

This is a vast subject, due its own book. There are now scores of research projects demonstrating the validity of planetary effects. *(Payne, Kolisko, Hill, Seymore, Polit, Kollerstrom, Thompson, etc.)*

It is thought and long espoused in Jyotish (the astrology of India), that the subtle cosmic light of the Lights and planets enter and exit vortexes (chakras) in a body of fine matter that surrounds and interpenetrates our physical body.

In the West, this invisible body has been given various names, presenting much confusion: astral body, etheric body, spirit body, aura. It is this etheric body that patterns and receives the energetics behind our dense physical body. Some assert there are many layers of fine-matter bodies, like an onion. Clairvoyants claim to see these bodies. Most of us do not.

Each planet emits its own cosmic color. It is the excesses and deficiencies of cosmic color that lead to health related imbalances. These imbalances are shown as tendencies in the natal chart.

In the yearly round, the current planetary transits exert pressures (more red, less green, etc.). If unattended, these excesses and deficiencies can manifest physically in predisposed charts. Hence, medical astrology! A more detailed explication is available in *Astrology & Your Vital Force: Healing with Cosmic Rays and DNA Resonance*. However, there are other theories to explain why the planets influence us.

The late physicist Buryl Payne, Ph.D. states:

"The protons of the body which are free to wiggle do so and then can produce tiny radio waves. These protons are at the center of hydrogen atoms constituting water molecules. The body has more hydrogen atoms

than any other type. This is the same effect which MRI or Magnetic Resonance Imaging makes use of. A few other elements in the body also exhibit this effect…. Possible changes in the light from the Sun produces effects on the DNA/RNA."

"The light from the Sun reflects the structure of the air and water which we breathe and drink. This can in turn effect our moods. This was observed in a series of experimental observations carried out for many years. The device used to do this was simple and can be verified by anyone."

In the traditional Western medical paradigm, intact through the late Renaissance, all forms and bodies were regarded as connected through vibrational affinity, much like octaves on a keyboard. Low C vibrates to high C in the same manner that peaches resonate Venus, or our adrenal gland vibrates to Mars. Some forms vibrate closely, and others not…but at base, all is One. The modern Western medical paradigm dismissed this entire paradigm as foolish superstition, and wind.

We have a similar problem with time. The original Western medical paradigm knew time as possessed of both quantity and quality. For instance, next Tuesday's Moon in Taurus possesses an inherent quality that is just perfect for planting lily bulbs.

Once again, the modern medical paradigm rejects this idea, continuing to book surgical procedures on eclipses. In the modern paradigm, time has only quantity. The astrologer's doctrine of *time quality* was regarded as useless nonsense until the recent advent of "Chrono Medicine." This new approach recognizes that the time of treatment has unexplained influences upon the healing process that can be harnessed for patient benefit. Strangely, the empirical observations of two millennia of medical astrologers are ignored.

The following extract from a reading given by the renowned medical psychic and prophet Edgar Cayce, regarding music, is especially relevant towards the understanding of the various planetary vibrations and their influence upon human health, and also, the traditional method of antipathetic treatment.

"Every entity is on certain vibrations. Every dis-ease or disease is creating in the body the opposite or discordant vibrations with the conditions in a body-mind and spirit of the individual. If there are used certain vibrations, there may be seen the response. In some it is necessary for counter-action, in some it is necessary for changes...." extract from reading 1861-12

Transit Orb

The word "orb" in this text refers to the distance necessary between any two planets to produce a valid influence. This word can also be used to simply mean any distance in degrees of ecliptic longitude between two celestial bodies.

Aspects between either natal or transit planets occur when two planets are within specific orbs to each other. The designation of the appropriate orb of influence is very important to an accurate interpretation of a chart. Yet the topic is complex. Therefore, **orbs are discussed individually within each chapter on the planets, Lights, and Lunar Nodes.** But first some rules for applying the information in those chapters:

• Determining the strength of an aspect is a matter of assessing the cumulative weight of several factors. There are many suggested "true orb" systems to be found in extant astrological literature, varying both according to the planets involved and the writer! In Jyotish (the horoscopic astrology of India), there is a consensus that any two planets in the same sign together are, in fact, conjunct. Western astrologers don't agree, some insisting on the exact orbs delegated by their preferred orb system.

• The primary rule of determining orb of influence is "the closer, the stronger." This practical method slices through all the confusion like butter. For example, the standard orb of the natal Sun conjunct natal Mars would be about 12° within a given sign. However, if they are exactly conjunct, then the influence would be most potent. As we move away from exactitude, the influence diminishes, with 5° showing far less power; and the influence at 12° being less still.

Interestingly, beyond the standard 12° orb, in this example, the influence of the Sun (or any planet) does not disappear, because the influence of a planet is felt throughout the sign it inhabits. Both East and West can keep their stake in the battle.

• The influence of a planet fades rapidly over a sign boundary (see discussion in section on Squares). Very close orbs still work well for two planets straddling either side of a sign boundary, such as Saturn at 29° Libra conjunct Mercury at 1° Scorpio. However, this influence is negligible at larger orbs.

• Orbs of influence vary by the type of aspect, as well as the size, distance and speed of the planet. For example, the large Ptolemaic planets, Saturn and Jupiter, as well as the Sun and the Moon, have effective orbs that can reach between 10 to 15°, especially when between one another. On the other hand, little Mercury and sweet Venus have relatively small orbs, with their conjunction working best within 3°. The transit of the outer planets Pluto and Neptune manifest mostly within an orb of 1°.

• For natal to natal aspects, the orb of the planet with the larger orb extension rules. In transit to natal aspects, the orb of the transit planet rules. This is one way that orbs can be different for exclusively natal and transit-to-natal aspects.

• There are other factors that are standard in Western astrology that affect the orb of influence. For example, the strength of an aspect increases when planets are in mutual application or mutual reception. The strength of an aspect is also amplified by factors that increase a planets strength, such as being stationary, in dignity, and on an angle.

A full discussion of these issues is not the province of this book. These rules can be found in most good beginner and mid-level texts on the subject. Should any planet enjoy multiple tendencies of strength, joy, fortification, or dignity, its impact will be potent!

THE CONJUNCTION (0°)

Conjunctions are often the **strongest felt** of medical aspects and by far the easiest to understand. Understanding the physical impacts of a given conjunction is the **gateway** for understanding the impact of the other major aspects. For this reason, this book focuses much of its attention on the delineation of conjunctions, with less text devoted to squares and oppositions.

During a conjunction, a transiting planet temporarily co-mingles its distinctive "beam" or vibration with the natal plant conjoined. This vibration is received primarily as temperature, moisture level, and speed.

In grammar school, we learn to combine the letters "t" and "h" to form the new sound "th." Astrology works the same way! Combining two different forces creates a third entity.

For example, when cold, slow, astringent transit Saturn conjoins the sensitive, emotional natal Moon, we enter a period of lowered fertility, constrained emotions and cold stomach (to name a few). Conversely, as hot transit Mars crosses over natal Luna, we might experience an acid stomach or temper tantrum.

As explained in the earlier *Chapter 1: Essentials*, one may frame conjunctions exclusive to the natal chart as "permanent," and the *transit* conjunctions to natal planets as "temporary." However, these can work in different ways. For example, a potential malady suggested by a permanent conjunction in the natal chart may lie dormant for years, be prevented, or if manifesting, be cured. Conversely, a malady brought forth by a transiting planet that temporarily conjuncts a natal planet could signal the onset of a chronic condition!

THE SQUARE (90°)

Squares create friction. Squares build. Squares force interaction in the physical universe. Squares demand either a decision or action. Squares are not always bad! They provide energy, lessons, and problems to solve.

In delineating the effects of a square aspect, we must consider the astrological *element* and *mode* of both the transiting planet and the natal planet it squares. These same considerations are useful in exclusively natal squares. Planetary sections in this book contain a section on squares specific for those bodies.

ELEMENTS: *(pertaining to squares)*

Understanding Squares by Element

Squares normally occur between planets that are positioned in signs of *conflicting* elements. This creates **four distinct types of squares**, each with their unique influence, occurring in one of the following pairs: *Fire-Water, Fire-Earth, Earth-Air,* and *Air-Water.* These are briefly summarized below.

Fire-Water Squares: Aries/Cancer, Leo/Scorpio, Sagittarius/Pisces

Fire-Water squares create boiling emotion and often raise energy. Creative, artistic, passionate! Emotional extremes result. Watch the Sagittarius/Pisces square for flights of fancy or hyper-religiosity. Sagittarius/Pisces is dominant in mental derangement, blood cholesterol issues, hip-foot alignment and sleep disorders (to name a few).

This square is dangerous for those who suffer schizophrenia. Aries/Cancer produces sudden shifts to hormones, moods and brain chemistry. In Leo/Scorpio squares, observe the colon-heart connection. This square is physically and emotionally volatile.

Fire-Earth Squares: Aries/Capricorn, Leo/Taurus, Sagittarius/Virgo

Fire-Earth squares frustrate energy by stultifying and/or suffocating the Fire element. However, this square provides both grit and determination. This square disturbs metabolism, burn-rate, bile flow, gallbladder function, and digestive enzymes. Drying to the mucous membrane.

The Taurus/Leo square is one of the most stressful squares of all for sufferers of heart problems, high blood pressure, gallbladder congestion and back-neck issues. Impacts thyroid, blood pressure, skin conditions, arthritis. Often the sufferers of natal Fire-Earth squares are ambitious, determined, capable, red-faced, and irritable.

In practice, Fire-Earth is extremely acidic. Many cases of GERD, hyperacidity and gallstones have come across my desk with Fire-Earth problems. Sagittarius/Virgo squares are associated with anxiety, panic attacks, and hyperthyroid.

Earth-Air Squares: Taurus/Aquarius, Virgo/Gemini, Capricorn/Libra

Earth-Air squares combine ideation with practical function, thus, bringing ideas into form. Taurus/Aquarius squares cause circulatory stasis, hypothyroid, and poor oxygenation and circulation. Virgo/Gemini amps up the nervous system, sometimes resulting in asthma, nervous exhaustion, or bowel dysfunction.

Air-Water Squares: Gemini/Pisces, Libra/Cancer, Aquarius/Scorpio

Air-Water squares produce energy or conflict between mind and emotions. This is an astral square, awkward for the mentally ill. This square can disturb lung function and oxygenation; increases potential for malnutrition and bone loss. Depression is symptomatic to this group. Gemini-Pisces evinces weak immunity, and lung sensitivity. Cancer/Libra is notable for hormonal-mental reactions.

Aquarius/Scorpio is associated with mental/emotional obsessions, brood-ing fixations; colonic stasis; rheumatic, circulatory, heart and thyroid issues, usually hypofunctioning.

MODES: *(pertaining to squares)*

The Rate of Matter in Motion
Understanding Squares by Astrological Mode (Quadruplicity)

Most squares occur in one of three astrological modes: *Cardinal, Fixed or Mutable.* The characteristics of each mode are important for understanding the physical effects of a square. Modes influence time. Also called "Quadruplicities," Modes indicate the rate of matter in motion. **Cardinal** is fast; **Fixed** is slow; **Mutable** is modulating, diffusing.

Cardinal Squares:

Cancer/Aries, Cancer/Libra, Aries/Capricorn, Capricorn/Libra

Cardinal signs produce impulse and energy. They act fast upon the body. Medically, these squares produce acute effects and are the fastest to resolve of all squares.

Fixed Squares:

Taurus/Leo, Leo/Scorpio, Scorpio/Aquarius, Aquarius/Taurus

Fixed sign squares represent slow, chronic, and deeply embedded issues. Medically, these squares are the hardest to resolve. If not resolved, issues commencing during fixed squares may sometimes last years or become permanent.

Mutable Squares:

Sagittarius/Virgo, Virgo/Gemini, Sagittarius/Pisces, Gemini/Pisces

Medically, all mutable squares produce lingering, fluctuating complaints that go latent, then recur. Many bugs that hide out in the nervous system or gut—awakening when the immune system is compromised—are indicated by mutable squares.

Squares between the signs *Sagittarius/Virgo* and *Virgo/Gemini* excite the nerves. Squares between the signs *Sagittarius/Pisces* and *Gemini/Pisces* stimulate the "higher" mind and imagination, and also weaken the lungs and immune system.

Squares Across Sign Boundaries

The very premise of a square is that of conflicting-element and same-mode. However, when the orb of the square brings us across a sign boundary, then the two squaring planets are not necessarily now both residing in signs with conflicting elements or **same** mode.

For example, with Mars at 29° Aquarius and Venus at 1° Gemini, we have a 92° aspect, well within the standard orb for any square. Yet the signs Aquarius and Gemini naturally *trine* each other! Thus, these squaring planets do not share the same mode and do not reside in conflicting elements (the whole premise of a square). Instead, they are now in the same element. **This weakens the square** because the two planets, although geometrically squared, are now factually in harmonious signs! *This same principle applies to other aspects across sign boundaries.*

THE QUINCUNX / INCONJUNCT (150°, 30°)

The quincunx and inconjunct aspects get their own chapter. Please see the extended discussion of these preeminent, yet least understood, health aspects in *Chapter 4: Quincunx!* There is a general feeling that the quincunx is more powerful than the inconjunct, although more research is certainly needed to determine this as fact.

Correlation of Transit Planet to its Natal Position

The nature of the transiting planet, plus this same transiting planet's own **natal** position in the birth chart must all be compared. For example, for transit Mars in opposition of natal Venus, also check the natal condition of Mars because any Mars transit carries those qualities specific to Mars that were fixed at birth, and also the meaning of his natal house position.

THE OPPOSITION (180°)

The planetary chapters in this book include sections with extended discussions of oppositions of specific planets. The current section discusses general, but important, considerations for interpreting the physical effects of this aspect. Each of these, when applicable, will influence the effects of a given opposition.

Planets of Opposite Nature

In an opposition, the two planets involved actively oppose each other. Should planets of **opposite nature** oppose, we have a battle! This would occur, for example, when transit Mars opposes either transit or natal Saturn or vice versa. Other examples of planets with decisively opposite natures would be Mars-Moon, Saturn-Moon, Saturn-Sun.

Although Jupiter and Mercury govern opposite signs, they both love knowledge; and Mars-Venus are lovers!

Saturn is opposite in nature to all other planets. His opposition slows, or even halts their function, at least temporarily.

Planets of Similar Nature

When planets of similar nature oppose each other, they create *more of the same* energy across the polarity. Note that this rule applies to physical effects, but may not be the case for non-physical uses. As examples, Mars and Jupiter oppositions excite great energy across the polarity involved. Venus opposing the Moon, sometimes brings stasis or may go unnoticed entirely. Jupiter oppose Moon and Jupiter oppose Venus are not disharmonious. An opposition of Jupiter shines his benefic ray on the opposite sign, and any planets therein!

Planet Opposing a Current Malady

When a transit planet opposes a natal planet representing a current malady, then regard your natal planet as being either faced with something coming from without or being weakened by the pull of the opposing plant. An opposition, in these cases, often indicates the arrival of a medical practitioner, an opinion, scare, rescue, or diagnosis.

THE SIX POLARITIES

Oppositions usually occur in one of six sign *polarities*. An opposition occurs when a transiting planet stands opposite a natal planet. These "poles" must be carefully considered in your deline-ation and combined with your understanding of the influences discussed above.

When oppositions occur with one planet outside of the boun-dary normally designated as "in polarity" to the planet opposed, (as discussed in the section on squares), then this opposition is greatly weakened, because the sign polarity no longer applies. The six sign polarities are discussed here:

Aries – Libra:

Influences all balances, such as acid-alkaline, potassium-sodium, and hormonal. It also influences the bodily regions ruled by the signs involved, such as the brain, eyes, adrenals, kidneys, and ovaries.

Taurus – Scorpio:

Influences the excretory, sexual and genital-urinary systems, and all other body parts governed by these signs. The hypothalamus-sex hormone connection.

Taurus is the food intake point (mouth), and Scorpio the waste exit point (anus). The ear-nose-throat (Taurus) reflexes off the colon (Scorpio). One can evaluate the health of the generative system and colon from the voice. Both signs influence the thyroid.

Gemini – Sagittarius:

Emphasizes the voluntary nervous system, central nervous system, peripheral nerves, mind, movement, arms, shoulders, hips and legs, inspiration/expiration (respiration), arterial system, capillaries, and all other body parts governed by these signs.

Cancer – Capricorn:

Emphasizes the nutritive and skeletal systems, such as absorption by the stomach and *assimilation* of nutrients. Influences pituitary function, mucous membranes, fertility, menstrual cycle, and all other body parts governed by these signs.

Leo – Aquarius:

Emphasizes the heart and circulatory system. There is also a considerable influence over the back, the spinal nerves and sheaths, and all other body parts governed by these signs.

Virgo – Pisces:

Emphasizes the immune system, the lymphatic system, the automatic nervous system, and all other body parts governed by these signs, most especially the upper digestive tract and organs, and the feet.

Chapter 4
QUINCUNX!
THE TWELVE MEDICAL QUINCUNXES
The Preeminent Health Aspect

A surprisingly small amount of material is available on planetary quincunxes, especially for their medical implications, both transit and natal. This literary dearth is strange indeed, considering that the quincunx is the preeminent health aspect! Could this be because this aspect is notoriously hard to evaluate?

A transit quincunx occurs when a transit planet stands 150° (or 210°) from a natal planet, within a very small orb. The quincunx is also called the "inconjunct," a term shared with the 30° aspect. A natal quincunx occurs as a permanent fixture of the natal chart. To understand transit quincunxes, one must first understand natal ones!

A key to working with the quincunx is to realize that **all "quincunxes" and "inconjuncts" occur between two signs sharing neither element nor mode in common.** Furthermore, the quincunx angularly corresponds to the three traditional malefic houses (6th, 8th, 12th). Thus, planets in quincunx share the same angular ratio between themselves as these houses do to the Ascendant of a horoscope. Perhaps the malefic nature of these houses is due, in part, to being positioned at quincunx angles to the ascending sign and therefore, sharing neither its mode or element. The unique vital force of the signs so positioned on these three malefic angles cannot be adequately absorbed by the body (as symbolized by the Ascendant). Thus, they make for weakened body zones.

A transit planet in a 30° aspect (inconjunct) is also weakening, if standing in the sign behind or prior to the sign of the natal planet. Note that the transit planet, in this case, is in the 12th house position to that natal planet.

Sections regarding the impact of the quincunx on surgery dates are included in detail throughout this book. However, it is worth stating up front: surgery is unwise should the natal planet representing the topic of surgery (hip, stomach, etc.) be quincunx from any transiting planet within 0-3°. This is especially true should either sign involved in the quincunx govern the bodily region concerned. Unfortunately, surgeries are often required at these times—in many cases **because** of the effects of this transit. The worst quincunx in this regard is that delivered from transit Mars. Therefore, the client must always consult the responsible physician on surgical timing.

The Impact of a Quincunx – *Missed Signals*

Quincunxes are hard to understand. Their impacts are often hidden, mysterious, and hard to detect. They may hide in latency waiting for their perfect moment to strike you by surprise. A quincunx may have profound effects on a native's life, but still go unnoticed and misunderstood. However, they are not mild aspects! In fact, they are "the" primary health aspect. Yet because of their sneaky nature, when a quincunx causes a physical malady, doctors rarely can figure out the cause! Hopefully, this chapter will assist with this problem.

Usually, a quincunx brings a *disconnection* between any two planets placed in an angular relationship of 150° (or 210°) distant from one another. In essence, a quincunx is a conspicuous *non*-aspect, the very meaning of another term for this aspect: the "inconjunct."

Planets in quincunx operate without any reference to each other. For example, let's take a natal Mercury-Moon quincunx. The native's mind and the emotional reactions are not communicating well. The owner of this quincunx will toggle between being all mental with no feeling *("I can't explain my feelings!")*, or conversely, all emotional with no logic *("No, I don't want to talk about it!")*.

A natal quincunx indicates two disparate sides to the nature expressing themselves in different life spheres, such as home/career, youth/adulthood, or that secret nightlife and concealed mistress. Astrologers learn that most of us have more than one personality!

Quincunxes can express business acumen with spiritual longing, restless adventurism with a nurturing nature, ruthless ambition and a compassionate heart. *"What to do?"*

Many people live out both sides of their quincunx every day. There are many fine examples of office tyrants who are tender spouses at home, and vice versa! Then there are those who live out just one side of their quincunx for years, then reverse the emphasis by switching to the other personality for other years. For example, Ray builds his business empire, then retires to a monastery; Betty dutifully raises a family, then travels the world.

Healthwise, the "quincunxed" natal planet temporarily can't easily "digest" the energy of the quincunxing transit planet. Think of each planet as carrying a necessary nutrient composed not of minerals, but *of cosmic color*. To be healthy, we require all the colors of the spectrum. The quincunxed natal planet is deprived of a needed *light nutrient!*

For a transit Mars quincunx, however, this rule is reversed. **Mars delivers a red-hot beam to any planet he quincunxes**, quite observable in practice. The Jyotish consider the quincunx as one of the strongest aspects of Mars! Indeed, this aspect is sometimes profoundly heating. For further discussion of the Mars quincunx, see *Chapter 12: Mars.*

Solving a Quincunx – *Good Luck!*

Quincunxes have a rotten reputation as a predicament that "cannot be solved." Rather, a quincunx shows a conundrum that *cannot be solved without invention, reason and experiment.* More precisely, quincunxes are rarely fully solved, but satisfactory cures, mitigations, workarounds, or partial cures may be found. *For those of us so fortunate to have natal quincunxes, we have a lifetime of practice doing just that.* I call the quincunx "the engineer's aspect" because people who solve difficult problems for a living often have several quincunxes in their birth charts!

To solve a quincunx, a deal must be struck between the two divorced functions. One can insert the missing function when operating in the other side. Returning to our example of natal Mercury quincunx—the natal Moon, one can practice remembering to feel emotions when studying or performing intellectual tasks and conversely, learn to verbally describe one's emotional states.

With respect to solving health-related quincunxes, a book could be written on it! So, by design, this book discusses the effects and possible solutions to medical quincunxes in each of the chapters on the planets. Should a cause of suffering be not readily obvious from a conjunction (first), or next, a square or opposition, then study any current or natal quincunxes to your target problem planet.

Quincunxes and inconjuncts evince a "secret," or puzzling quality, striking from left field. The hidden cause of an unsolved health complaint is so often revealed by a quincunx from transit or of natal Saturn, Mars, or any large planet, plus the bodily organs of the sign it inhabits. Resolve medical mysteries by considering the bodily functions of two planets in quincunx, and the bodily regions of the signs they tenant.

THE TWELVE MEDICAL QUINCUNXES

Author's Notes

These brief notes on the twelve sign quincunxes are by no means complete. I am forced to rely on my own limited observations and anecdotal findings because of the dearth of extant writing about the *medical* implications of this *profoundly medical aspect*. This topic invites research!

Aries – Scorpio:

Excessive circulatory hormones and/or dirty colon (Scorpio) express as facial acne (Aries). Smell and taste sensory disruption may be linked with sexual disinterest (involving Mercury and Mars in one case). Excessive testosterone, adrenalin (three cases, all involving Mars).

Aries – Virgo:

Chinese medicine notes that liver conditions (Virgo/Jupiter) outlet in the eyes (Aries). Migraine and diabetes sufferers often show Virgo-Aries quincunxes. The vagus nerve originates in the brain stem as the tenth cranial nerve (Aries region) and runs to the abdominal organs (Virgo), influencing the parasympathetic control of the digestive tract (Virgo), amongst other organs (heart, lungs).

This quincunx clearly plays a prominent role in what is called the "Brain-Gut Axis." Extreme jaundice (Virgo-Capricorn) can cause brain damage (Aries).

Taurus – Libra:

Taurus is stability and Libra is balance on all levels. Hence we see a relationship worth contemplating between these two signs. Physical balance and some glandular functions; the hypothalamus-ovarian hormone link. Taurus strongly influences the thyroid gland and ears; whereas Libra regulates the adrenal hormones (with Aries), acid-alkaline balance, salt-potassium balance, and the physical sense of balance.

Balance is controlled by the fluids in the semicircular canals of the ear, and the cerebellum at the back base of the brain—both located in Body Zone 2, Taurus.

Is it plausible that breast feeding and/or the quality of mother's milk, and/or early nurturing (Taurus-Cancer), has a later effect upon the ovaries and testes? Do neglected and/or bottle-fed babies suffer more hormonal extremes than happily satisfied babies?

Taurus – Sagittarius:

Taurus governs the region of the thyroid gland, and the thyroid is allotted by sign to Taurus (and to planets Venus, Mercury, and Edgar Cayce's stated assignment, Uranus). Sagittarius, a sign located at a quincunx angle to Taurus, governs "running wildfire" and the urge to move! In my empirical studies, persons born with Sun, Mars or Jupiter in Sagittarius (or strong squares between Sagittarius and Virgo), seem uniquely prone to hyperthyroid.

Gemini – Scorpio:

Bronchial-lung complaints (Gemini) are often suspiciously paired to colon issues (Scorpio). Bronchitis (Gemini) is linked to ulcerative colitis (Scorpio).

Gemini – Capricorn:

Asthma (Gemini) and eczema (Capricorn) are often linked. Rheumatoid arthritis (Capricorn/Saturn) and asthma (Gemini/ Mercury) are possibly linked.

Cancer – Sagittarius:

This combination is inexplicable to me, so I will pose a series of questions. These questions will demonstrate the gist of finding the hidden links between any two quincunxed signs!

Is there a link between the stomach absorption (Cancer) and hip issues (Sagittarius)? Do sentimental emotions (Cancer) influence the hip (Sagittarius)? Is hip dysplasia (Sagittarius)—a malady common in female infants, related to infant milk absorption (Cancer)? Are there emotional effects (Cancer) upon the lower spinal nerves, hips, locomotion?

How do our personal feelings (Cancer) influence the Central Nervous System (Sagittarius)? Does panic (Sagittarius) influence the stomach, milk production or fertility (Cancer)? Does excessive aerobic athletics, especially running (Sagittarius) reduce fertility and halt menses (Cancer)?

Do locomotive problems (Sagittarius) relate to family attachments or states of fear (Cancer)? Are spinal cord diseases (Sagittarius), largely inherited, perhaps from the mother's side (Cancer)? Are claustrophobia (Sagittarius) and agoraphobia (Cancer) both implicated in this quincunx (one or the other)?

Cancer – Aquarius:

Cancer implies motherly nurturing, and Aquarius the impersonal, intellectual approach. Could either a premature birth or a failure to be cuddled or nursed on breast milk (Cancer), produce circulatory or venous deficiencies (Aquarius), or social introversion, or discomfort with crowds (Aquarius), or a greater susceptibility to blood cell diseases (Aquarius)?

Leo – Capricorn:

Gallbladder malfunction (Leo, Capricorn, Mars, Saturn) has been linked to heart disease (Leo). Bad knees (Capricorn) can lead to bad back (Leo). Scoliosis and other structural spine anomalies (Leo) can create imbalance that wears down the knees (Capricorn).

Leo – Pisces:

Weak lymphatic function (Pisces) is linked to cardiac health (Leo). Heart failure shows in fluid buildup in lower leg and foot (Aquarius-Pisces). Poorly aligned feet (Pisces) can influence or cause back troubles (Leo).

Virgo – Aquarius:

Spleen malfunction (Virgo) contributes to leukemia (Aquarius). Could the solar plexus (Sun, Virgo) and lower abdominal nerve plexus (Virgo), be linked to a malfunction of the bodily electrical system (Aquarius)? This quincunx strongly impacts the health of the portal circulation.

Libra – Pisces:

Kidney failure (Libra) can compromise the lymphatic system (Pisces). Kidney related failure to excrete fluids and salt can cause edema and an overall phlegmatic state, commonly known to some Piscean types. Venus governs Libra and is exalted in Pisces. This quincunx influences excesses or imbalance of female hormones, and has a profound relation to sexual issues in both genders.

Chapter 5
THE PLANET IN TROUBLE

Any natal planet under *exceptional affliction* is more likely to express symptoms in the physical body. What conditions constitute an exceptional affliction? To determine the likelihood of physical symptoms, we assess the cumulative weight of various stressors on a natal planet, including extreme natal aspects, stressful transits, debility, malefic placement, temperature extremes, and house placement.

Stressful Aspects to Natal Planets

The stresses signified by the following planetary conditions contribute to the potential for physical symptoms. If three or more of the afflictions listed below concur, you can safely assume that you have a "planet in trouble."

Multiple Stressful Aspects

A natal planet is exceptionally stressed when it receives at least three stressful aspects, from either natal or transit planets. This includes squares, oppositions, and quincunxes from any planet. This may also include a conjunction, especially from a malefic planet. Visualize the hapless planet at the apex of squares, oppositions and quincunxes. Three will do!

Eclipses, Transit

Any natal planet that is positioned within 3° of a current eclipse might express physical symptoms. In practice, this planet may signify a relative, spouse or close friend rather than oneself.

Eclipses, Prenatal

At some time in the life, a natal planet may be hampered from carrying out its natural functions when it is positioned on the exact degree of either of the two most recent prenatal eclipses (those eclipses occurring just prior to the birth date, within one year).

Midpoint of Natal Malefics

Any natal planet situated at the midpoint degree between natal Mars and Saturn will feel substantial stress for the life of the native. One gets used to this over time; so although this distressed natal planet may play a role in disease causation, it is seldom experienced as the constant vise grip of that hapless natal planet, seated like a duck, midway between two transiting malefics. See the following first two points below.

Midpoint of Transit Malefics

Any natal planet situated at the midpoint degree between transiting Mars and Saturn will receive considerable stress for the duration of that transit.

"In the Bends," Transit

A natal planet receives an abundance of temporary stress when positioned at the midpoint of the transiting Lunar Nodes within an orb of 1°.

"In the Bends," Natal

A natal planet is extremely stressed when "in the Bends," i.e., when situated at the midpoint of the natal North and South Lunar Nodes (and thus in square to both), within an orb of 3°.

STRESSFUL NATAL CHART PLACEMENTS
Sign Debility

The natal planet is in *debility* when its sign position places it in its *detriment* or *fall*. These are classic terms dealt with in most basic texts, including *Medical Astrology: A Guide to Planetary Pathology*. **Detriment** indicates a planet in the sign(s) opposite to those it rules. **Fall** means that it tenants the sign opposite to its sign of exaltation.

A planet in debility is hampered from expressing its nature in a natural manner. This is not bad for all matters, because the universe has a good use for everything. However, the condition of debility is one testimony that this planet's natural functions may be debilitated in some way.

Excessive Strength

While strong natal planets are usually favorable to the native, a natal planet can also be **too** strong! This is especially true in the case of the Sun and Mars. Excess strength of a planet can occur in multiple ways, based on their placement in the natal chart.

One example is dignity; that's when a planet tenants the sign it governs or is in its sign of exaltation. Such a planet will carry out its own functions with force. This is also true for planets on the angles, closely conjunct the Ascendant, Midheaven, Nadir, and Descendant.

The great medical psychic Edgar Cayce remarked that the strongest position for any planet is within a few degrees above the Ascendant, visible in the sky at birth. I've found this rule to be unfailing. I allow an orb of 15° above the horizon, and a full 30° should no other planet be situated in the 1st or 12th houses.

Note: Be careful when considering the Descendant as a point of strength, because some planets are diminished here, rather than strengthened. After all, the Descendant is where sunset occurs each evening, dropping the vital force as the Sun sinks below the horizon.

Temperature Extremes

These rules have been explored more thoroughly in my previous books. However, they are so reliable that they bear reiteration here.

*Natal Mars and Sun are too hot when **all** of the following conditions are true: Positioned above the horizon, in a daytime birth, **and** in a masculine sign (especially the Fire signs Aries, Leo, Sagittarius).*

Some astrologers would include Jupiter with this merry group.

If unchecked, this excessive astral heat is sometimes productive of stroke, hypertension, insomnia, mania, heart attack, meningitis and similar conditions. Antipathetic treatment ideas are provided in my previous works.

*Conversely, natal Saturn is pathologically cold when all of the following conditions are true: positioned below the horizon, in a night birth, **and** in a female sign.*

Tradition says Saturn should be above ground to fulfill this rule, but this has not entirely born out in practice.

In the Earth signs this condition produces hard, dry tissue states, impaction, constipation, stiffness, tumors, "stuffy gallbladder," and a host of related chronic conditions.

In Water signs, he produces lymphatic sluggishness, trapped fluids, dry mucus membrane, emotional isolation, physical cold, morbid fears and related conditions. Antipathetic treatment ideas are provided in my previous works.

Note that the Sun is always above the horizon during day births, and below the horizon at night.

Retrograde

The retrograde natal planet works differently for the benefics than for the malefics. Traditionally, this condition is *weakening* to the benefics, Venus and Jupiter, reducing their ability to protect the native.

Unfortunately, retrograde is traditionally *strengthening* to any affliction presented by the *malefics* Saturn and Mars. The worst afflictions are often seen with a retrograde Saturn backing up to station within a week or two—visualize a truck loaded down with concrete blocks, backing up to stop. If ignored, this action is not auspicious for health.

Flanked by Malefic Planets

A natal planet is stressed when it is flanked by two or more malefic natal planets. Traditionally, when a planet is closely flanked by Mars and Saturn it is "besieged."

Malefic House Position

Natal planets in the traditionally health problematic 6th and 8th houses are *highly inclined to produce physical symptoms*. The malefic 12th house may or may not produce disease as its province is primarily *mental health*. However, this rule is certainly not invariable!

The signs governing all three malefic houses of the natal chart indicate a deficiency in the bodily regions or organs governed by these signs. This concept is illustrated in great detail, with classic remediations in my book *Astrology & Your Vital Force*.

Sign functions are different than planet functions, although related. As discussed in greater detail in *Chapter 1, Essentials*, the physical deficiency of *sign-ruled* functions is based on the relative angular (house) relationship of any sign to the birth Ascendant. Thus, best results in medical astrology are achieved in the "Whole Sign" house system, counting forward counterclockwise, with the house of the rising sign as "House 1."

Advocates of other house systems: *Please do not overlook the physical deficiencies noted for signs that are angularly placed 6, 8, and 12 signs from the Ascendant. Do so at your client's peril!*

A Natal Light or Planet Tightly Conjunct the Natal South Lunar Node
Traditionally weakening.

THE LIGHTS

Chapter 6

THE SUN
LIFE AND LIGHT

Properties, Rulerships and Actions
Rules: Leo

Exalted: Aries

Detriment: Aquarius

Fall: Libra

Metal: Gold

Minerals: Magnesium, Iodine *(Nauman, Jansky)*, Manganese *(Jansky)*

Vitamins: A, D *(Nauman, Jansky)*

Gem & Cosmic Ray: Red Ruby, Red *(traditional)*

Governs: The Yearly Cycle

Light: The Sun is light, the light of life.

The Sun represents the vital force itself, and our personal reserve battery of this force, also known as chi, ki and prana. The strength, quality and amount of the native's *innate vital force* is discerned from the condition of the natal Sun. It deserves mention that there are many types of prana, and several declared seats of vital force storage in the body, i.e. the medulla, spleen, lower abdomen, and *dantien* (a chi storage region of the body known to Chinese medicine). However, the Sun represents the spark of life behind them all!

Body Rulership & Organ Affinities: The heart and aorta, the right eye in males, the left eye in females, and the brain (shared with Mercury, Moon and Mars). Cornell cites the natal Sun as influencing the right ovary, right testicle, the nucleus of cells, the pons Varolii in the brain stem, and the "vital etheric fluid entering the spleen."

General Action: *Transit Sol governs the yearly cycle for all natal charts.*

Sol's transits are in a class of their own, working differently than "his" planets. The great light of the Sun imparts its influence through the distinctive cosmic colors of the various planets, as they reflect Sol's light with their own unique hues and effects. This is similar in how a prism refracts sunlight into the seven visible colors.

A transiting planet vibrates its unique temperature, moisture level and color frequency to the natal planets aspected. In the old Greek way of thinking, the transiting planets "hurled rays" and "commingled beams." Whereas each planet effuses a cosmic color, the Sun represents light itself, encompassing all colors. The twelve zodiac signs obtain their unique character via twelve qualities of Sunlight, caused by the Earth's varied positional angle to Sol in his seasonal round. The 12 tropic zodiac signs represent, in part, 12 distinct types of the Solar vital force.

Sol's cyclic transit through the natal chart provides more or less *vital force.* Throughout his yearly sojourn, *he either feeds or starves each planet in turn on specific annual dates of his dependable cycle.* The planets transiting at any given time will then either support or counteract the Sun's influence.

Although Sol is hot and dry, his transit doesn't necessarily heat nor dry the **sign** he journeys through nor the planet he aspects as one might expect. *Instead, Sol emphasizes the season's element or the distinct nature of that sign or planet.* For example, the Sun increases moisture when in Water signs, while increasing heat and dryness in Fire signs. See the section on temperature and moisture *(next page)* for a further discussion of this unique characteristic of transit Sun.

Unless accompanied by a transit Node, the transit Sun rarely produces the obviously acute events of Mars or the chronicity of Saturn. However, one must watch his yearly cycle closely in weak, elderly or convalescing persons. Several studies have shown that people statistically tend to die more often at certain astrologically relevant points in their personal yearly cycle.

For example, one study from the "Annals of Epidemiology" demonstrated that people of both genders are 14% more likely to die on their exact birthday, with a big wave approaching and departing the birth date by a week. A peak is also noted in the month opposing the birthday (the anti-birthday). The reader may be amused that astrology was left out of *all* explanations given.

Furthermore, the largest cause of birthday death in replicated studies was heart attack and stroke (Sun ruled events). Curiously, Sol rules the heart and brain, and he returns to his own position on the birth date, emphasizing these organs! I discovered that the famous guitarist Jerry Garcia died of a heart attack within days of his birthday in Leo, the sign ruler of the heart.

Astrologically, this all makes perfect sense. For exhaustive detail on the Sun's influence on the vital force, and how practitioners might work with it, see the book *Astrology & Your Vital Force: Healing with Cosmic Rays and DNA Resonance*

Positive: Strengthens, steadies, increases vital force.

Negative: The Sun itself is associated with heart disease, hypertension, brain issues, and eye problems. *Additionally, the Sun emphasizes the problems of any natally afflicted planet he conjoins, squares, opposes or quincunxes.*
For some types of squares, and all oppositions and quincunxes, *less Vital Force is available to the functions represented by that planet at these times.* This in turn increases the likelihood that the issues represented by the natal planet may act up.

Excess: Internal heat builds up, red faced, heart pounding, hot brain, pounding pulse, self-importance, bombast. It is rare that the transit Sun produces these effects, while an overly dominant natal Sun readily does!

Deficiency: Cold, weak, fatigued, failing, pale, lacks will power and confidence. Rarely does the transit Sun produce these symptoms. However, the weak natal Sun readily manifests these traits.

Temperature & Moisture Levels: Sol is hot, but he is the *heat of the life* seated in the nucleus of each cell. This heat is an expression of the *vital force! This expression is distinct from the heat of Mars.*

Sol's warmth is radiating whereas Mars' heat is focused and inflaming. While Mars is **felt** as directly heating to the bodily zone he transits, the Sun is not, unless in Fire signs.

Although the Sun is "hot and dry," the transit of Sol doesn't necessarily heat nor dry the sign he journeys through nor the planet he aspects as one might expect (unless in Fire signs). *Instead, Sol emphasizes the season's element or the distinct nature of that sign.* If this wasn't true, then everybody would be constitutionally hot and dry! Instead, we typically adopt the energetic quality of our birth sign's element, along with that of the Moon, Ascendant and ruling planet.

For example: The Sun increases moisture when in Water signs, expresses windy changes in Gemini, pleasant moderation in Libra and downright cold in midwinter's Aquarius! In the mid-spring Earth sign of Taurus, Sol produces a warming magnetism so different from the dryness expressed in the two remaining Earth signs Virgo and Capricorn.

Sol's passage is specifically **drying** in Fire signs, in the Earth signs Capricorn (ruled by dry Saturn) and Virgo, and also in Air sign Aquarius (also Saturn ruled). In a hot, dry natal chart, the transit of Sun through the Fire signs will definitely stir up excess heat and dryness. A natal Sun in Fire is sufficient to produce the typical fiery "pitta" constitution and body shape of Fire signs, provided opposing elements don't dominate the natal chart.

Transit Frame & Orb: The Earth orbits the Sun once every 365¼ days, which defines what we call a "year." *Because of the extra quarter day each year, there is a leap year of 366 days every four years. In the geocentric view of planetary motion, which is represented in the astrological ephemeris, the Sun moves through all twelve signs once every year, and therefore transits about one degree per day, and one sign in 30 days. A rapid and supremely regular progression.*

As always, the cardinal rule of orbs is "the closer, the stronger." However, there are some further considerations for the effective orb of a Solar transit. While the transit Sun emphasizes the entire sign he passes through, he influences planets therein within at least a 10° orb, as long as he remains within the sign's borders.

His transits are most obvious and very potent within a 3° orb. Thus, the effects of a Solar aspect typically manifest within a few days on either side of exactitude. However, it may manifest as long as seven days, should the transit Moon trigger the Sun's aspect by making a hard aspect to the natal planet.

If a transiting Node accompanies the Sun, then eclipses may take place nearby. If the eclipse is within a 3° orb of a natal planet (or square or opposed), then Sol's transit would strike with great force producing either a surge or outage of vital force to the planet. This impact could extend **in a cyclic manner** through one or even two years, as the eclipse degree is triggered when the Sun, Mars, or the planet ruler of the eclipse rolls around into hard aspect to that degree. (For detail on the distinctive medical effects of Solar and Lunar eclipses through each zodiac sign or when conjunct either transit or natal planets, see *Eclipses and You*.)

Special Discussion on Natal Solar Conjunctions: Cazimi, Combust, and "Under the Beams"

Readers interested in the Sun's **natal** orbs should familiarize themselves with three terms: *Cazimi, Combust* and *"under the Sun's beams."* Classical astrologers were aware of these three special circumstances related to Sol's conjunction with a natal planet at birth—for example, *"Edward was born with Venus in Cazimi."* In practice, many astrologers find that these distinctions do not reliably bear out. Still, it's good to note the tradition.

  • *Cazimi:* When a planet is conjunct the Sun within seventeen minutes (17') of ecliptic longitude, this planet is said to be Cazimi or "in the heart of the Sun."

Traditionally, this condition is held to be an extremely strong placement for this planet, as the ray of the planet shines through the orb of the Sun. However, nobody at the time studied the difference produced by which side of the Sun the planet stands, with respect to the Earth. Is it standing between the Sun and the Earth, facing the viewer as it were; or is the planet concealed behind the Sun, as if blotted out?

Certainly, the effects of these two types of Cazimi would be markedly different! Additionally, the planet's position by *declination* must be taken into consideration. A planet sharing the same declination as Sol (parallel) would certainly be in super-cazimi!

• *Combust:* A natal planet is combust when it conjuncts the Sun within 3° to 8°30' *(Nicholas Devore)*. While traditionally thought to be weakening to the planet, in practice the case is *most often reversed!* The efficacy of this rule remains a topic of debate. For example, could it influence only Mercury or in *what manner* would planets be weakened?

• *"Under the Beams":* A planet is under the beams when it is situated less than seventeen degrees (17°) of the Sun. This placement is traditionally considered unfavorable, although very often it does not bear out in practice! Venus and Mercury are frequently in this condition, and typically do not seem the worse for it. The efficacy of this rule remains a topic of debate.

Special Discussion: Transit Sun and North Node, Similarities

The reader will notice a great deal of similarity between the Sun's transit influence and that of the transit North Lunar Node. This is quite true. Both the Sun and the North Node transmit *extra vital force* to any natal planet conjoined.

However, the Sun's close transit is far briefer and inherently less impactful than that of the North Node. The Sun merely heightens the vital current for a brief time; whereas the North Node can signal a tidal surge lasting several months. Natally, and by transit, Sol and "The Dragon's Head" (North Node) are associated with different disease processes; for example, Sol is not linked to the cancer or skin diseases attributed to the North Node and Saturn. The Sun is hot whereas the North Node is very cold.

However, the two share an affinity to many maladies in predisposed charts when they are either natally placed or transiting through Fire signs, such as stroke, hypertension, brain issues, and glaucoma. In Earth signs both produce impactions, and stiff, dry conditions. In Water signs, both heighten fluidic pressure.

THE SUN THROUGH THE ELEMENTS & SIGNS

Health Potentials for Predisposed Nativities

Aspects do not always manifest as health concerns or benefits.

Applicable to both natal and transit charts, these partial lists of expressed symptoms apply only to predisposed nativities. These conditions are obviously uncommon and require multiple testimonies beyond the presence of the Sun.

Manifestation of symptoms may be enhanced by lifestyle choices, and taking preemptive measures can reduce, remove or prevent potential issues from manifesting. It is not possible to list all potential expressions.

Sun in Fire Signs

Aries: *The seasonal vital force moves more strongly to the head, brain and eye region.*

Increases pressure to head, eyes, brain. Sharp vision. Energy rises up fast. Possible negative effects include increasing natal tendency toward mania, rages, and sudden, high fever. In very rare cases, brain storms, glaucoma, brain problems, aneurism, and (with assist from Mars) meningitis.

Leo: *The seasonal vital force moves more strongly to the heart region. Internal heat increases (astrologically, this is the hottest season).*

Possible negative effects include increasing tendency to rapid heartbeat, heart attack, stroke, hypertension, aneurism, thrombosis, overheating, heatstroke, back pressure, mania, sunstroke, paralysis, back injury, temper fit.

Sagittarius: *The seasonal vital force moves more strongly to the hips, legs, muscles, arterial circulation, "higher mind" and lower spinal cord.*

Possible negative effects include increasing natal tendencies toward sciatica, hyperactive lower spinal nerves, paralysis, hyperthyroid, and injuries incurred from horses, dogs, driving, sports, risky behavior, firearms, or arrows. Increases stimulation to neuromuscular system, overactive motor nerves. Aggravates conditions of excess Fire, such as religious mania, hyperactivity, restlessness, insomnia, hypertension, heart attack, stroke, aneurism, and seizures.

Field Note: Amongst my natal case studies are three persons with hyperthyroid so severe that all required their thyroids removed. All three persons were Sagittarians, born with the Sun conjunct Jupiter in prominent aspect to Mars. Two of the three were born as the Sun-Jupiter conjunction squared Mars in Virgo.

The Sun in Earth Signs

Taurus: *The seasonal vital force moves more strongly to the lower head, jaw, ears and neck area. Magnetism increases.*

This lovely season produces the highest magnetism of the year, bringing sweetness, good appetites and high libidos. Taurus is demonstrably one of the three most fertile signs of the zodiac. Muscle, bone and fat build more readily during Sol's transit through this mid-spring sign.

Possible negative effects include increasing typical Taurus maladies in predisposed charts: neck injury, throat inflammation or infection, tongue inflammation, tonsillitis, ear obstruction, deafness, ear injury, eating disorders and addictions, gorging, choking, suffocation, difficulty swallowing, blockages in general, heavy metal poisoning from dental fillings, tooth impactions, abscessed teeth, bruxism, TMJ, infected salivary glands, overeating, vocal polyps, tongue, mouth or throat cancer, cancer of upper esophagus, excessive masturbation, vocal cord inflammation or infection, lower brain pressure, lower brain tumor or thrombosis, cysts, injury to cervical vertebrae, boils, swollen palette.

Virgo: *The seasonal vital force moves more strongly to the liver, pancreas, spleen, and upper intestine. Drying.*

This season speeds up the nervous system and increases mental acuity. If negative, it potentially emphasizes typical Virgo maladies in predisposed charts: indigestion, poor appetite, abdominal hernia, appendicitis, duodenitis, pancreatitis, colitis, diverticulitis, splenitis, intestinal worms or parasites, liver flukes, parasites in gall or liver ducts, liver diseases, intestinal blockages, intestinal aneurism, liver injury, hepatitis, sclerotic liver, appendicitis, jaundice, swollen spleen, ruptured spleen (with both Nodes), injury to upper digestive organs, cancer or tumors of liver, pancreas, duodenum or intestine; obstructed colon, colitis and Crohn's disease (with Scorpio); yoga and diet extremes, "dying to be healthy."

Capricorn: *The seasonal vital force moves more strongly into the bones, skin, knees, tendons and ligaments. Drying and hardening.*

Capricorn is one of the best seasons for building (or rebuilding) bone mass. However, Capricorn is also one of the best fasting signs. This season's energy is astringent, and tightens up the periphery.

Possible negative effects include emphasizing typical Capricorn maladies in predisposed charts: skin changes or potential skin cancer, itchy skin, excessively oily or dry skin, plugged skin ducts, plugged bile duct, parasites in gall or liver ducts, eczema, psoriasis, pituitary excitation, excess bile production (jaundice) knee injury, bodily stiffness, strong knee (if positive), tendinitis at knee, the retention of toxins in joints, arthritis, rheumatism or gout.

Stomach issues and nausea (reflex to cancer-causing acidic stomach), poor appetite, dental carries, vomiting, lead poisoning, bone infections, bone spurs, mineral deposits in joints, gallbladder or kidney; may contribute to cellular changes in skin or bone; influences kidney function; stimulates anterior pituitary, especially near 4°.

Sun in Air Signs

Gemini: *The seasonal vital force moves more strongly to the peripheral nerves, shoulders, arms, hands, bronchial tubes, lungs, speech center, scapula.*

Accelerates speech and gesticulation. Possible negative effects include the increase of any natal tendencies toward insomnia, boredom, restlessness, excessive talking, nervous complaints, asthma, bronchitis, bronchial and lung issues. May be implicated in some types of seizures.

Libra: *The seasonal vital force moves more strongly to the kidney, ovary and lumbar area.*

This season produces a relaxing, effect, tending towards stasis. Negatively, this season can increase natal tendencies toward kidney issues, (typically inactivity), ovarian or testicle complaints, hormonal imbalances, edema, diabetes, copper-iron imbalance, acid/alkaline imbalance, venous issues, adrenal fatigue or hyperactivity, lumbar pressure, lumbar issues. Increases the love of sugar and wine.

Aquarius: *The seasonal vital force moves more strongly to the venous circulation, electrical body, spinal cord and lower leg. Internal cold increases.*

Possible negative effects include the increase of any natal tendencies toward depression, mysterious blood disorders, blood poisoning, circulatory disorders, low blood pressure, carbon monoxide poisoning, auto-intoxication, lower leg thrombosis, cold extremities, varicose veins, ankle issues, restricted Achilles, excitation to spinal nerves, heightens electrical impulses through spinal nerves, ankle or calf emphasized, neural pain in lower leg, nutritional deficiencies, rare diseases of the spinal nerves, bites of venomous creatures.

Note: Aquarius is an extremely cold, Saturn ruled, mid-winter sign. Thus, astrologically speaking, it is incorrectly conflated with the "hot, moist" Sanguine "humor." Astrologers have woefully conflated the four elements with the four humors, regardless of the fact that they are not the same thing. Signs are **not** humors!

Sun in Water Signs

Cancer: *The seasonal vital force moves inward to the breast and stomach. Moisture increases.*

Energy pools inward toward the memory, emotions, home and hearth. Cancer is one of the three most fertile times of the year with increases in estrogen or progesterone.

Possible negative effects include increasing natal tendencies toward fluidic pressure, breast cysts or tumors, plugged breast ducts, leaking poison from breast implants, breast injury or surgery, emphasis to breastbone; mood swings, depression, tears, ulcers, food cravings, insatiable appetites, food addiction, nausea, stomach and diaphragm issues, pleural effusion, emotionalism, waterborne parasites, shortsightedness. Family pattern issues, strong allergic response, fluid to lower lung, lung tumors, agoraphobia, heightens any phobia. Emphasis on meninges or pericardium. Stimulates posterior pituitary, especially near 4°.

Although Pisces is the sign "ruling" the lymphatics, Cancer is equally implicated through its rulership of the thoracic duct and armpits. For predisposed persons, lymphatic pressure and toxicity may increase when the Sun transits through either sign.

Scorpio: *The seasonal vital force moves more strongly to the genitals, bladder, nose, excretory system and colon. Moisture and excretion increase.*

Sexual appetites increase, more energy flows to the sexual chakra. Activates the nose, bladder, sweat glands and colon. Scorpio's regenerative powers can work real miracles. This season greatly activates the excretory system. Gentle assistance may be required lest the lymphatic system and/or bloodstream become overburdened with toxic matter, resulting in acne, body odor, etc. Because the Scorpio season activates all releases, this is perhaps the best sign of all for recovery from impossible conditions!

Possible negative effects include increasing natal tendencies toward diarrhea, diuresis, sweat, skin disease, excessive menses. An increased tendency exists at this time for STDs, vermin, candida, fungus, mildew, viruses, venomous bites or stings, acne, boils.

Pisces: *The seasonal vital force moves more strongly to the feet, lymphatic system and interstitial fluids. Cold moisture increases.*

This season seems to make folks sleepy and increases appetites for food or sex. What else could ancient people do in late winter? Imagination increases. Alcohol and drugs may impact the bloodstream and body far more than average. Psychically sensitive people may be advised to strengthen their psychic boundaries at this time because the season of Pisces lowers them.

Possible negative effects include the increase of natal tendencies toward foot issues, lymphatic overload, wasting or lingering viruses, pneumonia, fatigue, and psychic complaints. This month is problematic for depression sufferers, the lonely, and those with mental illness. Feet issues may occur. The lymphatic system may require more attention as it may overload at this time.

THE SUN'S TRANSIT OF NATAL PLANETS
Health Potentials for Predisposed Nativities
Transits do not always manifest as health concerns or benefits.

Applicable to both natal and transit charts, these partial lists of expressed symptoms apply only to predisposed nativities. These conditions are obviously uncommon and require multiple testimonies beyond the presence of the Sun.

Manifestation of symptoms may be enhanced by lifestyle choices, and taking preemptive measures can reduce, remove or prevent potential issues from manifesting. It is not possible to list all potential expressions.

For guidance on timing, please refer to the discussion earlier in this chapter on *Transit Frame & Orb*.

The Master Cycle of the Year
Transit Sun Aspects to the Natal Sun
On his annual sojourn around the ecliptic plane, Sol makes various exact angles to his *natal placement (the birth date)* at approximately the same times each year. This regular sequence provides our personal yearly cycle of vital force circulation. To know this cycle is so essential to practitioners that I've devoted the first chapters of *Astrology & Your Vital Force* to this one topic! For the reader's convenience I will reiterate a brief amount of that material in this present work, and hope I am not faulted for so doing.

The Sun's cycle is divided into twelve seasons called "signs." These zodiac signs are further divided into thirty-six periods of ten days each known as "decans" or "decanates." Thus, each sign has three decans. For example, Taurus is divided into 3 decanates by zodiacal degree in this manner: 0°–9° 59'; 10°–19° 59'; and 20°–29° 59' of Taurus. The basics of the Solar cycle are outlined below, followed in the next sections by a discussion of Sol's transits of the signs and natal planets.

Orb for the Sun's Transit to Natal Sun

Please see the earlier discussion of *Transit Frame & Orb* for a more complete discussion. However, unique to transit-Sun-to-natal-Sun aspects, the influence reverberates nicely within the full decanate, but manifests best within an orb of 3°. The exception is the quincunx, which is generally felt only within an orb of 3°.

Transit Sun Conjunct Natal Sun:

The few days around one's birthday can be a time of very important health events. *(See General Action, pages 52 and 53).*

Transit Sun Square Natal Sun

This period presents friction to the native Vital Force. This friction sometimes lowers one's internal battery, and in other cases stimulates it, producing an energizing effect! See the discussion on types of squares by sign and mode in *Chapter 3: Aspect Mechanics.* This is a prime few days to enhance and protect the vital force. Avoid early hospital release and if convalescing, continue to do so.

Because of their natural surplus of life force, healthy, vital people rarely notice this aspect.

Transit Sun Trine Natal Sun

Unless counteracted by other testimonies, this period offers the native a superior supply-line toward increased vital force. This is a perfect time to refuel one's inner battery. This is a wonderful time for vibrational healing work. The effects may be only subtly felt but results are typically sure. The "sextile" aspect is very good too, but not as strong.

Transit Sun Quincunx Natal Sun

These few days are *distinctly weakening* to the vital force, as less Solar energy fuels the native's life battery. This internal energy-lowering effect is not too noticeable in healthy people.

Caution is extended however, to strong individuals who may "blow out their circuits" by remaining on high drive at this time. This is a sneaky aspect, often creating an unforeseen action between the bodily organs governed by the sign of the transiting Sun *secretly pulling upon* those governed by the sign of the natal Sun.

The vital force absolutely needs raising. It is wise to be very alert to one's health around this time within an orb of 3°. Because of their natural surplus of life force, healthy, vital people rarely notice this aspect.

Should either transit Node be simultaneously present in the same sign of the transit Sun, look for an eclipse occurring within two weeks on either side. If an eclipse quincunxes the natal Sun within an orb of 3°, the impact can extend in a cyclic manner through one or even two years! During this time, if any malady arising concurs with symptoms classic to the two signs involved in the quincunx, or to the Sun itself, then heightened precautions should be taken.

Surgical and Medical Tips: If the responsible doctor agrees, avoid all surgical procedures at this time. This would be doubly so for surgery to the heart, brain, or eye. Convalescence should never be hurried at this time, and early hospital release is unwise. Frail individuals can learn to pull more "prana" into their personal reservoir of vital force during these periods.

Herbal Note: A professional herbalist might use gently strengthening cardiac herbs, and also foods high in prana at this time. Do not self-treat.

Field Note: This author has observed many sudden and unexpected deaths and health crises when eclipses occur at quincunx to the Sun, or shortly following. If convalescing, do not ignore this aspect. This is a poor time for hospital release.

Transit Sun Opposite Natal Sun

The anti-birthday or half-birthday is the nadir of anyone's personal Solar year. The Sun, our beacon of vital force supply, is now standing on the opposite side of the ecliptic plane from where it stood on the day you were born! Sometimes people feel fatigued near their anti-birthday. Convalescing persons should take it easy at this time and not overdo things. This debilitating effect may not be obvious should the Ascendant or natal Moon be in the same sign as the transit Sun. Because of their natural surplus of life force, healthy, vital people rarely notice this aspect.

THE SUN'S CONJUNCTION
Health Potentials for Predisposed Nativities
Transits do not always manifest as health concerns or benefits.

Transit Sun Conjunct Natal Sun:
> See *General Action (page 52)* and *(page 62) The Master Cycle of the Year.*

Transit Sun Conjunct Natal Moon

This transit emphasizes everything the natal Moon means for that person. Possible generic areas of emphasis include: moods, emotion, stomach, breasts, fluids, fertility, birthing, allergy sensitivity, and appetite. People are more sensitive at this time.

Surgical and Medical Tips: Fertile! Multiple births are likely if the woman is taking fertility enhancement drugs at this time. A trine or conjunction of Jupiter doubles this testimony.

Transit Sun Conjunct Natal Mercury

This transit emphasizes everything the natal Mercury means for that person. Increases mental powers and function. Potentially, could add pressure on the brain, sensory nerves or ears; prone to moles or warts on the hands or fingers; may engorge bronchial tubes or lungs. For epileptics, a "red alert" potential. If positive, this transit enhances Mercurial function by providing more vital force to the nerves of the region governed by the natal sign of Mercury.

Herbal Note: Practitioners should watch for an increase in neurologically related symptoms and antidote accordingly.

Transit Sun Conjunct Natal Venus

This brief transit emphasizes everything the natal Venus means for that person. Heightens blood sugar, estrogens and copper. Possibly a "red alert" time for diabetics. Temporarily increases libido and attractiveness. Brings temporarily heightened fertility.

Negatively, this transit can lead to a dangerous rise in blood sugar or estrogen levels. Can increase venous pressure or sluggishness, varicosities, swollen ovaries or testes, impacted or engorged kidneys, kidney obstruction. cysts.

If positive, this transit enhances magnetism and calm providing more vital force to Venus. If the native's natal Venus is pleasant, then female healers are beneficial at this time.

Herbal Note: There are excellent herbs available to offset varicosities (Sage, Mullein, Horse Chestnut, Rue, etc.). Cysts respond well to Cleavers, Poke Root, Red Clover. Do not self-treat.

Transit Sun Conjunct Natal Mars

This brief transit emphasizes everything that natal Mars means for that person. In most cases, strong transits to Mars excite to action. However, in symptoms of a deficient natal Mars, one occasionally notices an increase of the negative symptoms such as anemia.

Typically though, this transit temporarily promotes available energy to rise; strengthens the muscles; increases testosterone, adrenalin and iron; improves blood cell count, and is hemorrhage and accident-prone. Can produce excesses of "Martian" themes with consequential hyperactivity, anger control issues and mania. Potential for sudden burns, fevers, excretions, and sweats.

Other temporary changes may include insomnia, excessive libido, obsessions, increased sperm count and male potency, impactions (of sweat glands, urethra/ureters, or testes), genital infections, nose bleed, hemorrhage, strokes and aneurysms (with added pressure from Sun, Jupiter and/or Mars). This transit can produce an unmanageable surge of temper or aggression, especially in Fire signs.

Surgical and Medical Tips: If having a medical procedure, there is a heightened potential for hemorrhage, stroke, infection, mistakes or suddenly rising blood pressure. Therefore, it's wise to check other testimonies.

Herbal Note: Herbalists can treat skin inflammation and burns with Dr. Kloss' burn ointment; or alternatively, Aloe Vera, Calendula, Slippery Elm, etc. Marshmallow and Chickweed are wonderful for internal inflammation of the intestinal tract and urinary canal.

Cayenne pepper can stop external bleeding in its tracks. Yarrow, as Matthew Wood calls "the master of the blood" allays internal bleeding and threatened stroke. Nettles, Beets and soaked Black raisins assist with blood related asthenic conditions. However, due to Mars' wide array of seriously acute issues, it is best to refer to Wood's *Earthwise Repertory of Herbal Medicine*. Do not self-treat.

Field Note: Renowned comedienne and television producer Lucille Ball died 8 hours after surgery of a dissecting aortic aneurism as the transit Sun stood between her natal Mars and North Node (in the 5th house of the heart); also loosely squaring her natal Sun in Leo (sign of the aorta), in the 8th house of death; while simultaneously opposing her natal Jupiter within 1°.

Any and all interconnects between Jupiter-Mars-Sun-North Node—either natally, or by transit to the natal chart— are renowned for aneurism, stroke, hemorrhage heart attack, or heart issues of all kinds.

Transit Sun Conjunct Natal Jupiter

This brief transit emphasizes everything the natal Jupiter means for that person. This transit is stimulating to the arterial circulation and accelerates both blood pressure and liver function. Invigorating and athletic. Energy rises, and some people feel great!

The liver is emphasized for one to three days. Portal circulation may increase slightly. This may be concerning to those with liver disease or engorgement. This aspect may temporarily increase weight, fat, edema or swelling (depending on the element). Stimulates the pituitary gland, with odd results caused by hormone increases, such as hot flashes, swollen breasts, and high libido. Temporarily heightens fertility. This is a positive aspect for desired weight gain or pregnancy!

Generally warming to the body. Especially in Fire signs, this transit heats and pressurizes the arterial blood, heightening any inherent tendency to stroke, heart attack, thrombosis, or sunstroke. Those with liver disease should note that this transit temporarily increases liver function.

Influences the blood. There is some potential for increased glycogen release and consequential changes in blood sugar levels. Blood cholesterol may unexpectedly soar. May cause a plethora of blood in the bodily region ruled by the sign of natal Jupiter. Migraine prone.

Hope and joy are enhanced—a great assist to *victims of depression.* Conversely, this transit is a potentially dangerous stimulant for individuals suffering bipolar, mania, panic, anger control issues, or ADHD.

In some cases, this transit signals a miraculous health intervention, beneficial information or angelic help. Prayers are effective at this time! Medical insurance can also come through.

Surgical and Medical Tips: Women who do not wish multiple births at this time should be wary of fertility enhancement drugs that are known to cause them. Excellent for the commencement of aerobic and movement therapies provided the patient has a good cardiovascular system and strong heart (as determined by the responsible physician).

Field Note: Those who have courageously battled a long mortal illness may welcome this conjunction. A few days on either side can bring either a miraculous cure or relief from suffering. The rock singer Freddie Mercury, suffering from AIDS, died the day the transit Sun arrived over his natal Jupiter. This is not untypical. Don't worry, we all live through this conjunction once yearly and typically it is quite a positive experience.

Herbal Note: Gentian and Agrimony are *cooling* bitters useful for sudden liver-related distress or engorgement that sometimes occurs at this time. Yarrow, Linden and Hawthorne are three of many choices known to relieve fast building hypertension or threatened stroke. Do not self treat.

Transit Sun Conjunct Natal Saturn

This brief transit emphasizes everything the natal Saturn indicates for that person. This aspect is briefly positive for calcium absorption, strengthening to the entire body structure; positive for strengthening weak tendons and ligaments. It is strengthening to the elderly and convalescing, and excellent for the onset of nutritive therapies. However, if someone is failing, this conjunction can be the proverbial "straw that breaks the camel's back."

This transit is briefly cold and drying (emphasizing Saturn). It can be productive of sudden bone spurs, broken teeth, arthritic attack, rheumatic episode, teeth impactions, ear impactions, spasm, hemorrhoid, miscarriage, suffocation, choking, falls, and broken bones. Beware of ice, caves, mines. The elderly must guard against falling.

The Sun conjunct natal Saturn is so often a "bad day." However, the reverse conjunction, the conjunction of transit Saturn to natal Sun, is lengthy and far stronger.

Urgent Medical Note: This brief transit strongly inclines to amass toxins to a dangerous level. Sudden obstructions may occur to unrelieved organs: appendicitis, blocked or twisted intestine, choking or perhaps the sudden blockage of a ureter. Prior to Sol's yearly visit of natal Saturn, it would seem wise to actively cleanse and relax the bodily regions governed by the sign he tenants in the birth chart!

Field Note: The wildly popular diva, Whitney Houston, died within a few days of the transit Sun's conjunction of her Saturn-in-Pisces, 12th house. Pisces is a Water sign. Both the 12th house and Pisces are implicated in mysterious deaths, coma, sleep and drowning. Houston tragically drowned in a bathtub under the influence of multiple drugs in the bloodstream.

Star Wars' "Princess Leah," Carrie Fisher, died unexpectedly as the transit Sun conjoined her natal Saturn-in-Pisces within one or two degrees. Many other transits, of course, were adding stress in both these examples. Remember, we all experience this transit once yearly and, if you are reading this, you probably have not died!

Herbal Note: The warming, oxygenating, blood clearing "alternative" herbs can offset a pending "Saturn event" at this time (arthritis, et al). Reduce stiffening and improve circulation to the bodily region indicated by natal Saturn's sign. Do not self-treat.

Transit Sun Conjunct Natal Uranus

This brief transit emphasizes everything the natal Uranus means for that person. Potentially, this transit can stimulate a surge of electrical activity in the body or other unexpected surprise. Negatively, this period can cause electrical shock, inexplicable spasm or paralysis, electrical storms in the heart or brain, seizure, and very strange "undiagnosable" events. A 'red alert' for epileptics!

Surgical and Medical Tips: Salt influences electricity and so do crystals; salt is a crystal. The ancient Europeans had fascinating cures for epilepsy involving the drinking of water poured over crystals, or water laid out in copper bowls under Lunar eclipses.

Epilepsy is a condition thought to be caused by little understood electrical brainstorms. It appears that some sort of electrical-charge reversal is involved, transferred to the sufferer via the charged water. Normally, however, one should *never* drink water left out under any type of eclipse!

Field Note: A remarkable traveler I met at the sacred headwaters of Mt. Shasta imparted that soon after being persuaded by a healer to drink "eclipse water," he fell chronically ill and has remained so for several years.

Herbal Note: Herbalists should have well on hand their anti-spasmodic herbs at this time, especially for patients with obvious symptoms of cramps or seizures: Lobelia (specific to the vagus nerve), Catnip, Cramp Bark, Skullcap, etc. Do not self-treat.

Transit Sun Conjunct Natal Neptune

This brief transit emphasizes everything the natal Neptune means for that person. Miracles can happen! This conjunction enhances any native clairvoyant or clairaudient faculty. (This phenomenon is more noted for the reverse aspect, the long-term transit of transit Neptune conjunct natal Sun.)

This brief conjunction also increases any tendency towards drug and alcohol abuse. Issues can arise regarding viruses, mold, mildew or poisons. Some people experience this period as relaxing and sleepy whereas others feel fatigued. This aspect can be significant in charts of those clinging to life by a thread.

Prayer is unusually effective at this time, provided the natal Neptune is strong and positive. Relax. Mark the day before, of, and after this transit and note its effect on sleep and dreams. Many feel sleepy, sleep soundly, or have amazing dreams during this transit!

Field Note: Popular singer Amy Winehouse died of alcohol poisoning on the day when the transit Sun plus transit North Node conjoined her natal Neptune-South Node conjunction on her Descendant in close orb.

Surgical and Medical Tips: Watch out for possible misdiagnosis or medication errors in prescription or dosage. Alcohol, drugs and anesthesia may have far stronger effects than anticipated. Highly effective during this time are vibrational therapies, such as homeopathy, Bach Flower Essences, music therapy, aromatherapy, and shamanic healing.

This short transit is also useful for hypnotherapy provided the native has a therapist who can be trusted with control of their subconscious! Always avoid hypnosis entirely should either the natal or transit Neptune be conjunct the natal South Node!

Herbal Note: Red alert! Any relaxants will theoretically work double strength during the one-to-two days of Sol's exact conjunction to natal Neptune. Never combine drugs with alcohol—but especially not now!

Transit Sun Conjunct Natal Pluto

This brief transit emphasizes everything the natal Pluto means for that person. Because Pluto is indicated in poisoning (along with Mars, Neptune, Saturn, the Nodes and certain signs), this conjunction can testify to blood, chemical or food poisoning as much as the famous Mars-Neptune combination. Danger of drug overdose.

May suggest the entry of dangerous bacteria into the bloodstream through needles, bites or medical carelessness. In wound cases, there exists a heightened potential for sepsis or gangrene. This transit could signal the reception of HIV, STDs, and the like. Be extra careful of parasite infestation, especially if natal Pluto is in an Earth or Water sign.

Those with hex wielding enemies should psychically shield themselves during this time. In rare cases, and with multiple testimonies, this transit could warn of spirit control for weak or submissive persons, especially if occurring in the 8th or 12th house. This is not the week for anyone to fool around with spirit entities.

Surgical and Medical Tips: This conjunction is dangerous through either overdose or heightened responsiveness (or even drastic responses) to procedures such as hormone therapies, stem cell transplants, organ transplants, and blood transfusions. Potentially dangerous because of drastic responses to drugs, herbs, lasers, and the like. Chemotherapy or radiation-therapy would be extra-effective at killing cancerous cells while simultaneously more potent in damaging healthy tissue too. If concerned, and the responsible physician agrees, clear this conjunction by at least three days on either side.

Conversely, this aspect could suggest a highly effective day for these same drastic treatments—the whole chart must be consulted in this case. Pluto rules destruction **and** regeneration! Potentially, no planet can turn around a desperate case as effectively as can Pluto! This transit is hopeful for those awaiting organ transplant, especially if Jupiter chimes in!

Transit Sun Conjunct Natal Ascendant

This aspect is generally vitalizing, unless the natal South Node shares this same sign. Sun's transit of the Ascendant degree suggests an awakening, following a month of rest, spiritual work or confusion so typical of the Sun's transit of the 12th house!

This week could lift the vital force, particularly if the transit Sun simultaneously trines the natal Sun or Moon. In the yearly Solar cycle, the Ascendant degree marks the "personal New Year" for each nativity. At this point, the native begins his/her cycle of *the rotating emphasis of twelve spheres of life activity, famous as the twelve astrological "houses."*

Transit Sun Conjunct Natal North Node

Solar energy enters strongly for a few days around this transit event. However, should eclipses occur during this week, the influence can hold for a year or more, being triggered when the Sun, Mars, or the planet ruler of the eclipse sign come in hard aspect to the eclipse degree!

On these few days, Solar energy rushes into the bodily regions governed by the sign of the natal North Node (for good or ill). Positively, this transit is strengthening to the constitution (unless square, opposed or quincunx the natal Sun) and can present the native with positive lifestyle choices.

This transit renews interest in self-improvement. However, this period could be worrisome if the natal Sun is too strong, or should a patient suffer from high blood pressure, aneurism, glaucoma, migraine, mania, brain tumor, or heart disease. In these cases, it would be important to reduce Solar pressure. (See remediation suggestions for physicians in *Astrology and Your Vital Force*).

Herbal Note: Should circulatory or fluid pressure build in the body system governed by the natal North Node, refer to that body system in Matthew Wood's *Repertory of Herbal Medicine* for herbal selection. Do not self-treat.

Transit Sun Conjunct the Natal South Node

Solar energy exits strongly for a few days around this transit event. However, should an eclipse occur during this week, the influence can hold for a year or more, being triggered by the Sun, Mars, or the planet ruler of the eclipse sign coming into hard aspect to the degree of that eclipse!

For good or ill, energy drains from the bodily regions governed by the sign of the natal South Node. This period could be worrisome should the natal Sun be weak, or should a patient suffer from anemia, fatigue, low blood pressure, or drug addictions. In these cases, it would be important to increase Solar energy, and fortify the body parts governed by the natal South Node. (See remediation suggestions for healers in *Astrology and Your Vital Force*.)

Any negative habits of "self-undoing" may be highlighted around these dates. Those undergoing drug or alcohol detoxing must be exceptionally vigilant to avoid temptation or relapse.

Field Note: The renowned 20th century magician Houdini died shortly after a man attempted to test one of Houdini's famous stage tricks of taking a sledgehammer to the stomach and being none the worse for it. Sadly, Houdini was caught unawares by the prank. The transit Sun was exactly conjoined his natal South Node that very day (the proverbial "point of self undoing"), while transit Mars simultaneously conjoined his natal North Node, opposite. Translation: Mars (attack) vigorously entered Houdini's life, the precise day when the performer was most vulnerable.

Surgical Tip: Theoretically, this is never the best day one can choose for surgery. Unless your situation is acute, and/or your physician insists on an immediate surgery, it is best to clear this aspect by a few days on either side.

Herbal Note:: First, discern the innate weakness suggested by the natal South Node. Then, tonify. Do not self-treat.

THE SUN'S SQUARE
Health Potentials for Predisposed Nativities
The Square does not always manifest as health concerns or benefits.

Many writers conflate all "hard aspects" under the same heading of influences. This is only partly true, and lazy.

Squares are unique from conjunctions and oppositions *(see Chapter 3, Aspect Mechanics).*

Surgical, Medical and Herbal Notes, as are given in the sections for Sun Conjunctions and Sun Quincunxes, are often applicable to Sun Squares.

Transit Sun Square Natal Sun:
Discussed earlier in this chapter, section: *Master Cycle of the Year, Transit Sun Square Natal Sun.* Note the discussion of the square mode of Cardinal, Fixed, and Mutable *(earlier in this chapter).*

Transit Sun Square Natal Moon
The tension created can disturb or mark a brief adjustment point for the emotions, menstrual cycle, brain, absorption process, stomach, breasts, and progesterone.

Transit Sun Square Natal Mercury
The tension created can create a brief adjustment point for the peripheral nerves, communication, thinking processes, bronchial tubes, or hands. This square is experienced as increased stress and demand upon the mental functions—either useful or exhausting. It is especially strong in the Mutable signs.

Transit Sun Square Natal Venus
The tension created may indicate a brief adjustment point for the libido, estrogen, kidney function, veins, sugar metabolism, copper. The resultant stress can increase or decrease these functions depending on the two elements involved. Relationships are in an adjustment zone this week.

Transit Sun Square Natal Mars
The tension created can signal a brief adjustment point for the libido, available physical energy, pizzazz, muscles, male potency, adrenal gland, iron, red blood cells. The resultant stress either enhances or lowers these functions, depending on the two elements involved. The Fire-Water squares may excessively stimulate Mars. The reverse occurs should natal Mars be in Earth and the transit Sun be squaring him from Fire, causing frustration.

Transit Sun Square Natal Jupiter
Presents a brief adjustment time for the liver functions, pituitary gland, arterial circulation, and possibly the blood. The resultant stress either enhances or lowers these functions, depending on the two elements involved. A watch-week for diabetics and liver disease patients, and those with aneurysm, arterial disease or blood pressure challenges.

Transit Sun Square Natal Saturn

This aspect can signal a brief adjustment time for the mineral assimilation, bones, teeth, ligaments, tendons, skin. The resultant stress either enhances or lowers these functions, depending on the two elements involved. A watch-week for elderly patients (falls), and those with dental, skin or bone challenges. Sometimes this square is a positive game changer, forcing lifestyle decisions by laying reality squarely in one's lap.

Transit Sun Square Natal Uranus

Presents a brief adjustment time for bodily electrical functions. Possible electrical outages or surges. The thyroid gland is influenced, especially in the case of Fixed squares. The resultant stress either enhances or lowers these functions, depending on the two elements involved. Especially in Air or Fire signs, a watch-week for epileptics, migraine sufferers or persons with electrical-surge issues. A good time for medical revelation.

Transit Sun Square Natal Neptune

The tension created can signal a brief adjustment time for sleep and the parasympathetic nervous system. Viruses, poisons, mold, anesthesia, drugs, or alcohol. The resultant stress either excites or reduces these issues. A watch-week for sufferers of narcolepsy, sleep disorders, psychiatric issues involving psychic openness, drug addicts and alcoholics. Viruses take a turn.

During this week, one may see more clearly into the cause of mysterious, "undiagnosable" fatigue or wasting ailments, because squares expose things!

Transit Sun Square Natal Pluto

Catalytic. Can affect malignant diseases, bacterial infections, and also those receiving transplants or transfusion. The resultant stress can either signal a crisis, a miraculous technical intervention, or provide an accurate diagnosis. The effect is dependent on the two elements involved. A watch-week for anyone in critical care or suffering a potentially mortal illness or drastic infection.

Pluto can also turn around impossible, hopeless cases like no other planet save Jupiter! Spiritual willpower is generated by this square—use it! This is a perfect time for strong lifestyle choices— "I'm quitting cigarettes!"

Transit Sun Square Natal Nodes

The transit Sun is now in "the bends" *(see page 46)*. This suggests an ideal time for lifestyle realignment and important spiritual choices. Sometimes these decisions relate to health, and sometimes to other matters. This transit is experienced as increased stress.

THE SUN'S OPPOSITION

Health Potentials for Predisposed Nativities

Oppositions do not always manifest as health concerns or benefits.

Many authors cite all hard aspects as behaving in the same manner. However, the opposition has distinctive qualities. Foremost, a transiting planet both *confronts and pulls* upon the vital force of the natal planet opposed. The exact outcome is often hard to define.

What we do know is that an energy drain is applied from the opposite sign. Also, the pull is weakening because it pulls from the *opposite side* of the circle of ecliptic longitude. The opposition can be best understood by observing the "pause point" in the forward swing of a pendulum. A pendulum swings forward to full extension, pausing, just before it starts to swing back.

The houses and signs involved in the transit opposition of a Sun's natal planet opposition are essential to note. It is beyond the scope of this text to discuss all sign and polarity combinations.

Here's a helpful formula to use.

Opposition Interpreting Formula:

Transit Sun in sign _____ *(give sign)*, and the bodily regions ruled by this sign _____ *(give sign's body regions)*, will pull upon the planet he opposes _____ *(name planet)*, and its bodily functions _____ *(describe bodily functions)*, in the bodily regions ruled by sign of the natal planet _____ *(list body regions)*.

The resultant Solar "pull" lowers the energy of the natal planet so opposed, being the low point in its own personal yearly cycle from the horoscope's viewpoint.

Sometimes this transit indicates a *diagnosis* related to the functions of the planet opposed. Also, it can indicate the arrival of medical news or test results of the nature of the planet opposed. For example, transit Sun opposed to natal Mars would bring a temporary low swing to the yearly energy cycle (which is ruled by Mars). However, should there be an existing Mars-related health complaint, this is a time when diagnosis can be made.

Surgical, Medical and Herbal Notes given in the section *Transit Sun Quincunx Natal Planets* are also applicable to oppositions from transit Sun. My reasoning is that both the Sun's opposition and quincunx weaken the vital force provided the natal planet. Therefore, solutions would be similar (strengthen the planet).

THE SUN'S QUINCUNX
Health Potentials for Predisposed Nativities
A quincunx doesn't always manifest as health concerns or benefits.

The quincunx aspects (150°, 210°, and 30°) are the preeminent health aspects because they correspond angularly to the three traditional malefic houses (6th, 8th, and 12th). These health-related houses are positioned at these same angles relative to the natal chart's Ascendant.

Quincunxes are sneaky and hard to diagnose as they represent a disconnection between the two planets involved. **Indicative of the disconnect between such planets, all quincunxes occur between two signs *sharing neither element nor mode in common*.** For a fuller discussion of the twelve quincunxes, see *Chapter 4, Quincunx.*

The natal planet quincunxed by the transit Sun is temporarily unable to "digest" enough Solar prana (vital force). Thus, this signals a few days of *reduced functioning* of the quincunxed natal planet. This may often pass unfelt. However, sometimes this is no small matter! Surgery is unwise should the planet representing the topic of surgery be receiving an exact Solar quincunx, especially if either sign involved coincides with the bodily region concerned.

Typically, quincunxes have tiny orbs and are best at 0-1°. See the discussion in this chapter on Solar transits: *Transit Frame & Orb*.

Transit Sun Quincunx Natal Sun

See *The Master Cycle of the Year, Transit Sun Quincunx Natal Sun (page 63)*.

Surgical Tips: If the responsible physician agrees, avoid all surgical procedures during this week. This would be doubly so for surgery to the heart, brain, or eye.

Herbal Note: During this time, the professional herbalist may consider cardiac herbs and foods high in prana. Do not self-treat.

Transit Sun Quincunx Natal Moon

Briefly reduces the flow of the vital force to breasts, fertility, lungs, and stomach absorption. The momentary transit could affect brain chemistry in ways hard to diagnose (look to the signs of transit Sun and natal Moon); disturb the timing of menstrual cycles and most monthly bodily rhythms; brings strange moods. The circulation of the vital force throughout the body is compromised, lowering energy.

Surgical Tips: If the responsible physician agrees, avoid all surgical procedures during this week. This would be doubly true for surgery to the stomach, breast, lung, eye, brain or womb. The orb of clearance should be at least three days.

Herbal Note: During this brief time, the professional herbalist may find useful herbs for female support, lymph clearing herbs, lung herbs, mucus membrane demulcents, uterine support, and stomachics. Do not self-treat.

Transit Sun Quincunx Natal Mercury

Briefly reduces the flow of vital force to the peripheral nerves, senses and neural connectivity. Can influence neurological and mental complaints. The flow of neural current and information through the nerves may be briefly "off." Sensory information may be addled. This may cause clumsiness, lack of hand coordination, or momentarily exacerbate neurological conditions. Nerves may be strained.

Surgical Tips: If the responsible physician agrees, avoid all surgical procedures to the nerves, lungs, hands, any tubes or blood vessels, and ears when this aspect is within 3°, and sometimes more.

Herbal Notes: During this brief transit, the professional herbalist may consider nutritive nervines. Nerve and lung support are useful now. Do not self-treat.

Transit Sun Quincunx Natal Venus

Briefly reduces the flow of the vital force to the ovaries, kidneys and veins. For most people, this transit is insignificant. However, these few days is a red alert for diabetics. Kidney hormones may slow, producing electrolyte or fluidic imbalances. Estrogen or copper levels may temporarily lower.

Surgical Tips: If the responsible physician agrees, avoid all surgical procedures to kidneys or ovaries when this aspect is within 3°, and sometimes more.

Herbal Note: During this brief transit, the professional herbalist may consider estrogenic herbs, copper-rich herbs, kidney support, and venous herbs. Do not self-treat.

Transit Sun Quincunx Natal Mars

Briefly reduces the flow of the vital force to the muscles, and motor nerves. Some may experience fatigue. For most people this is insignificant and goes unnoticed.

Because Mars rules the red blood cells, this aspect could be dangerous for anemics or hemophiliacs. For athletes, this aspect could impair timing or reduce spunk, just enough to lose that race! Timing and muscular coordination and contraction may be slightly "off."

Although this aspect is brief, and for most people insignificant, it can produce first rate accidents! Be careful with equipment, driving and risky sports. Hypothetically, could correspond with stings, insect or reptile bites, animal bites and plant toxins.

It is never advised to be off in the woods alone when expecting an exact quincunx to natal Mars from the Sun or any transit planet or, worse, from transit Mars to any natal planet!

Potentially can signal a sudden bite, mishap, or in rare cases an unforeseen infection, such as appendicitis. Note the bodily regions ruled by the signs of both the transit Sun and natal Mars for clues on where issues can manifest.

Can temporarily upset the output of adrenal hormones or the normal excretion of toxins. For males, sexual performance issues may occur.

Surgical Tips: This brief transit, when in exact orb, constitutes a first-rate surgical danger, especially for Mars-ruled body parts. If the responsible physician agrees, avoid all surgical procedures when this aspect is within 3°, and sometimes more.

Herbal Note: The professional herbalist may consider iron rich herbs, male support, muscle herbs and stimulants.

Warning: The effect of the quincunx to Mars sometimes produces effects opposite to those expected by revving up Mars instead of reducing him! Study symptoms carefully. Do not self-treat.

Transit Sun Quincunx Natal Jupiter

Briefly reduces the supply of the vital force to the liver, pituitary gland and arteries. The liver and gall bladder may be more sensitive to fats during these dates. This is a nice time to eat light.

Surgical Tip: If the responsible physician agrees, avoid liver, pituitary or arterial surgery at this time. Clear the exact transit by at least three days.

Herbal Note: The professional herbalist may consider hepatics, cholagogues, arterial cleansers and blood pressure regulating herbs. Do not self-treat.

Transit Sun Quincunx Natal Saturn

Briefly reduces the flow of the vital force to the bones, ligaments, tendons, and bodily structure. Possible sudden instability, "trick knee," falls, or spinal subluxations. Dental issues. Earache. Elderly persons would be more prone to falls and fractures. Joint pains of unclear origin might arise. Regulation and timing of bodily processes may be "off."

Be alert for ingestion of heavy metals, especially lead. Diagnosis occurring at this time may be off. For most people, this transit is insignificant.

Surgical Tip: If the responsible medical professional agrees, avoid bone, skin, ear or teeth work within at least three days of exactitude.

Herbal Note: The professional herbalist may consider mineral rich nutritives, skeletal system support, and a possible missing nutrient. Do not self-treat.

Transit Sun Quincunx Natal Uranus

Possible electrical malfunction or danger for a few days.

Herbal Note: For convulsion, seizure: Lobelia, Mistletoe, Blue Vervain. Do not self-treat.

Transit Sun Quincunx Natal Neptune

Briefly reduces the flow of the vital force to an already lax natal planet! A mysterious complaint could surface. Very subtle symptoms should not be ignored. A virus could take advantage of the weakened environment, especially in the body region ruled by the sign of natal Neptune. Anesthesia, alcohol or drugs could have unforeseen effects. Should this brief aspect correspond to insomnia, look to a deficiency of sleep hormones.

Surgical Tip: This aspect warns of unforeseen effects of anesthesia and possible errors concerning medication or dosage. Blood transfusion may have secret consequences.

Herbal Note: The patient under this transit may fail to disclose the drugs or medications they are using, creating danger in herbal or medication prescription.

Transit Sun Quincunx Natal Pluto

This brief aspect may be indicated in snake bites, bee stings, animal bites, plant venoms, secret radiation exposure, poisons and deliberate poisoning. The brevity of this aspect belies its potential dangers.

This is the time when the doctor insists on yet another high radiation mammogram. There may be innocuous but potent dangers (possibly addiction) inherent in hormonal treatment, prescribed medications, or herbal regimes commenced at this time, especially within two days of exactitude.

Surgical and Medical Tips: Quincunxes suggest that something odd could go wrong, something nobody expected or noticed, always catching us by surprise. Pluto governs transplants, transfusion, cadavers and all manner of body-sharing technologies.

This brief transit suggests that it is wise to wait a few days on commencing these types of procedures, as well as hormone therapies, with the concurrence of the responsible physician.

Chapter 7

THE MOON
The Herbalist's Companion

Properties, Rulerships and Actions
Rules: Cancer

Exalted: Taurus

Detriment: Capricorn

Fall: Scorpio

Metal: Silver

Minerals: Fluorine *(Jansky)*; Potassium *(Jansky, Nauman)*

Vitamins: B2 *(Jansy, Nauman)*

Gem: Pearl, Moonstone

Cosmic Color Ray: Orange *(traditional Jyotish)*

Herbs: (see *Herbal Notes* throughout this chapter)

Governs: Luna governs monthly cycles, and the rate and manner of the distribution of the Sun's vital force current. Dr. William Davidson emphasized that the Sun was the vital force itself, whereas the Moon indicated the distribution of this force. He likened this to amperage and voltage of electrical current.

Luna cycles through all 360 zodiacal degrees of the natal chart every 27.3 days, passing over each **natal planet** once in this time frame. This is known as her *sidereal cycle*.

However, she completes her *synodic cycle* (a full orbit relative to the Sun) every 29.5 days. Thus, the Full Moon and her other phases, being governed by the synodic cycle, occur regularly every 29.5 days, while her regular transit of a planet, governed by the sidereal cycle, occurs every 27.3 days.

Obviously, Luna governs "menses." She also influences all manner of daily and monthly rhythms including our sleep cycles, sexual receptivity, daily habits and changing moods. The Moon holds considerable influence, along with Jupiter and Pisces, over the coordination of the glands.

You can palpably experience the regular repetition of the sidereal cycle for yourself by tracking the recurrent "complaint cycles" of friends and family for at least one year. Perhaps you will find that your friend who suffers insomnia each month does so when the Moon transits through Gemini and Sagittarius, or that your relative is predictably nauseous at every month's return of the Virgo Moon.

Conversely, our larger life cycles and physiological changes are ruled by Saturn (puberty, menopause, old age). It is fascinating to note that Saturn and the Moon govern opposite signs Capricorn and Cancer! Together, they govern the lesser and greater circles of life rhythms.

Body Rulership & Organ Affinities: The female menses and other monthly cycles; absorption; breast, stomach, lung (with Gemini and Cancer), protective organ coverings (meninges, pericardium), female hormones (with Venus), water (our bodies are about 60% water), mucous membranes, mother's milk, lactation, the womb when pregnant. Additional and more complex listings for Lunar body-sign correlations are found in Cornell's *Encyclopedia of Medical Astrology.*

General Action: Cold, moist, fluidic, changeable, sensitizing, nourishing, nurturing, feeling, softening, and unstable. Because Luna moves with great speed, her transits are viewed (and used) in a different manner from those of the planets.

The Moon pulls fluid to the area of the body ruled by the sign she transits, spending approximately two and a half days in each sign. She also transmits magnetic currents to the region. In a similar manner, she transfers current to any transit or natal planet she currently aspects (especially by conjunction).

The sign of transit Moon must be carefully noted at the onset of treatments. Traditionally, one "cuts not with iron" (avoids surgery) to the body part governed by the sign she passes through. However, one can successfully nourish this region because of the temporarily increased flow of blood and magnetic current.

Luna also brings the best times each month for collecting, decocting and administering herbal medicines by elemental need. She is our essential monthly time clock!

The list of herbal remedies is structured to reflect the importance of sign and element in the section *Luna Through the Signs*. This is essential knowledge for herbalists.

Throughout this book, the focus is on the implication of current *transiting planets to natal planets*. However, the Moon's transit aspects to fellow *transiting* planets traditionally have essential medical uses all their own!

I've detailed these previously in *Astrology & Your Vital Force*. However, for the convenience of fellow herbalists, I've briefly reiterated Luna's specific uses by *transit* conjunction to *transit (not natal)* planets for the express purpose of herbal harvest, decoction and administration (in the planetary sections of this chapter). The decision to capitalize mentioned herbs is in veneration of their conscious individualities.

Please note that the herbal sections included for the Moon are for general knowledge and for herbalists who appreciate astrological herbalism. This information is not to be construed as medical directive, advice, opinion or prescription. Therefore, I've reiterated after each section: "Do not self-treat."

Positive: A happy natal Moon gives contentment and good memory; strong stomach and good appetite; cycles are normal; the body is fertile and neither too fat nor thin.

Negative: A correct delineation depends on whether Luna is excess or deficient in the natal chart. Expressions range from malnourished and depressed-phlegmatic to convivial. See below.

Excess: Phlegmatic. Emotion overwhelms logic; acts from instinct, overeats; fluidic issues, menorrhagia, highly fertile, large or excessive breasts, brain chemistry or hormonally influenced mood swings. Menorrhagia. Fertile, social. Edemic and cyst building.

Deficient: Uterine cysts or tumors, infertility, poor appetite, loneliness, depression, thin or dry mucous membranes, weak stomach, small breasts, difficult lactation. Amenorrhea, infertility. Depression.

Temperature & Moisture Levels: Luna's influence by sign and element far outweighs the fact she is "moist and cool." *Rather, she stirs up the element of the sign she passes through.* For example, when in Fire signs, she stirs up heat, despite herself being moist and cool by nature! This works the same way in the natal chart. For instance, folks with natal Leo Moons are not emotionally moist and cold, rather the reverse! Because of this fact, I've given special attention to *Luna Through the Elements & Signs (next pages).*

Transit Frame & Orb: As described at the beginning of this chapter, Luna cycles through all 360 zodiacal degrees of the natal chart every 27.3 days; one sign roughly every two and a quarter days; and one degree about every two hours. Thus, the Moon's exact transit of any planet by one degree on each side lasts about four hours. While subtle effects can reliably be felt during these brief passages, most of the time, Luna's aspects go unnoticed on the physical level. If this were not true, few of us would keep well all month!

The transit Moon does not possess the large orb of the natal Moon, unless she is at her full, new, or quarter phase, or involved in either a Solar or Lunar eclipse. While the natal Moon can command an orb of influence of 15° within the sign boundary, the transit Moon's conjunction of a natal planet is maybe 5° for symptom triggering, and of course stronger within 1°. Its actual extension in time is really a matter of feel.

The Lunar phases are another matter. The New or Full Moon occurring over a natal planet can sometimes produce a month of effects in relation to that specific planet's functions. Eclipses work like triple strength Full or New Moons, capable of heralding in a year or more of ongoing effects, undulating through the year (see my book, *Eclipses and You*).

Sans full Moons and eclipses, it is observably true that neither the Sun nor Moon can best Mars or Saturn for expectable health events due to any one aspect. Rather, the two Lights set the underlying energetic stage for seasons, months, weeks and days.

Astrologers disagree on whether a closely *applying* aspect is stronger than a recently departing or *separating* aspect. In some branches of astrology only the application is considered valid. However, Medical Astrology accepts that the Moon's physical influence works for a time on both sides of exactitude.

Chemist Frau Lily Kolisko proved this as a fact. She photographed metal salt solution reactions on filter paper made during Lunar conjunctions of the planets traditionally assigned to these metals. Invariably, the strongest response was ten minutes following the exact conjunction.

This "tail wind" of the Moon's conjunction has sure surprised me many times! Never relax your guard until Luna clears her exact conjunction of a planet by one or two degrees (two to five hours).

LUNA THROUGH THE ELEMENTS & SIGNS
Health Potentials for Predisposed Nativities
Aspects do not always manifest as health concerns or benefits.

Applicable to both natal and transit charts, these partial lists of expressed symptoms apply only to predisposed nativities. These conditions are obviously uncommon and require multiple testimonies beyond the presence of the Moon. Manifestation of symptoms may be enhanced by lifestyle choices, and taking preemptive measures can reduce, remove or prevent potential issues from manifesting. It is not possible to list all potential expressions.

Moon in Fire Signs

Herbal Note for Fire Signs: Fire-sign Moons are best for harvesting, decocting and administering hot-dry herbs (to counteract cold-damp), heart, eye and brain tonics, arterial and muscular stimulants, male potency herbs, and adrenal support.

Aries: At this time, the body fluids and electromagnetic energies pull readily to the head, eyes, brain, upper jaw, teeth nerves, adrenals (with Libra, Mars) upper teeth (with Saturn), and mandible (with Taurus). The Aries Moon is notably hot and dry, bursting forth.

This Moon stimulates the adrenal glands, enhancing action, temper and increasing the need for muscular movement. Excites brain, blood flow to head. Avoid light in eyes or excessive Sun on head. Dehydrates.

Herbal Notes: This is a fine time for the professional herbalist to decoct or administer stimulating brain stimulants, iron rich herbs, adrenal support herbs, adaptogens, eye-strengthening herbs, and herbs for muscular energy and aerobic movement. See also, in this chapter: *Transit Moon Conjunct Natal Mars.* Do not self-treat.

Surgical and Medical Tips: Heat rises suddenly, so watch fevers and tempers. Aries is fast acting and hemorrhage prone. If the responsible physician agrees, avoid surgery to Aries bodily regions listed above. However, these few days are good to nourish and heal these same regions, provided they are deficient. One never wants to overstimulate fire!

Leo: At this time, body fluids and electromagnetic energy pull readily to the upper back, spinal cord sheaths, upper spinal cord, heart, gallbladder (with Capricorn, Saturn and Mars), and wrist.

Leo is the hottest Moon sign, and dry (though warmly affectionate). Enhances muscular strength and command. Hot and drying. Impacts the blood pressure, heart, gallbladder, and back. Heats the blood and organs. Dehydrates! Increases patient willfulness, affection, temper. A pleasure Moon.

Herbal Note: This is a fine time for the professional herbalist to harvest, decoct or administer stimulating herbs for muscular energy and aerobic movement. Excellent for decocting and administering warming, drying herbs, and cardiac tonics. See also, in this chapter: *Transit Moon Conjunct Natal Sun.* Do not self-treat.

Surgical and Medical Tips: Avoid surgery to the Leo bodily regions noted above, unless the responsible physician advises otherwise. However, the Leo Moon is good for nourishing these same regions provided they are weak.

Sagittarius: At this time, the body fluids and electromagnetic energies flow readily to the hips, thighs, gluteals, sciatic nerve, spinal cord (with Leo), lower spinal nerves, hip and thigh muscles, coccyx and sacrum (with Scorpio).

Influences arteries and the arterial circulation. With opposite sign Gemini, co-governs the coordination of the nervous system, with Sagittarius emphasizing the voluntary nerves, and central nervous system (Sagittarius), and Gemini governing the peripheral nerves. In rare cases this transit can relax hip ligaments, throwing the femur out of alignment.

The action of this Moon is restless (both mentally and physically), and stimulating. Activates the motor nerves. Stimulates the sciatic nerve and the muscular system of legs. This Moon excites all "red" mental illnesses in those prone, including mania, paranoia, panic, schizophrenia, claustrophobia, insomnia, grandiosity, hysteria, PTSD, MPD, ADHD, and hyperactivity. This Moon stimulates need for large muscle movement and aerobics. Animals run off. Insomniacs may require calmatives.

Herbal Note: This is a fine time for the professional herbalist to harvest, decoct or administer stimulating herbs for muscular energy and aerobic movement. Sagittarius Moon is also a wonderful time to nourish the arterial system, leg muscles or lower spinal nerves.

Know your soporific herbs for those that find it impossible to sleep during Sagittarius Moons!. See also (in this chapter): *Transit Moon Conjunct Natal Jupiter.*

Surgical and Medical Tips: Unless the responsible physician advises otherwise, avoid surgery to Sagittarius' bodily regions listed above. However, these days are fine for nourishing these same regions, should they be hypo-functioning or weak.

Moon in Earth Signs
Herbal Note for Earth Signs: Earth sign Moons are best for harvesting, decocting and administering strengthening herbs, nutritive

bone builders, hemostatics and astringents (especially Capricorn). Earth signs considerably vary from one another in their herbal application, so read closely the descriptions by sign. Traditionally, emesis (vomiting) is more likely when medicine is taken during the Moon's transit through the three Earth signs.

Taurus: Taurus is neither dry nor cold as are Earth signs. This sign holds and generates comfortable warmth. This sign is relaxed, sensual and affectionate (unlike Capricorn or Virgo).

At this time, body fluids and electromagnetic energies pull readily to the throat, ears, neck, lower brain, lower jaw, tongue, mouth, trachea, upper esophagus, thyroid (with Uranus – *Edgar Cayce*), teeth (with Saturn), mandible (with Aries, Mars), and cervical vertebrae. Mucus is prone to build in the ears, nose and throat. Rarely, are children born at the time of a Taurus Moon not prone to ear, nose, throat and tonsil infections, clogs and impactions.

Fixes form. Taurus is the most magnetic sign, warm, and slow. Its influence is grounding, stabilizing, calms, pleasant, relaxing; magnetizing, beautifying; aphrodisiacal, sensual, anxiety relieving. Enhances senses. Strengthens, nutrifies, concentrates, builds, swells, pools; impaction prone, masses pressure or toxins and can produce obstructions. Anodyne. Gourmand's Moon. Food tastes better and appetites are strong.

Herbal Note: Excellent for harvesting, decocting, and administering galactagogues and fertility herbs (unlike fellow Earth signs). Also good for throat herbs, aphrodisiacs and anodynes (pain killers).

Traditionally, a time to avoid administering medicines as they are thought to vomit up. Earth sign Moons (including Taurus) are traditionally avoided for onset of a course of medicine. Because Taurus loves to eat, perhaps this rule is more appropriate to Virgo and Capricorn.

Surgical and Medical Tips: If the responsible physician agrees, avoid surgery to thyroid, neck, lower teeth and jaw, ears, mouth, tongue, upper esophagus. However, these couple of days are good to nourish these same regions if weak.

Virgo: At this time, body fluids and and electromagnetic energies pull readily to the upper intestines, pancreas, liver, spleen, fingers (with Gemini), abdomen, solar plexus. Boosts immune system and smell sensitivity.

This Moon sign is quite drying, especially to the hair, skin and mucus membrane. Virgo also stimulates the Beta brain waves, contributing to insomnia, anxiety and overwork. Quickens nerves and blood sugar reaction. Sensitizes the digestive organs, (intestine, liver, pancreas, gall bladder). Avoid fried fats, alcohol and chemical medicines at this time.

Herbal Note: This Moon sign is good for harvesting, decocting, and administering herbs for strengthening and assisting the liver, gallbladder, pancreas, spleen and upper intestine, hepatic circulation.

Surgical and Medical Tips: Unless the responsible physician advises otherwise, avoid surgery to the Virgo bodily regions listed above. However, these couple of days are good for nourishing these same regions.

Capricorn: At this time, body fluids and electromagnetic energies pull readily to the knees, skin, ligaments, tendons, nails, bones (in general, with Saturn), anterior pituitary gland (with Jupiter), and gallbladder (with Leo, Saturn and Mars). Natally, productive of uterine fibroids. Davidson states that laxatives taken at this time won't work!

Drying, cold and brittle. Enhances planning, goal achievement, hard work, physical and character, strengthening, accepting parenthood, durability, order making, reality, authority or responsibility. Slows liver and gallbladder. Avoid chemical medicines as this Moon vibration is associated with heightened vomiting response.

Drying to mucous membranes, uterus and stomach. Sensitizes skin, knees, cuticles, ligaments, tendons. Increases allergic responses. A strong time for nutritive bone building and general strengthening.

Herbal Note: A fine time for harvesting, decocting, and administering the nutritive, bone building herbs. Also excellent for astringents. See also, in this chapter: *Transit Moon Conjunct Natal Saturn.*

Surgical and Medical Tips: Avoid surgery to the knees, bones or skin, unless the responsible physician advises otherwise. However, these couple of days are good for nourishing these same regions. Avoid Earth sign Moons for onset of a course of medicine (emesis prone). This is the best fasting Moon.

Moon in Air Signs

Herbal Note for Air Signs: Air sign Moons are best for harvesting, decocting and administering the strengthening nervines, mental and neural stimulants and nutritive neural tonics.

Gemini: At this time, body fluids and electromagnetic energies pull readily to the shoulders, arms, hands, bronchial tubes, upper lungs, peripheral nerves, speech. This Moon quickens neural connections, alertness, curiosity, mental alacrity, language skills, playfulness, improvisation, dexterity. Awakens. Stimulates the mind, hands and verbal centers. Not the best time for insomniacs! Good where flexibility or speed is lacking. Erratic. Gemini energy resembles fast-changing breezes. Warm/Cool (changeable). Avoid EMF fields.

Herbal Note: This Moon sign is good to harvest, decoct, tincture and administer neural tonics, and circulatory herbs to increase capillary function; e.g. Hawthorne Leaf, Prickly Ash, etc. Also, the bronchial and lung supporting herbs and expectorants (Coltsfood, Mullein, Osha, Horehound, Inula, et al.). See also, in this chapter: *Natal Moon Conjunct Mercury.*

Surgical and Medical Tips: Avoid surgery to the Gemini bodily regions listed above, unless the responsible physician advises otherwise. However, these couple of days are useful for nourishing these same regions. Traditionally, one avoids chemical medicine, intravenous procedures and bleeding of the patient at this time.

Libra: At this time, body fluids and and electromagnetic energies pull readily to the kidneys, ovaries, lower back, waist, and adrenals (the adrenals are co-ruled with Aries and Mars).

Libra Moon is useful for pain relief and also for quelling excessive histamine response, (or at least for harvesting or tincturing medicines for that purpose). Magnetic. Affects acid-alkaline balance and balance of hormones, electrolytes, and salt. May increase kidney filtration or urination. Increases vertigo in those prone and also desire for sugar and alcohol. A pleasant, sociable and relaxing influence. Anodyne. Calms aggression.

Herbal Note: A good time for the professional herbalist to harvest, decoct or administer kidney, vein and ovary nourishing herbs. See also, in this chapter: *Transit Moon Conjunct Natal Venus.*

Surgical and Medical Tips: Avoid surgery to the Libra bodily regions listed above, unless the responsible physician advises otherwise. However, these couple of days are good to nourish these same regions, provided they are hypo-functioning.

Aquarius: At this time, body fluids and electromagnetic energies pull readily to the shins, ankles, electrical body (little is known of this body), and spinal nerves (with Sagittarius). There is some relation to eyesight (with Aries), circulation of blood, blood issues, veins (with Venus), and oxygenation.

Cold, spastic. The Moon's transit of this sign imparts the greatest electrical charge of the month, and results are unpredictable. Great for stimulating ideas and imagination. Excellent for philanthropy and idealized vision, odd projects, invention, intuitive discovery, science. Enhances sense of humor and imagination. Friendly. Depression prone, light deficient.

Sources vary on the attribution of cold or hot to this sign. However, traditional Aquarius health complaints lean cold, as do those of this sign's ruling planet Saturn. Midwinter is also the coldest time in the northern hemisphere.

This is the most extreme period of the month for electromagnetic and barometric effects that are hard to diagnose and unpredictable. If you don't believe this, try getting a haircut at this time. Fatigue. Influences circulation, spinal nerves, blood quality (anemia, etc.), oxygenation of blood, neural impulses.

Natives with this Moon sign may require more vitamins, minerals and oxygen then do natives of other signs and often crave salt and open windows while sleeping.

Herbal Note: The Aquarius Moon is a fine time for the professional herbalist to harvest, decoct and administer medicines to treat venous insufficiency, sub-oxygenation, and circulatory sluggishness—Rosemary, Hawthorne berry and leaf, Sage, Yarrow, Mullein, Ginkgo, etc. Aquarius is also fine for working with blood building herbs: Nettles, Dulse, Kelp, Beets, Sesame Seeds, et al. Do not self-treat.

Heightens neurological sensitivity. Energies are unpredictable, and reactions can be extreme to medications, hormones and homeopathic remedies. Hypothetically, Aquarius-Moon-made remedies have a strong negative or positive influence on spasm, paralysis, epilepsy, and insanity (but can go either way).

Surgical and Medical Tips: Avoid surgery to ankles or veins, unless the responsible physician advises otherwise. However, these couple of days are good for nourishing and strengthen these same regions. Chemical medicines may have unforeseen or extreme results if taken at this time. This sign produces unpredictable results for intravenous procedures.

Moon in Water Signs

Herbal Note for Water Signs: Water sign Moons are best for harvesting, decocting and administering cold, damp herbs to moisten and hydrate and/or counteract dry or hot conditions.

Although all three Water signs play a part in excretion and lymphatic action, each has its own specialty. Cancer absorbs at the stomach and strongly influences the lymphatics of the breast as well as governing the thoracic duct. Scorpio is cathartic throughout all excretory orifices, and Pisces rules the lymphatics in general, the inter- and extrastitial fluids, and possibly the "matrix." Energy flows inward and down, then out!

Cancer: Energies turn inward. At this time, body fluids and electromagnetic energies pull readily to the breasts, ribs, sternum, elbow, arm pit, stomach, lower lung, spleen, thoracic duct, posterior pituitary gland (with Jupiter), and gums (with Taurus).

This sign has some influence on brain fluid level. Stimulating to lactation, sound sensitivity, and the memory. Cool and moist. This is a phlegmatic, mucous producing sign. Swells, bloats, edemic. Fertile!

Stimulates emotions, maternal tenderness, tears, memory, sentiment. People prefer to stay home, sleep, eat, cuddle. Highly fertile. Suggestion: Allow only pleasant images and sounds to enter the mind. Nurtures self or others. Increases allergic response.

Herbal Note: The Cancer Moon is traditionally excellent for the harvest, decoct and administration of most herbal remedies. Specifically, good for stomachics, galactagogues, fertility enhancement and herbs cleansing to the lymphatic system of breasts and brain. Dandelion Root, Red Clover and Poke Root are specifics for cleansing the lymphatic tissue of the breast. Useful for emmenagogues.

Surgical and Medical Tips: Avoid surgery to the breasts, stomach, lower lung, pancreas, thoracic duct, pituitary, hypothalamus, elbow or armpit, unless the responsible physician advises otherwise. However, these couple of days are useful for nourishing these same regions.

Scorpio: At this time, body fluids and electromagnetic energies pull readily to the genitals, bladder, anus, rectum, prostate, pelvis, colon, uterus, cervix, nose (increasing smell sensitivity), sweat glands, sacrum and coccyx (with Sagittarius), and prostate.

Cold and moist, though passionate! Fertile. Aphrodisiacal, increases intense emotion and desire. A potent healing Moon. Strongly cathartic, stimulating the excretory functions. Immune system ramps up. Laxatives work doubly strong.

Herbal Note: Great for harvesting, decocting, fermenting and tincturing most herbs, especially potentatizes vermifuges, antibiotics, antivirals, antifungals and cathartics. This is the best Moon for removing worms and parasites! This Moon is expulsive. Useful for emmenagogues, aphrodisiacs and uterine strengthening herbs (such as Red Raspberry leaf).

Scorpio Moon is perhaps the best time for working with alterative, "blood cleansing," herbs, diuretics, sweating herbs, cathartics and potent antiviral and antibacterial herbs: Tea Tree, Eucalyptus, Chaparral, Oregano, etc. If administered, these will work extremely strongly at this time so doses must be lowered!

Matthew Wood has brought to our attention the miraculous wonders of chewed Sassafras for one recent case of extreme "undiagnosable" nose and anal bleeding with the expulsion of alarming clots. Both bodily regions are governed by Scorpio. It would make sense then, to harvest and decoct this notorious "blood cleansing" herb at the time of the Scorpio Moon!

Avoid if pregnant. Do not self-treat. Also see *Transit Moon Conjunct Mars* (as well as Pluto) in this chapter.

Surgical and Medical Tips: Avoid surgery to Scorpio's bodily regions listed above, unless the responsible physician advises otherwise. However, these couple of days are good to nourish these same regions.

Pisces: At this time, body fluids and electromagnetic energies pull readily to the feet, lymph system (with Cancer ruling the thoracic duct), duodenum, cecum, immune system. This sign strongly affects glandular coordination. Highly productive of phlegm. Highly fertile.

Moist, cold, meandering. Sleepy, relaxing, letting go, accepting. Spiritually sensitizing, lowers psychic boundaries. Not helpful for depressed or phlegmatic cases, or for persons who oversleep, or those with low psychic boundaries. Mucous-producing, edemic and highly fertile.

This Moon strongly stimulates the parasympathetic nervous system. Energy meanders. Sensitizes feet, glands; increases sound sensitivity. Avoid exposure to contagion, crowds, ghosts and loud noise. This is the strongest Moon for hypnosis and past life recall.

Herbal Note: The Pisces Moon is traditionally considered to be one of the best for harvesting, tincturing, decocting and imbibing most medicinal teas. Pisces has a special affinity with lymphatic assisting herbs, and herbs that globally balance the glandular system. Also excellent for soporific (sleeping) herbs, anesthetics, relaxants, hypnotics, opioids and dreaming herbs. *See also Transit Moon Conjunct Neptune* in this chapter.

Surgical and Medical Tips: Tradition warns to avoid all surgery to the feet, lymph nodes or pituitary, unless the responsible physician advises otherwise. However, this is the most receptive Moon both psychically and physically, and thus a good candidate for transplants and transfusions where rejection is of concern. Also, one can pamper and strengthen the feet at this time.

LUNAR TRANSITS OF NATAL & TRANSIT PLANETS

Applicable to both natal and transit charts, these partial lists of expressed symptoms apply only to predisposed nativities. These conditions are obviously uncommon and require multiple testimonies beyond the presence of the Moon. Manifestation of symptoms may be enhanced by lifestyle choices, and taking preemptive measures can reduce, remove or prevent potential issues from manifesting. It is not possible to list all potential expressions.

THE MOON'S CONJUNCTIONS

Health Potentials for Predisposed Nativities

Conjunction does not always manifest as health concerns or benefits.

Luna's transit of any natal planet last only a few hours and is usually not physically relevant unless occurring for seriously ill or frail persons or on full Moon or eclipses. However, should the natal planet already be under significant transit stress, then the Moon's passage can act as the second hand of a clock, triggering an event! This triggering action usually occurs within a tight orb. At full phase, and eclipses, the Moon can certainly trigger significant health events!

The Moon provides a most significant time clock in a less direct way. The previous New or Full Moon appears to "set up" the events that play out in anyone's life in the following two to four weeks.

One commonly witnesses a health malady arise within one month relating to any planet afflicted by a previous New or Full Moon, or any afflicted natal planet that received the conjunction, square or quincunx of a previous New or Full Moon (or eclipse), within 3°.

There is another category of Moon lore to consider. The ancient ones well knew that Luna's transit aspects to fellow transiting planets have their specific uses for the harvest, decoction and administration of medicinal herbs. Herbalists can use these same relationships today to amplify the effectiveness of their herbal preparations.

These are discussed in the *Herbal Note* section for each planet below, and in greater detail in *Astrology and Your Vital Force: Healing with Cosmic Rays and DNA Resonance.*

Transit Moon Conjunct Natal Sun

Normally, the Moon's monthly conjunction with the Sun slightly raises the vital force and we feel good. However, should one suffer Solar maladies, such as heart, brain or eye complaints, this conjunction could swing either way, because energy pulls to the these organs. Similarly, should one experience the maladies of their Sun sign, these are emphasized at this time.

Transit Moon Conjunct Transit Sun

The New Moon! A time of beginnings. Considered unwise for surgery within 24 hours. However, if one is getting rid of something permanently (e.g. worms, tumors, bad teeth), the period of two days prior to the New Moon is perfect, allowing for 24 hours clearance.

Some sources say the New Moon reduces swelling-bleeding, while others say it causes more of same. Emergency room nurses could resolve this debate!

Herbal Note for Transit New Moon: It's good to avoid the New Moon by one, or even two days, allowing her to emerge, waxing from her congress with Sol. It was not thought prudent to harvest at the Balsamic Moon, the day or two just previous to the New Moon.

Transit Moon Conjunct Natal Mercury

Normally, the Moon's monthly conjunction with Mercury stimulates the mind and speech. However, should one suffer neurological, speech, lung, hand, arm, finger or mental complaints, the effects of this brief conjunction could swing either way, because this transit emphasizes Mercury.

Luna's one day passage over natal Mercury can briefly impact the breath, bronchial tubes, and lungs through her fluid attracting tendencies. This is notable should someone be in the throes of bronchitis, or suffer serious lung complaints already.

Field Note: A friend suffering with a bronchial cold thought she was almost well and was dismissed from the doctor's office. However, I noticed that the coming transit Moon-Mercury conjunction was due in exactly two days to conjoin her own natal Mercury-Saturn conjunction. This would occur exactly as many other distressing aspects were also coming due in Gemini (sign of bronchial tubes and upper lungs).

I staunchly warned her to return in haste to her doctor and obtain a aspirator to be kept on hand at all times. This saved her life! Precisely as the conjunction came due, she experienced a violent asthma attack so intense that she would have perished had she not had her aspirator quite literally in hand.

Herbal Note for Transit Moon Conjunct Transit Mercury: This is an ideal time for the professional herbalist to harvest, decoct or administer herbs to quicken or nourish the peripheral nervous system, speech, hearing, hands or mental acuity. Milky Oat Seed and Alfalfa are examples of nutritive herbs that assist burned-out nerves. See Wood's *Earthwise Herbal Repertory*.

In the case of bronchial or lung complaints, respiratory herbs may be needed now to open the tubules and relieve congested fluids. For this purpose, it is traditional to combine Peppermint with either Elder lowers, Yarrow flowers or Linden flowers. There are many other fine lung assisting herbs ("expectorants"), each with a distinct action: Osha, Coltsfoot, Mullein, Horehound and Black Horehound, Yerba Santa. Do not self-treat.

Transit Moon Conjunct Natal Venus

Normally, the Moon's monthly conjunction with Venus arouses feelings of love. However, should one experience ovarian, kidney, venous, blood sugar, diabetes or female sexuality problems, the effects of this conjunction could swing either way, because this transit emphasizes Venus. Fertile!

Herbal Note for Transit Moon Conjunct Transit Venus: This is an ideal time for the herbalist to harvest, decoct or administer herbs to arouse the female libido, increase copper, strengthen veins, assist ovaries, breast or kidneys and in some cases to balance blood sugar levels. This is an ideal time for working with anodynes, relaxants, emollients and soothing demulcents. Venus' ray is strongly anti-spasmodic and thus useful for working with anti-spasmodic herbs (Lobelia, Catnip, Black Cohosh, etc.). Do not self-treat.

Transit Moon Conjunct Natal Mars

Normally, the Moon's monthly conjunction with natal Mars arouses energy, temper and libido. Sometimes we experience extremes of energy, or heightened adrenal response. Iron or testosterone levels may spike. Mennorraghic.

Increases potential for parturition. This aspect speeds excretion, influences male functions, and arouses temper, or inversely, panic.

Stimulating to histamine response, rash, hives. This transit briefly heightens any extant acidic or caustic condition: ulcer, fever, inflammation, etc. Infants respond strongly to all hard Mars aspects: fuss, cry, fever, colds, etc.

Unless stationing, this aspect is brief, but can be acute. Transit Mars conjunct the natal Moon generally has more clout.

Herbal Note for Transit Moon Conjunct Transit Mars: This is an ideal time for the herbalist to harvest, decoct or administer herbs to arouse the libido, strengthen the muscles, and increase iron, testosterone, male virility, red blood cells energy and athletic prowess (Nettles, Beets, Black Raisins, etc.). Excellent for working with stimulants (Cayenne, Horseradish, Garlic, Onions, spices.)

This transit is also a great choice for working with vermifuges, anti-parasitical, antibacterial and antiviral herbs Wormwood, Olive Leaf, Black Walnut, Cloves, Papaya seeds, etc. If the system temporarily overheats, use your cooling herbs, organ specific. Do not self-treat.

Field Note: Here is a strong example of Luna's powers to "trigger a landslide." Within the exact half-hour period that a full Moon (by transit) conjoined a client's natal Mars-in-Capricorn square his natal Mercury-in-Aries (with a simultaneous transit of Mars-in-Cancer opposing his natal Mars-in-Capricorn and the transit Moon); he collapsed at the gym while lifting weights, and was rushed to the emergency hospital with heart palpitations. This spun off into months of intense yet clinically undiagnosable pain with multiple symptoms including severe nausea.

Field Note 2: The aorta is governed by 0° Leo. A total Lunar eclipse occurred on a senior lady's natal Mars on this exact degree. Although in perfect cardiac health, she experienced a sudden aortic dissection within two weeks of this event. The eclipse (and her natal Mars) were also situated at precise quincunx to her natal Sun (heart). This is an example of a natal weakness lying dormant for years, then triggered by an astrological event.

Transit Moon Conjunct Natal Jupiter

Normally, the Moon's monthly conjunction with Jupiter stimulates the liver. This also influences the blood, as the liver dumps more glycogen, bile, and minerals. This aspect also increases arterial expansion and should be noted in cases of hypertension, and aneurysm.

Because this transit emphasizes Jupiter, the effects could swing either way, should one be overweight or underweight, or have diabetes, blood clots, arterial fat, liver problems, high blood pressure, growth disorders or pituitary problems.

Herbal Note for Transit Moon Conjunct Transit Jupiter: This is an ideal time for the professional herbalist to harvest, decoct or administer nutritive herbs to gain weight or strengthen a poorly functioning liver. This period is also perfect for working with the nutritive oily herbs (as Matthew Wood says "Bear Medicine"), and for your protective adaptogens. Burdock and Fenugreek comes to mind as useful "Jupiterian" favorites. Do not self-treat.

Transit Moon Conjunct Natal Saturn

Normally, the Moon's monthly conjunction with Saturn tightens, cools and dries tissue, while at the same time it dampens down enthusiasm! Because this transit emphasizes Saturn, the effects could swing either way should one experience Saturn related maladies, such as bone or dental issues, skin disease, malnutrition, constipation, sub-oxygenation, arthritis or any other chronic hardening, dry condition. Be on the alert in cases of pneumonia.

Herbal Note for Transit Moon Conjunct Transit Saturn: This is an ideal time for the professional herbalist to harvest, decoct or administer nutritive bone building herbs, such as Oat Straw, Nettles, Alfalfa, and Comfrey. This is also a perfect time for working with astringents, and useful for ligament and tendon strengthening herbs, such as Solomon's Seal root, Teasel, and Boneset. Do not self-treat.

Field Note: A friend who drinks an excess of alcohol, regularly complains of "nausea" for one day each month, just as the transit Moon conjoins her natal Saturn and South Node conjunction in Virgo. One would think the culprit was not the stomach, but either the liver, pancreas, upper intestine or gallbladder (because all these organs involve either Virgo or Saturn). As the Moon travels through Virgo, the liver gets touchy! Always ask the location of someone's "stomach" discomfort. A surprising amount of people will point to their lower belly or liver!

Transit Moon Conjunct Natal Uranus

Normally, the Moon's monthly conjunction with Uranus is mentally stimulating yet unpredictable. However, should one already experience seizures, cramps, spasm or extreme hormonal shifts, then the effects of this conjunction could swing either way, because this transit emphasizes Uranus.

The electrical system of the body gets boosted during these hours. Air and Fire signs channel Uranus' energy more intensely through the nerves (Air), or Muscles-heart-brain (Fire). Water signs typically respond emotionally to this event, whereas Earth signs can usually ground the subtly increased electrical charge.

Herbal Note for Transit Moon Conjunct Transit Uranus: This would seem an ideal time for the professional herbalist to harvest, decoct or administer herbs to awaken nerves, brain or muscles lacking electrical stimulus; for example in cases of stroke or paralysis. However, I generally avoid choosing Uranus for any herbal work because the influence of this planet is so unpredictable. To offset seizure or spasm occurring under this aspect, know your antispasmodics. Do not self-treat.

Transit Moon Conjunct Natal Neptune

Normally, the Moon's monthly conjunction with the Neptune is felt as sleepy. However, if one is already experiencing fatigue, psychic overwhelm, depression, wasting or addiction, then the effects of this conjunction could intensify these matters because this transit emphasizes Neptune.

Field Note: The popular diva, Amy Winehouse, passed away by self-induced alcohol poisoning eight days following an eclipse conjoined her natal Neptune-South Node conjunction on the Descendant (a traditional death point). Her progressed Moon was also there, positioned right between her natal South node and natal Neptune! Neptune rules alcohol. A traditional meaning of the South Node was "the point of self-undoing." Astrology speaks.

Herbal Note for Transit Moon Conjunct Transit Neptune: This is an ideal time for the professional herbalist to harvest, decoct or administer your soporific (sleeping) herbs and sedatives. This transit would potentize Passion Flower, Scullcap, Lemon Balm, Cannabis, Hops and alcohol. Neptune is antispasmodic and thus useful for working with antispasmodic herbs, such as Lobelia, Catnip, and Black Cohosh. Your dreaming herbs are best harvested and tinctured at this time as well, Mugwort, etc. Do not self-treat.

Transit Moon Conjunct Natal Pluto

Normally, the Moon's monthly conjunction with the Pluto, if noticed at all, intensifies emotional extremes. However, since this transit emphasizes Pluto, if one experiences sepsis, bacterial invasion, parasites, radiation, chemotherapy or X-rays, the effects could swing either way.

Herbal Note for Transit Moon Conjunct Transit Pluto: This is an ideal time for the professional herbalist to harvest, decoct or administer vermifuges (Wormwood, Olive Leaf, Black Walnut, Cloves, etc.); cathartic herbs: Senna, Cascara Sagrada, Butternut, Rhubarb, etc.; homeopathic poisons, poisonous plants and venoms; or strong antivirals (Olive Leaf, Chaparral, Eucalyptus, Oregano). Theoretically, Pluto may evince a strong affinity with the more potent anti-carcinogenic herbs and lymphatic cleansers, such as Poke Root. Do not self-treat.

Transit Moon Conjunct Natal North Node

Normally, the Moon's monthly conjunction with the natal North Node is a time of positive connections or events. However, should one already experience symptoms related to the body region of natal North Node, this brief transit could add fluidic pressure, creating impaction, boils, swelling, and the like.

Because the North Node as the "Dragon's Head" is a major entry point for celestial energies, sometimes the head, mouth or throat are literally emphasized.

Herbal Note for Transit Moon Conjunct Transit North Node: These few hours are generally positive for harvesting, decocting or administering herbs intended to nourish and strengthen the bodily regions governed by the sign of the transiting North Node. However, if the body zone is experiencing pressure, impaction, obstruction or tumor growth, do not use.

Additionally, the elemental qualities of the sign that this conjunction occurs in are greatly intensified. For instance, if you are looking for more Fire energy, you will get what you ask for! Never self-treat.

Transit Moon Conjunct Natal South Node

Normally, the Moon's monthly conjunction with the natal South Node is to be entirely avoided for most medical purposes. This is not invariably the case, but a good rule of thumb.

Herbal Note for Transit Moon Conjunct Transit South Node: Herbs harvested at this time may be "unhappy." Decoctions made or administered at this time may have unintended negative effects or be ineffectual.

This period is particularly dangerous time for experiments with psychotropics and "dreaming herbs." Do not self-treat.

Field Note: Every month like clockwork, when the Moon transits my client's natal South Node in Cancer, he draws inward, feels hypersensitive, antisocial and sleepy. This lasts about one day. Luna's passage of the South Node signals a natural rest period within each month.

Transit Moon Conjunct Natal Ascendant

First, be certain the Ascendant degree is really true. This aspect is generally sensitizing to the body, most especially to the regions governed by the Ascendant's sign. Traditionally this day is a time to avoid all medical procedures, unless the responsible physician says otherwise.

THE MOON'S SQUARE

Health Potentials for Predisposed Nativities

The square does not always manifest as health concerns or benefits.

These transits last only a few hours and are usually not relevant to health except in the seriously ill, frail, or if occurring at the full Moon or on an eclipse.

A conflictual energy field, or friction is briefly set up between the two elements involved. This energy activates and emphasizes the functions of the natal planet. The emphasis is traditionally regarded as "negative" although this is not invariably true in practice.

Squares are far more reactive than trines or sextiles and seek action to resolve. For delineating square type, see *Chapter 3:*

Aspect Mechanics. Remember, Luna's transits do not always express themselves as medical issues, and do so only a small percentage of the time, and only in some cases.

A square is useful for mitigating stasis or torpor. Squares also expose problems by bringing them to light. To interpret a square, read the general information for planetary rulerships in the chapter sections for that planet. Also, refer to the section on square types by paired elements in *Chapter 6, The Sun.* Alternatively, refer to keywords listed in the *Transit Moon Conjunct Natal* and *Transit Planets* section above.

THE MOON'S OPPOSITION
Health Potentials for Predisposed Nativities

Please note that not everyone responds excessively to Luna's brief oppositions. Transits do not always express themselves as health issues, and in fact, do not do so in the majority of cases.

Luna's opposition to a natal planet lasts only a few hours and is usually not relevant to health unless occurring for seriously ill or frail persons, or at full Moon or eclipses.

When the Moon opposes a natal planet, she pulls against its "permanent vibrational resonance imprint" that is somehow embedded at birth in our energetic blueprint. Typically, this weakens the opposed natal planet's functions. Traditionally, oppositions are deemed "negative," although this is not invariably true in practice. Sometimes an opposition provides a necessary balance. When we are too hot, we require cold, and vice versa!

The transit Moon's monthly opposition of the natal Sun is weakening to the vital force. For the healthy and young this is no big deal. However, a brief lowering of prana can be a serious matter for the frail elderly and convalescent.

To define the planetary functions in the natal chart that are briefly weakened (or balanced) by the Lunar opposition, read the general information for planetary rulerships in the sections for the planet of interest. Alternatively, refer to keywords listed in the

Transit Moon Conjunct Natal Planets section above. Then, think "briefly weakened." For delineating oppositions by sign polarity, see *Chapter 3: Aspect Mechanics.*

TRANSIT MOON QUINCUNX NATAL PLANETS
Health Potentials for Predisposed Nativities
A quincunx does not always manifest as health concerns or benefits.

These transits last only a few hours and are usually not relevant to health unless occurring for seriously ill or frail person, or at full Moon or eclipses. We experience two Lunar quincunxes to each natal planet every month (four if we include "inconjuncts," too). Yet, somehow we survive!

When the Moon quincunxes a natal planet, she briefly weakens, confuses or disturbs its natural function. This is rarely problematic unless this natal planet has already been experiencing substantial stress. In rare cases, the Moon's quincunx is the proverbial "straw that breaks the camel's back."

Quincunxes can let you know when the doctors have either missed the cause of symptoms or don't understand them! Quincunxes have a concealed influence, confounding diagnosis. Look for causal clues stemming from the sign of the transit Moon as applying to the body rulerships of the sign of the natal planet, as well as the functions of that planet. For ideas on how a specific quincunx might work, see *Chapter 4: Quincunx!*

As an example of exploring a hidden cause, a male friend had a dangerous blood sugar swing. You wish to see what was going on with his birth chart. Venus rules sugar and Virgo governs the insulin-producing Isles of Langerhans in the pancreas. You discover that at the time of the event, a transit Moon-in-Virgo exactly quincunxed his natal Venus in Aries.

This scenario would indicate either a slowed or, conversely, a heightened reaction of the pancreas (Virgo), influencing the blood sugar (Venus), in the sign of the adrenals and brain (Aries). Perhaps your friend had been angry or had consumed an excess of caffeine!

If you feel lost while interpreting a quincunx, don't despair, because you have company. Quincunxes are the most mysterious, least understood and most difficult to define aspect in medical astrology!

To define the planetary functions in the natal chart that are weakened or flummoxed, read the general information for planetary rulerships in the sections for that planet. Alternatively, refer to keywords listed in the *Transit Moon Conjunct Natal & Transit Planets* section above.

For delineating quincunx types by the two signs involved, see *Chapter 4*. **Please note that not everyone responds excessively to Luna's quincunx.**

TRANSIT MOON TRINE & SEXTILE NATAL PLANETS
Health Potentials for Predisposed Nativities
Aspects do not always manifest as health concerns or benefits.

These transits last only a few hours and are not usually relevant to health, though mildly helpful to seriously ill or frail persons.

Normally the trine and sextile are "nice" and present no health issues. However, there are occasions where a trine Moon allows a situation to continue in an unwanted pattern. For instance, a trine from the transit Moon to Venus will seldom block someone from indulging in excessive sugar or wine! Similarly, the Moon's transit trine to Mars or Uranus will not halt a panic attack or seizure.

In most cases, Luna's trine briefly raises the energy of the natal planet's function. This is especially nice in the case of the Sun. Twice monthly, for a few hours, our energy raises slightly as the transit Moon trines our natal Sun.

To define the planetary functions in the natal chart that are briefly enhanced by these "soft" aspects, refer to the general information for planetary rulerships in the sections for that planet. Alternatively, refer to keywords listed in the *Transit Moon Conjunct Natal & Transit Planets* section above in this chapter.

THE LUNAR NODES

Chapter 8

THE NORTH LUNAR NODE
POWER SURGE, STRENGTH, IMPACTION
The Doorway to the World

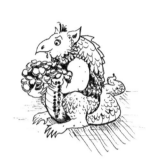

Alternate Names: The Dragon's Head,
The Head, Cauda, Rahu *(Jyotish)*

Properties, Rulerships and Actions
Sign Rulerships: The North Node rules no signs. However, there are two traditions for the exaltation of the Lunar North Node: Gemini and Taurus. He is happiest in these signs.

Metal: None cited

Gem: The Hessonite is the gem that is traditionally believed to refract the ultraviolet light of the North Node.

Cosmic Ray: Ultraviolet, *(traditional)* whereas Saturn's cosmic ray is visible violet.

What are the Lunar Nodes?
The North and South Lunar Nodes rotate exactly opposite to one another backward through the ecliptic plane in "ecliptic longitude." The two Nodes designate the intersection of the Moon's orbit with the ecliptic plane, i.e., the apparent path of the Sun though the sky.

The North Node is the junction where Luna moves northward above the ecliptic in her monthly orbit.

All eclipses occur either very near, or exactly conjoined either the North or South Node. The Lunar Nodes are therefore supremely important in astrology because they have the power to swallow both the Sun and Moon! I write more extensively about Eclipse influences in my book *Eclipses and You.*

In the natal chart, the North Node or "Dragon's Head" functions as a major celestial entry portal for planetary energies. By transit, the North Node represents an incoming tide of celestial force. This celestial tide is dependably delivered to any sign traversed or natal planet conjoined.

On the positive side, this brings an extra supply of strength! This empowering effect is enjoyed by the bodily regions ruled by the sign the Head is passing through or provided to the functions of the natal planet conjoined. For the transited natal planet, the North Node creates an surplus of incoming vital force, in turn creating a wide array of possible maladies.

Body Rulerships & Organ Affinity: The head and mouth. This may explain why some assign Taurus as the exaltation sign of the North Node, because Taurus also rules the mouth, and the medulla area, the portal for incoming vital force, according to Paramahansa Yogananda. The North Node is associated with brain related issues.

Hormones: Unknown. However, both Nodes appear to influence the growth hormones.

Genetics: In Jyotish, both natal Lunar Nodes are significators of inherited diseases.

Field Note – The Nodes' Impact on Growth Extremes: Astrologer George White discovered that the Lunar Nodes influenced height extremes when ascending, or in the 1st house. Could they influence the pituitary gland? White associated the South Node with dwarfism and the North Node with giantism. However, my one case of dwarfism has it reversed! Another unusually tall client was born with the South Node ascending, again reversing his finding. Nevertheless, it does appear that height extremes are influenced by the Nodes to some degree!

General Actions: Traditionally, the Dragon's Head is aggressive, invading, gobbling and greedy. These mechanisms produce impaction, blockage, swelling, bursting, invading, massing, gorging and productive of autoimmune diseases. The North and South Nodes are both associated with genetic diseases, the paternal side being more linked to the North Node.

The North Node is also sclerotic, stiffening, hardening and tissue building, similar to Saturn. The Jyotishi (astrologers of India) say "he" is extremely cold, and thus linked to Saturn. Both give rheumatic complaints. However, the North Node shares Jupiter's penchant toward excess and engorgement. Additionally, the Head also shares some of Pluto's pathological associations: aggressive pathogens, sepsis, gangrene, disfiguring diseases, bacterial invasion, genetic disease.

Both the North Node and Pluto produce great physical strength. They are also both noted when found in the birth Ascendant for producing "mysterious loner" types. They also share a temperature with a twist: North Node is extremely cold, whereas Pluto blows frigid cold and boiling hot!

A minority of Jyotishi associate the North Node with cancer, boils, parasites, skin diseases, paralysis, addictions and insanity, whereas the majority assign these same diseases to the South Node! If we view the North Node's pathological expressions as arising from excess, (and the South Node's arising from deficiency), we can better understand their roles in these ailments.

In this chapter, we will explore how both Nodes can create similar effects from reverse mechanisms! The North Node brings insatiable desires and is specific to unnatural, premature or violent deaths, and the Jyotish have specific preventative measures for these indications.

For example, the North Node's toxin-amassing and growth-generating properties would appear causative to cancer. Indeed, the "Head" is the predominant Node in most observed cases. Conversely, for cancers that have pathogenic etiologies, the South Node's weakening influence provides a sweet invitation for invading pathogens by lowering immune resistance.

Although a unique force unto itself, it is fair to state that the North Node can exhibit the extremes of Saturn, Pluto and Jupiter combined!

Positive: Strengthens, increases vital force. The transiting North Node signifies an energy surge.

Negative: Produces a dangerous piling up of fluid, prolific blood, excess vital force, tissue growth, impaction, obstruction, fluidic swelling or hardening, (depending on the element it is transiting through).

Disease Associations: Acidosis, parasite and bacterial invasion, dysentery, cholera, fluidic or blood pressure, glaucoma, aneurism, eclampsia, bursting vessels or organs, appendicitis, overwhelmed lymphatics, auto-toxicity, poisoning, plugged ducts.

Some types of cancer, growths, tissue hardening, leprosy, lupus, glandular and uterine swellings, suffocation, addictions, bites, skin disease, leprosy, poisoning, polyps, gluttony, stroke, heart attack, snake bite, high blood pressure, sclerosis of any organ or vessel, piles, mineral deposits, constipation, brain disease, brain tumor, mania, viscous addictions, insanity, and paralysis.

Autoimmune disease and spirit possession may have a connection to the North Node; the insatiable Dragon's Head gobbles up anything in its path! However, these issues appear related to both Nodes.

Transit Orb: The North Node is strongly felt when transiting a planet within 1°. However, because the Dragon's Head heralds a year-and-a-half eclipse season in any sign he transits through, his orb works in a general way throughout his passage through any sign, and upon any natal planet tenanting that same sign.

Cycle: The North Node will transit over a natal planet approximately once every 18.6 years.

Temperature: Very cold. In Jyotish tradition, the North Node's influence resembles that of Saturn.

NORTH NODE THROUGH THE ELEMENTS & SIGNS
Health Potentials for Predisposed Nativities
Nodal aspects do not always manifest as health concerns or benefits.

These conditions are obviously uncommon and require multiple testimonies beyond the presence of North Node.

Manifestation of symptoms may be enhanced by lifestyle choices, and taking preemptive measures can reduce, remove or prevent potential issues from manifesting. It is not possible to list all potential expressions.

North Node in Fire Signs

Aries: *Surplus vital force enters the head area.*
Mania, rages, high fever. Increases pressure to head, eyes, brain. Sharp vision. In very rare cases, brain tumor, glaucoma, or hemorrhagic stroke.

Field Note: A dear friend born with the North Node exactly rising in Aries enjoyed 20-10 vision until over age forty. She later died of a suddenly arising brain tumor (glioblastoma).

Leo: *A surfeit of vital force enters the heart area.*
Accelerated heartbeat, heart attack, hardening heart muscle, sclerotic heart vessels, thrombosis, heart or brain blockages, stroke, back pressure, back injury, spinal sheath problems, tumors in heart or back, hypertension, mania, heatstroke, spinal cord inflammation, paralysis.

Sagittarius: *Excess vital force enters the hips, legs, muscles and lower spinal cord.*
Hyperactivity, mania, athleticism, strong hips and thighs, sciatica, injury to lower spinal nerves, hips or thighs, femurs, etc., paralysis, pain in lower spinal nerves, hips or thighs, overactive motor nerves, injury's incurred from horses, dogs, driving, sports, risky behavior, firearms, arrows. Increases stimulation to neuromuscular system, excessive or pathological sexual desire in men, satyriasis, religious mania, hypertension, heart attack, stroke, seizures.

North Node in Earth Signs

Note: The reader may note that North and South Nodes will share some of their pathological expressions in Earth signs. However, the reasons for these shared symptoms have opposite mechanics! For example, a potential for appendicitis is listed under both Nodes in Virgo. Should symptoms suggest it, the North Node in Virgo could signal an impacted appendix gone toxic, whereas a South Node appendicitis might reveal an unchecked infection caused by weak bodily defenses!

These subtle differences between Nodal action, once understood, allow the practitioner a refinement of diagnosis. **"North Node in/ South Node out."**

Taurus: *Excess vital force enters the lower head, jaw, ears and neck area.*

Neck injury, throat inflammation or infection, infected salivary glands, vocal polyps, tongue, mouth or throat cancer, cancer of upper esophagus, vocal chord inflammation or infection, swollen tongue, tonsillitis.

Cysts, boils, swollen palette, heavy metal poisoning through dental fillings, tooth impactions, abscessed teeth, TMJ, bruxism, eat-ing disorders and addictions, overeating, gorging, choking, suffo-cation, difficulty swallowing, ear obstructions, deafness, ear injury, blockages in general; excessive masturbation, pressure in the lower brain, lower brain tumor or thrombosis, injury to cervical vertebrae.

Virgo: *Surplus vital force enters the liver, pancreas, spleen, and upper intestine.*

Abdominal hernia, appendicitis, duodenitis, pancreatitis, colitis, diverticulitis, splenitis; intestinal worms or parasites, intestinal blockages, obstructed colon (with Scorpio), intestinal aneurism, colitis and Crohn's Disease (with Scorpio); liver diseases, liver flukes, parasites in gall or liver ducts, liver injury, hepatitis, jaundice, sclerotic liver; swollen spleen, ruptured spleen (both Nodes), injury to upper digestive organs, cancer or tumors of liver, pancreas, duodenum or intestine; yoga and diet extremes; "dying to be healthy."

Capricorn: *Excess vital force enters the bones, skin, knees, tendons and ligaments.*

Skin changes or potential skin cancer, itchy skin, excessively oily or dry skin, plugged skin ducts, eczema, psoriasis; plugged bile duct, parasites in gall or liver ducts, excess bile production (jaundice), knee injury, strong knee (if positive), tendonitis at knee, the retention of toxins into joints—warning of arthritis, rheumatism or gout; stomach issues or nausea (reflex to Cancer causing acidic stomach), vomiting; bodily stiffness.

Dental carries, lead poisoning; bone infections, bone spurs, mineral deposits in joints; gallbladder or kidney, may contribute to cellular changes in skin or bone.

Influences kidney function, pituitary excitation, stimulates anterior pituitary, especially near 4° Capricorn.

Field Note: The natal conjunction of North Node and Mars in Capricorn appears to cause excretion (Mars) to be obstructed at the surface (Capricorn).

Over time, this can preclude skin conditions. A recent case of vitiligo (loss of pigmentation of the skin) presented this combination, with several other supportive testimonies.

North Node in Air Signs

Gemini: *Surplus vital force enters the nerves, arms, hands, bronchial tubes, lungs and speech center.*

Pressure-related neuralgia anywhere possible, but specific to shoulders, arms, hands, fingers, scapula, clavicle; plugged bronchial tubes or lungs, asthma, cystic fibrosis, tuberculosis; injury to shoulders, arms, hands or nerves; insomnia, mental obsessions, some types of seizures, nervousness, accelerates speech and gesticulation.

Field Note: One client born with the North Node conjunct Saturn in Gemini (sign of the hands) had a form of lupus that was causing her fingers to "turn into stone."

Libra: *A surfeit of vital force enters the kidney and lumbar area.*

Kidney cysts or tumors, kidney stones and blockages, ureter obstruction, ovarian or testicular cysts or tumors, adrenal tumors, adrenal hyperactivity, hormonal excesses, lumbar pressure and stenosis.

Aquarius: *Excess vital force enters the circulation, electrical body, spinal cord and lower leg.*

Mysterious blood disorders, blood poisoning, carbon monoxide poisoning, auto-intoxication, phlebitis, lower leg thrombosis, ankle stenosis, restricted Achilles tendon, circulatory disorders, excitation to spinal nerves, heightened electrical impulses through spinal nerves, electrocution, ankle or calf injury, neural pain in lower leg, cysts, tumors or skin lesions of lower leg, rare diseases of the spinal nerves, bites of venomous creatures.

North Node in Water Signs

The reader may note that North and South Nodes will share some of their pathological expressions in Water signs. However, the reasons for these shared symptoms have opposite mechanics! For example, "dirty blood" is listed under both Nodes for Scorpio and Pisces. In Water signs, the "greedy" Dragon's Head (North Node) dumps fluids in and then dams them up. Conversely, the "releasing" Dragon's Tail (South Node) dumps them out, into the blood, bladder, nose, colon, etc. **North Node in/South Node out!**

Nodal mechanics in Water work in this manner: The North Node in Water could suggest that the normal toxins entering the bloodstream cannot adequately exit, hence "dirty blood."

Conversely, the South Node would indicate an excessive dumping of lipids or hormones into the bloodstream from overstuffed lymphatics. Alternatively, the South Node could indicate a weakness in the normal blood filtering systems, contributing to toxic blood.

While the symptoms of "dirty blood" may be identical the North Node impedes blood clearance through obstruction, whereas the South Node poisons the blood through excess release or functional weakness. These subtle differences between nodal action, once understood, allows the practitioner a refinement of diagnosis.

Cancer: *Surplus vital force enters the breast and stomach.*

Fluidic pressure, breast cysts or tumors, plugged breast ducts, leaking poison from breast implants, oversized breast tissue, breast injury or surgery, excess estrogen or progesterone; acidic stomach, stomach tumors, ulcers, irritable or inflamed mucous membrane, sclerotic stomach membrane, insatiable appetite, food addiction, food cravings, nausea due to inflammation, vomiting, stomach surgery; tendency to abortion and miscarriage.

Injury to ribs, breastbone, breasts, stomach, diaphragm; pericarditis, pleural effusion, pleurisy, waterborne parasites, infection of lower lung, tuberculosis, lung tumors, inflammation of marrow; emotional coldness, alcoholism and drug addictions, family pattern issues, strong allergic response. Stimulates posterior pituitary, especially near 4° Cancer.

Although Pisces is the sign ruling lymphatics, Cancer is equally implicated through its rulership of the thoracic duct (the largest lymphatic duct), armpit and breast. For predisposed persons, lymphatic pressure and toxicity may increase when the North Node transits through either sign.

Field Note: A recent client born with the Moon conjunct the North Node in Cancer suffered severe edema throughout her tissues.

Scorpio: *Excess vital force enters the genitals, bladder, nose, excretory system and colon.*

Sex addiction, nymphomania, sexual obsessions, STDs (especially syphilis), HIV, genital fungus, genital yeast, vaginal infection, injury to genitals, abortion, infected penis or testes, jock itch, "dirty blood," extreme genital odor; plugged sweat glands, foul smelling sweat; colorectal cysts, polyps or cancer, colorectal parasites, candida, worms, bloodworm, parasites, hemorrhoid, inguinal hernia, rectal bleeding, cystitis, bladder cysts, bladder cancer, blocked ureters, gravel, blocked ureter, enuresis, anal thrombosis, colon blockage, colectomy, injury to anus, rectum, colon, bladder, genitals.

Plastic poisoning, hormone poisoning, stings of all kinds, snakebite, bedbugs (with Mars, Mercury), plant venoms, vermin-caused disease, Lyme disease; fecal or urine contamination, contaminated water and waterborne parasites; chronic nasal infection, obstructed septum of nose, broken nose, smell problems, Appendicitis (with Virgo), colitis and Crohn's disease (with Scorpio), acne.

On the positive side, North Node in Scorpio can provide miraculous powers of regeneration!

Note: Many of these items are shared with the South Node in Scorpio, but by different mechanisms. Scorpio and the South Node both rule excretion and release. Both govern the anus, Scorpio specifically so, and the South Node in principle.

This may be one reason why the South Node is considered as exalted in Scorpio, the sign governing the excretory system! However, the action of the South Node is far more unconscious and involuntary than is the North Node. For example, we could say that abortion is a North Node in Scorpio action, while miscarriage is a South-Node-in-Scorpio or Cancer event.

Pisces: *Excess vital force enters the feet, lymphatic system and interstitial fluids.*

Foot pain, bone spurs, increases foot strength, injury to feet or toes, hot or cold feet, lymphatic toxicity, engorged lymph nodes; onset of psychical problems, mental illness, weird or engrossing dreams, psychic invasion (entities or magical attack), hypnosis.

Inability to process alcohol, problems from mixing drugs and alcohol, drug overdoses; blood chemistry issues, blood toxicity, heated blood; plastic poisoning, water pathogens, hormone poisoning, bloodworm.

Increases or decreases lymphatic action (good unless other toxin-clearing systems are down); STDs, sexual addictions, seductions; boils, watery cysts, carbuncles, hot-wet rashes, dyes allergies.

NORTH NODE TRANSIT OF NATAL PLANETS

Applicable to both natal and transit charts, these partial lists of expressed symptoms apply only to predisposed nativities.

These conditions are obviously uncommon and require multiple testimonies beyond the presence of North Node. Manifestation of symptoms may be enhanced by lifestyle choices, and taking preemptive measures can reduce, remove or prevent potential issues from manifesting. It is not possible to list all potential expressions.

Orb & Duration: The North Node transits are most obvious within an orb 0-3° and very potent within an orb of 1°. Since the progress of the Nodes through the ecliptic is fairly regular, that gives a transit lasting about 60 days, with special intensity for about 20 days. However, eclipses may occur over a planet within about 10 months of the nodal transit itself. Should a Light or any planet be eclipsed within an orb of 3°, the impact is powerful and may last a year or longer.

Extensive detail on eclipses occurring conjunct all natal planets is provided in the advanced back-section of my book *Eclipses and You*.

THE NORTH NODE'S CONJUNCTIONS
Health Potentials for Predisposed Nativities
Transits do not always manifest as health concerns or benefits.

Transit North Node Conjunct Natal Sun
Energizing! If the natal Sun is strong, this transit boosts vitality and some people feel fantastic. Potentially invigorating to weak persons. A weak vital force rises. Some danger of excessive heart stimulation, stroke, heart attack or hypertension (especially in Fire signs). Pressure builds in brain, heart or eyes. Glaucoma alert. Danger of heart attack or stroke, or bursting vessels, sunstroke, or snow blindness especially in Fire signs. Can coincide with accidents to head, brain or eye. Increases heat throughout the system, muscle, nerves, and spinal cord. A feeling of self-importance can bloat in susceptible persons, and temper rises. Rare: meningitis.

Herbal Notes: Rosemary, Cayenne equalize circulation, diffusing extra pressure building in the brain. Sage has a reputation for preventing thrombosis in those so prone, and Yarrow is believed to break up clots. Never self-treat!

Surgical and Medical Tips: Elderly or weak persons should be careful of excessive sun, or heatstroke, stress, or aerobic activity under this transit.

Transit North Node Conjunct Natal Moon

One of the strongest testimonies of heightened fertility. Fluids enter faster than they exit. Increases swelling and edema, especially in the body part governed by the natal Moon (especially so in Water signs or Taurus). Heightens natal tendencies towards swelling, cysts or tumors in the breast, lung, stomach, ovaries or uterus. The lymphatic system may be overtaxed, or lymph nodes engorged.

A dangerous aspect for those with fluidic lung conditions. Potentially, raises blood pressure. This transit can be extremely challenging for emotional and mental health, but not invariably so.

Field Note 1: On more than one occasion, I've comforted a client suffering protracted infertility with the news that the transit North Node would soon be conjunct their natal Moon. Sure enough, they conceived just as expected at that time! Other testimonies of enhanced fertility include: North Node's transit conjunction of natal Venus; Jupiter's transit conjunction over the natal North Node, or Moon.

Field Note 2: Today, while speaking with a phone client, I noticed that he was born with a natal North Node tightly conjunct to both his natal Moon, and Saturn, in Aries, the sign of the head and eyes. This suggests a surplus of intraocular pressure. "By any chance do you have glaucoma?" I asked. "Yes," he replied.

Surgical and Medical Tips: Fertile! Multiple births are likely if the woman is taking fertility enhancement drugs. A trine or conjunction of transit or natal Jupiter doubles this testimony.

Herbal Note: This aspect responds well to diuretic herbs: Watermelon Seeds, Burdock, Cornsilk, Cimex (a homeopathic remedy), Dandelion Leaf, etc. It may be necessary to relieve lymphatic congestion of breasts (Dandelion Root, Poke Root). Mullein is specific for glandular and testicular swelling. Herbs for dropsy may all be considered. Each case is unique; never self-treat.

Transit North Node Conjunct Natal Mercury

Increases and improves mental powers and function. Potentially, could add pressure on the brain, sensory nerves or ears. Prone to moles or warts on the hands or fingers, may engorge bronchial tubes or lungs. For epileptics, a "red alert" potential.

Transit North Node Conjunct Natal Venus

Heightens blood sugar, estrogen, and blood copper levels. Increases libido and attractiveness. One testimony of temporarily heightened fertility! (See *Field Note* for *Transit North Node Conjunct Moon.*) This is an excellent time to tonify weak kidneys, veins, or hair.

Negatively, this can be a 'red alert' time for diabetics. This transit can cause estrogen-related cysts and tumors; swollen ovaries or testes, venous pressure or sluggishness, varicosities, impacted or engorged kidneys, kidney obstruction, kidney stone, cystic kidneys.

At this time, women are beneficial to the native, which is really nice if you have feminine nurses.

Herbal Note: In kidney congestion, this aspect is offset by diuretic herbs (do not self treat). See North Node conjunct the Moon. Should symptoms suggest, check for kidney or ovarian cysts.

Transit North Node Conjunct Natal Mars

Strengthens the muscles and increases testosterone, adrenalin and iron. Available energy rises. Can produce excesses of these hormones with consequential hyperactivity, anger control issues and mania. Blood iron levels may rise. There can be changes in blood cell counts, or the blood cells. Most especially in Fire signs, this aspect can cause an unmanageable surge of temper or aggression.

Other potential changes include insomnia, excessive libido, obsessions, impacted sweat glands, impacted urethra or ureters, impacted testes, genital infections, nose bleed, hemorrhage. Influences blood cell count, raises sperm count and male potency. Possible strokes and aneurisms, (with added pressure from Sun, Jupiter, and/or Mars).

Excellent for the commencement of aerobic movement therapies provided the patient has a good cardiovascular system and strong heart (check with a physician). A good blood-building aspect (if needed).

Field Note: One female client born with the North Node conjunct Mars in Fire, likes to "shred" violent music on her electric guitar.

A friend born with this conjunction in the Fire sign Sagittarius was possessed of a supernatural level of muscular strength plus an unfortunately violent temper triggered by trivial offenses.

Surgical and Medical Tips: If one requires surgery, an excellent surgeon could enter the scene. However, if negative, he/she may be too aggressive.

Herbal Note: Chaste Teaberry is a traditional monk's herb for reducing excessive libido. The cool and moist Lunar herbs traditionally balance Martian complaints: Chickweed, Marshmallow Root, etc. Venus' herbs are also good antidotes for Mars (the pleasantly warming or moderately cooling, sweet demulcents).

The great Renaissance physician Blagrave felt that Solar herbs should be included in all herbal mixtures for Mars' inflammatory maladies (because the Sun is exalted in Aries, a home sign of Mars).

Saturn's cold, astringent herbs can be useful in specific Mars-ruled conditions. Moistening astringents would be best unless the conjunction occurs in a Water sign (Witch Hazel, White or Yellow Pond Lily, etc.). It may be important to assist excretion. Do not self-treat.

Transit North Node Conjunct Natal Jupiter

Invigorating, cheerful, hopeful and athletic. Energy rises, and some people feel great! If convalescing, don't overdo it too soon! Accents Jupiter, and all he means in the natal chart. In some cases, this transit signals a miraculous health intervention, beneficial information, or angelic help. Prayers are especially effective during this transit! Medical insurance can also come through.

Generally warming to the body. Stimulating to the arterial circulation and accelerates both blood pressure and liver function. Heats, thins and pressurizes the arterial blood. Heightens any inherent tendency to stroke, heart attack, thrombosis, and sun stroke especially in Fire signs. Migraine prone. Internal hemorrhage prone. May increase weight, fat, edema or swelling, depending on the element. Can be productive of tumors in the liver or increased liver sclerosis.

Stimulates the pituitary gland, with odd results caused by hormonal increase, such as hot flashes, swollen breasts, and high libido. Some potential for increased glycogen and consequential changes in blood sugar levels. Blood cholesterol may unexpectedly soar. May cause excess proliferation of blood in the bodily region ruled by the sign of natal Jupiter.

A potentially dangerous aspect for individuals suffering bipolar, mania, panic, anger control issues or ADHD. Conversely, hope and joy are enhanced, a great assist to victims of depression.

Temporarily heightens fertility. A positive aspect for desired weight gain or pregnancy!

Medical Tip: At this time, women who do not wish multiple births should be wary of fertility enhancing drugs that are known to cause them.

Herbal Note: Portal circulation decongestant herbs and liver-clearing herbs may be beneficial at this time, such as: Gentian, Agrimony, Burdock, Holy Basil, Linseed tea, etc. Do not self-treat.

Transit North Node Conjunct Natal Saturn

Strongly positive for calcium absorption and bone building. Strengthening to weak tendons and ligaments, and the entire body structure. Strengthening to elderly and convalescing persons. Excellent for the onset of nutritive therapies. However, this aspect can cause mineral deposits in joints, blood vessels, gallbladder, kidneys. Blocked gall ducts are common, and constipation.

Productive of skin diseases, skin cancers, moles or warts, fibrous growths, arthritis, rheumatism, bone spurs, bone cancer (rare), teeth impactions, ear impactions, and deafness.

Note: This transit strongly inclines to mass toxins, creating stiffness and the conditions fertile for cellular change. Knowing this, the practitioner can devise a means to relax and cleanse the effected region prior to and during this transit. Diffuse off accumulations!

The body parts ruled by the sign of natal Saturn point the way; or look to Saturn's natural significations. The wise physician begins work well before this aspect's exactitude.

Herbal Notes: The relaxing, warming, moistening herbs of Venus are useful for the onset of Saturn's cold, stiff conditions. Hot Martian herbs are equally useful, all depending on the exact nature of the malady.

Should symptoms arise, gravel removal herbs for the kidney or gallbladder are appropriate should symptoms arise: Gravel Root, Chamomile, Parsley, etc. Bile-moving herbs: Dandelion, Agrimony, Yarrow, Butternut, Burdock, Spanish Black Radish, etc. Select warm or cool herbs by noting the element of natal Venus. Select for moderate temperature, unless symptoms suggest otherwise.

Skin opening and lubricating herbs are useful, such as olive or sesame oil, Oregon Grape, Yellow Dock, Burdock et al.

This is the best possible aspect for treating osteoporosis or atrophy with nutrient herbs: Oatstraw, Nettles, Alfalfa, Fenugreek, et al. Do not self-treat.

Transit North Node Conjunct Natal Uranus

Brings surges of electrical activity in the body. Negatively, can cause electrical shock, inexplicable spasm or paralysis, electrical storms in the heart or brain, seizure, and very strange "undiagnosable" conditions. For epileptics, a 'red alert'.

Herbal Notes: Antispasmodics (Lobelia, Catnip, Cramp Bark, Prickly Ash, Blue Vervain, Black Cohosh et al.) Sedatives may be called for if Mars or Mercury are involved: Scullcap, Lemon Balm, Catnip, Passion Flower, Hops, Lavender, Blue Vervain, et al. Do not self-treat.

Medical Tip: Salt influences electricity and so do crystals (salt is a crystal). The ancient Europeans had diverse treatments for epilepsy involving the drinking of water either poured over crystals, or water laid in copper bowls under Lunar eclipses. It appears that some sort of electrical-charge reversal is involved, transferred to the sufferer via the charged water.

Normally however, one should never drink water left out under any type of eclipse! (See *Field Note,* page 148.) However, this does seem an ancient technology for healing epilepsy, a condition thought to be caused by little understood electrical brainstorms.

Field Note: A recent client was seized with an epic amount of painful gripes and upper gut and stomach gas following a North Node eclipse loosely conjunct her natal Uranus in Cancer, the sign of the stomach (Uranus rules spasm).

Transit North Node Conjunct Natal Neptune

Neptune's meaning in the personal natal chart is highly potentized under this transit! One can become more psychic or receive psychic information. Miracles can happen, and dreams come true. This is a very useful aspect for many vocations, (musicians, photographers, wine sales, and the like), but we are talking about health.

Increases tendency to drug and alcohol addiction and also their availability. Can signal the onset of cellular change or invigorate a hidden virus, fungus or mold. In predisposed charts, this can coincide with the onset of rare psychiatric conditions. Possibly tumor prone, usually hidden. When symptoms arise under Neptune-Node contacts, keep looking.

During this transit, vibrational therapies are highly effective, including homeopathy, Bach Flower Essences, music therapy, aromatherapy, and shamanic healing. Prayer is especially effective at this time, provided the natal Neptune is strong and positive.

This aspect is also useful for hypnotherapy, provided you have an impeccable therapist whom you trust to control your subconscious! However, hypnotherapy is never recommended if the natal Neptune is conjunct the natal South Node!

In rare cases, this conjunction increases potential for drowning, but not nearly as much as the transit South Node–natal Neptune contact. Increases mucous lymphatic congestion and potentially can act to commence cellular changes or tumor growth.

Herbal Notes: Should symptoms present or precancerous conditions arise, lymph moving herbs might greatly alleviate the situation. Poke Root (phytolacca americana), Violet, Dandelion Root, Burdock, Red Root (ceanothus), Blue Flag, Red Clover, grapes. Never self-treat!

Transit North Node Conjunct Natal Pluto

The Head's transit to natal Pluto may be unclear and not felt in all nativities. Because both the North Node and Pluto govern poisoning (along with Mars, Neptune, Saturn, South Node, and signs Scorpio, Aquarius and Pisces), this conjunction can testify to poisoning as much as does Mars-Neptune.

Danger of drug overdose. Potential sepsis or gangrene. May suggest the entry of dangerous bacteria into the bloodstream through needles, bites or medical carelessness. Could signal the reception of HIV, STDs, etc. Be extra careful of parasite infestation, especially if natal Pluto is in an Earth or Water sign.

This transit offers one supportive testimony for those suspecting that their recent health problem might be hex involved. Although very rare, and requiring multiple testimonies, weak or submissive persons could be subject to spirit-control, especially if this transit occurs in the 8th, or 12th house. This is not the time to fool around with spirit entities!

Plutonium poisoning or disruptions caused by various medical rays and lasers.

Field Note: One friend was experiencing this conjunction exactly, with an attendant eclipse occurring upon the exact degree of her natal Pluto. Sitting innocently under a tree and minding her own business, a tic or spider fell down and bit her arm, creating what appeared to be a classic Lyme Disease "bull's eye."

Medical Tip: This conjunction is dangerous through either overdose or over responsiveness to procedures such as hormone therapies, stem cell transplants, organ transplants, and blood transfusions.

Chemotherapy would be extra-effective at killing cancerous cells while simultaneously more potent in damaging healthy tissue.

Drastic responses to drugs, herbs and lasers would be typical. Inclines to excessive damage or side effects caused by radiation therapy, lasers, chemotherapy.

Conversely, this could suggest a highly effective time for these same drastic treatments. Therefore, the whole chart must be consulted in this case. Pluto rules destruction and regeneration! Potentially, no planet can turn a desperate situation around as effectively as Pluto.

This transit is hopeful for those waiting to receive an organ for transplant!

Herbal Notes: Blood cleansing herbs might be considered for Plutonian conditions. Sassafras, Sarsaparilla, Burdock, Ceanothus, Yellow Dock, Oregon Grape Root, Beets, Garlic, and Onions.

Antiviral and antibiotic herbs may be useful in specific cases. These include: Oregano, Olive Leaf, Rosemary, Eucalyptus, Grapefruit Seed Extract, Chaparral, Garlic, Bay Laurel, Thyme, Thuja, etc.

Should parasites present, Vermifuges and anti-parasitic herbs may be called for: Olive Leaf, Black Walnut, Cloves, papaya seeds, etc.

Should poisoning or insect/snake bites be extant, the herb must be matched to the poison. Plantain, Echinacea Gentian, and Black Snake Root all have poison-clearing reputations.

Transit North Node Conjunct Natal Ascendant

Many report a significant rise in physical energy for several weeks or months around this important transit. Remember, the given birth time (that signifies our Ascendant degree) is almost always recorded 10-15 minutes late, according to the great astrologer Robert C. Jansky who worked in obstetrics wards! This is a good time for strengthening the body.

THE NODAL SQUARES
Health Potentials for Predisposed Nativities
The square does not always manifest as health concerns or benefits.

The Lunar North and South Nodes are always opposite. This means that as one Node squares any natal planet, both Nodes do! Any natal planet posited at the exact midpoint of a transiting Nodal square is temporarily "in the bends" *(see page 46),* experiencing pronounced stress. Study the function and body affinities listed for each planet to determine how this stress may be contributing to your patient's symptoms. Study the sign and element of the natal planet receiving the impact. Then, study the sign polarity of the transiting Nodes.

Orb: Very strong at 0-1°. This seldom lasts more than a few weeks, and sometimes much less, depending on the current speed of the Nodes.

THE NODAL QUINCUNX
Health Potentials for Predisposed Nativities
A quincunx does not always manifest as health concerns or benefits.

Case studies indicate that an exact 0-1° quincunx to any planet by a Node will add significant weight to other disharmonious transits that the planet may be concurrently receiving. Symptoms sometimes result. Additionally, a close quincunx (0-3°) to Sun, Moon, or Ascendant is dangerous within one month to one year, if simultaneous testimonies concur.

Chapter 9

THE SOUTH LUNAR NODE
POWER OUTAGE, WEAKNESS, DEFICIENCY
The Doorway to the Spirit

Alternate Names: The Dragon's Tail,
    The Tail, Cauda, Ketu *(Jyotish)*

Properties, Rulerships and Actions

Sign Rulerships: The Nodes rule no signs. However, there are two traditional candidates for the "exaltation" of the Lunar South Node: Sagittarius and Scorpio. Scorpio seems the best fit, because amongst other body parts, Scorpio literally governs the colon/anus, and their expulsion of toxic matter. This is similar to the action of "The Dragon's Tail," the preeminent exit point for celestial forces.

    Important! The Lunar Nodes are always are exactly opposite one another in ecliptic longitude. Eclipses invariably take place in conjunction to one Node while simultaneously opposing the other. Either Node, having the power to eclipse the Lights, is immensely powerful by transit, and should never be ignored (as so often occurs).

Metal: None cited

Gem: Chalcedony, Cat's Eye

Cosmic Ray: Infrared Red *(traditional Jyotish)*

Body Associations: The anus. There may be some logic to linking "The Tail's" influence to the genitals (with Scorpio, Venus and Mars). The South Node is also associated with the soles of the feet, normally the province of the sign Pisces.

Action: Depleting, fatiguing, leaking, draining, excreting, unconscious. Helpful to the release of toxic matter, gravel, weight, etc. If pathological, a passage of the Dragon's Tail depletes vital force of the planet or Light it conjoins, in turn creating a panoply of symptoms.

Natally, the South Lunar Node, or Dragon's Tail, functions as a major celestial exit portal for planetary energies. By transit, the South Node signifies the outgoing tide of Solar-Lunar forces.

By transit, this out-pulling "celestial tide" dependably weakens the natural function of all natal planets conjoined, excepting Mars' excreting force. In this case, Mars is either weakened or strengthened—yes, its hard to know! Why? Because Mars excretes and so does the South Node. Logically, this could intensify excretions, and indeed hemor-rhage is observed in some cases.

Conversely, the transit South Node weakens any planet it conjoins. Obviously, this could act to weaken Mar's excreting powers! Much would depend on the condition of natal Mars.

In Jyotish tradition, the South Node's influence resembles that of Mars. However, this regards only his excreting function, because the South Node is likewise excreting.

In most other respects, they are opposite in nature. South Node weakens whereas Mars strengthens. Mars is a warrior, whereas Cauda is timid. Mars' action is extroverted, whereas the South Node turns inward, being a notable spiritual gateway in the natal chart. All told, the South Node's action strongly resembles that of Neptune more than any other planet!

Positive: Releases toxins and karmic accretions; allows "letting go."

Negative: Produces a dangerous draining and leaking, fatigue. Behaves unconsciously. Releases leaks of disturbing memory from the deep subconscious, and all this may imply.

Disease Associations: Fatigue; anemia; starvation, deficiencies of all kinds; blindness; wasting illnesses; suicide; chronic depression, fear; loneliness, speech disorders, blindness, low immune defenses; eruptive diseases; boils, ulcers, plagues; contagion, mysterious diseases that weaken; diseases of filth and vermin; contagion; parasites.

Bleeding; victimization by magic or supernatural attack; skin disease; ulcers; boils; draining; leaking; excess excretion; hyper-sexuality or the opposite, low libido—this is the Dragon's Tail, after all! Anal problems; drug addiction, spirit-possession, weak self-confidence and nervous breakdown. The South Node is associated with extreme body heat and acidic conditions.

Genetically inherited disease (both Nodes). The South Node is associated with the maternal side. Autoimmune disorders may have a connection to either Node, although the North Node makes more sense.

Tuberculosis and wasting diseases of all kinds; internal bleeding, menorrhagia; blindness; senility; dependency; excessive bodily excretion of all kinds and subsequent exhaustion; loneliness; sorrow; and past life memory induced illness. Strange, "undiagnosed" viruses.

Both Nodes have association with poisons (as do Saturn, Mars, Neptune and Pluto). The "drag tide" effect of the Dragon's Tail weakens the bodily functions of any planet conjoined, and also the sign it tenants.

Useful Tip: For natal charts, note the sign of the natal South Node for a lifetime weak spot in the body that needs to be strengthened. Likewise, support the functions of any natal planet conjoined a natal South Node. You will not be unrewarded.

Both Lunar Nodes play a role in the development and onset of cancer (as do Saturn, Jupiter, Neptune, Uranus, Pluto and Mars). Jyotish writers are divided on *which* of the two Lunar Nodes causes cancer. Many define cancer as the specialty of the South Node, the logic being that cancer is a "hot" disease—and what is more deeply heating than the South Node's infrared light?

However, many forms of cancer are formatively "cold" in that they are caused by a slow accretion of toxic matter and/or lack of circulation and oxygen to the disposed region. This is more the action of the North Node and Saturn, brilliantly displayed in multiple cancer cases. We must keep in mind that there are many varieties of cancer, and many causes!

The Nodes' Influence on Growth Extremes: See *Notes* in *Chapter 8: The North Lunar Node (page 112).*

Temperature: Very hot (Jyotish tradition). However, the heat of the South Node varies from the heat of Mars. The South Node weakens, drains and fatigues, whereas Mars energizes and excites! Both entities stimulate excretion.

Hormones: Unknown. Possible influence on the pituitary gland, due to an influence on height extremes discovered by George White.

Time Frame & Orb: The South Node transits are most obvious within an orb 0-3° and very potent at 0-1°. However, should a Light or any planet be eclipsed within an orb of 3°, the impact of this event may last at least one year, sometimes longer. However, the transit conjunction is so important that it will be felt to some degree by any planet tenanting the sign that the Tail transits through for the entire transit of approximately a year and a half.

Cycle: The South Node will transit over a natal planet approximately once every 18.633 years.

All eclipses will occur very close to one or both Lunar Nodes. Any eclipse occurring within 3° of any natal planet or angle will produce striking effects (related to that planet, and its sign and house) within one year. For a detailed description of effects other than medical, see my book *Eclipses and You*. Extensive detail on both North and South Node eclipses occurring conjunct all natal planets is provided in the advanced back-section.

Possible medical effects by transit are listed in this present book under Chapters 8 and 9, which are devoted to the North and South Nodes. More natal-based medical effects are addressed in *The Astrological Body Types* and also in *The Lunar Nodes, Your Key to Excellent Chart Interpretation*.

SOUTH NODE THROUGH THE ELEMENTS & SIGNS
Health Potentials for Predisposed Nativities
Nodal aspects do not always manifest as health concerns or benefits.

Applicable to both natal and transit charts, these partial lists of expressed symptoms apply only to predisposed nativities. These conditions are obviously uncommon and require multiple testimonies beyond the presence of South Node. Manifestation of symptoms may be enhanced by lifestyle choices, and taking preemptive measures can reduce, remove or prevent potential issues from manifesting. It is not possible to list all potential expressions.

South Node in Fire Signs *(natal or transit)*

Aries: *Vital force is draining from the head region.*
Weakens brain function and eyesight, brain fatigue.

Leo: *Vital force is draining from the heart area.*
Weakened heart muscle, fatigue, weakened back, spinal sheath demyelination (rare, can occur for either Node).

Sagittarius: *Vital force is draining from the hips, legs, muscles and lower spinal cord.*
Weakened legs, weakened hips or femurs, fatigue, genetic spinal cord and neuromuscular disease (rare), seizures, visions, involuntary mental states.

South Node in Earth Signs *(natal or transit)*

Note: The reader may note that North and South Nodes will share some of their pathological expressions in Earth signs, true. However, the reasons for these shared symptoms have opposite mechanics!

For example, a potential appendicitis is listed under both Nodes for Virgo. The North Node in Virgo could preclude an impacted appendix gone toxic; whereas a South Node appendicitis might occur through an unchecked infection caused by weak bodily defenses. Hypothetically, a South Node appendicitis would be more readily cleared out then the North Node variety!

These subtle differences between Nodal actions, once understood, allow the practitioner a refinement of diagnosis. **North Node in/South Node out.**

Taurus: *Vital force is draining from the lower head, jaw, ears and neck area.*
Weakened neck, neck injury, slipped atlas bone, throat inflammation or infection, excess ear wax, weakened hearing, deafness, ear

injury, eating disorders and addictions, difficulty swallowing, heavy metal poisoning through dental fillings, loose or cracked teeth, weak teeth, cavities, abscessed teeth, bruxism, TMJ; infected salivary glands, malnourishment, diet-produced nutritional deficiency, diet extremes, poor appetite (sometimes reversed).

Vocal polyps, tongue, mouth or throat cancer (rare), cancer of upper esophagus (rare), weakened voice, vocal cord inflammation or infection, tongue inflammation, tonsillitis, lower brain issues, lower brain tumor or thrombosis (more typical of North Node), cysts, injury to cervical vertebrae, boils.

Virgo: *Vital force is draining from the liver, pancreas, spleen, and upper intestine.*

Abdominal hernia, appendicitis, duodenitis, pancreatitis, colitis, diverticulitis, splenitis, intestinal worms or parasites, liver flukes, parasites in gall or liver ducts, liver diseases due to insufficient action or malfunction, intestinal weakness, weakness of abdominal wall, intestinal aneurysm, liver injury, hepatitis, appendicitis, jaundice, swollen spleen, ruptured spleen, injury to upper digestive organs.

Cancer or tumors of liver, pancreas, duodenum or intestine, colitis and Crohn's disease (with Scorpio, Virgo), yoga and diet extremes "dying to be healthy," poor immunity due to insufficient action or number of white blood cells, inherited genetic disease of the Virgo-ruled organs (rare).

Capricorn: *Vital force is draining from the bones, skin, knees, tendons, connective tissues, ligaments weakening these structures (unless remediated).*

Insufficient skin protection, skin changes or potential skin cancer, pigmentation issues, itchy skin, excessively oily skin, plugged skin ducts due to excess oil, plugged bile duct, parasites in gall or liver ducts, eczema, psoriasis, excess bile production (jaundice) or conversely, insufficient bile.

Weak knees, knee injury, osteoporosis, tendonitis at knee, weak or "slippery" ligaments, over-elastic tendons, stomach issues and nausea (by reflex to cancer). Dry mucous membrane, dental caries, tooth decay, cavities, vomiting, lead poisoning, poisoning incurred through vocational activity, bone infections, disturbed mineral assimilations (e.g. weak bones with bone spurs), calcium deficiency, excessive excretion of minerals, cellular changes in skin or bone (rare), influences kidney function, stimulates anterior pituitary, especially near 4°; weak nails, thin, dry or brittle hair, dandruff; inherited genetic disease (rare).

South Node in Air Signs *(natal or transit)*

Gemini: *Vital force is draining from the nerves, arms, hands, bronchial tubes, lungs and speech center.* Weak lungs, poor inspiration, poor oxygenation, capillary insufficiency, weakened arms or hands, slowed neural response, nervous breakdown, nervous fatigue, malnourished nerves, speech impediment, trouble speaking or hearing, poor judgment, learning disabilities, disturbed coordination, dreamy, overly distracted, may be implicated in some types of seizures, epilepsy.

Field Note: One client born with the South Node conjunct Mercury, (with her Sun and Moon in Gemini in her 6th house) was epileptic and also paralyzed in one arm.

Another client born with Mercury closely conjunct the South Node in Aries in the 3rd house was born without one hand. A third client with a close Mercury-South Node conjunction was born missing one finger.

Libra: *Vital force is draining from the kidney and lumbar area.*

Excess secretions of salt or potassium, weak kidney filtration, excess or deficient release of adrenal or ovarian hormones, excess urination, poor bladder retention, weak lumbar spine, poor balance.

Aquarius: *Vital force is draining from the circulation, electrical body, spinal cord and lower leg.*

Mysterious blood disorders, blood poisoning, carbon monoxide poisoning, auto-intoxication, phlebitis, lower leg thrombosis, stretched or torn Achilles tendon. Circulatory disorders, varicose veins, deficient activity of spinal nerves, reduces electrical impulses through spinal nerves, paralysis, cramps, electrocution, ankle or calf injury, lower leg and ankle weakness, neural pain in lower leg, skin lesions of lower leg, rare diseases of the spinal nerves, weak cones of eye, color blindness.

South Node in Water Signs *(natal or transit)*

Note: The reader may note that North and South Nodes will share some of their pathological expressions in Water signs, true. However, the reasons for these shared symptoms have opposite mechanics!

For example, "dirty blood" is listed under both Nodes for both Scorpio and Pisces. In Water signs, the "greedy" Dragon's Head (North Node) dumps fluids in and then, dams them up; whereas the "releasing" Dragon's Tail (South Node) dumps them out. For a more detailed description of these mechanics, see *Chapter 8, The North Node: North Node in Water Signs.*

Cancer: *The vital force is draining from the breast, stomach, uterus, and lymphatics.*

Breast sensitivity, leaking poison from breast implants, delayed breast development, hormonal issues influencing water retention, deficient lactation for nursing mothers, immune and emotional problems stemming from not having been nursed, lowered estrogen or progesterone.

Weak stomach, ulcers, irritable or inflamed mucous membrane, malnourishment due to poor appetite, anorexia, food cravings, nausea, vomiting, tendency to miscarriage, injury to ribs, breastbone, breasts, stomach, diaphragm, pericarditis, pleural effusion, pleurisy, loss of breast tissue. Emotional distress or fear, paranoia, waterborne parasites, alcoholism and drug addictions, family pattern issues, strong allergic response.

Influences the posterior pituitary (especially near 4°); weak lung action, infection of lower lung, tuberculosis, lung tumors, depression, inherited genetic disease, past-life memory caused phobias.

Although Pisces is the sign "ruling" the lymphatics, Cancer is equally implicated through its rulership of the thoracic duct, armpit and breast. For predisposed persons, lymphatic pressure and toxicity may increase when either Node transits through either sign (but for opposite reasons)!

Scorpio: *Vital force is draining from the genitals, bladder, nose, excretory system, and colon.*

Sex addiction, nymphomania, plugged sweat glands, foul smelling sweat, excessive discharges of all kinds possible, colorectal cysts, polyps or cancer, bloody discharges, colorectal parasites, candida, genital fungus, sexual obsessions, STDs (especially spirochete origin).

Worms, bloodworm, parasites, chronic nasal infection, acne, plastic poisoning, hormone poisoning, stings of all kinds, snakebite, bedbugs (with Mars, Mercury); plant venoms, HIV, Lyme disease, dirty water, fecal or urinary contamination, vermin caused disease, contaminated water and waterborne parasites.

Smell problems, nasal infection, broken nose, vaginal infection, abortion, genital yeast, hemorrhoid, inguinal hernia, rectal bleeding, infected penis or testes, jock itch, "dirty blood," extreme genital odor, cystitis, bladder cysts, bladder cancer, blocked ureter, gravel, enuresis, colectomy, anal thrombosis, prostate issues.

Weakness or prolapse of anus, rectum, colon, bladder or vagina; lowered male potency, sperm viability issues, excessive nocturnal emission, genital development and size issues, appendicitis (with Virgo), colitis and Crohn's disease (with Scorpio), insufficient or excessive peristalsis.

Note: Many of these items are shared with the North Node in Scorpio, by different mechanisms. Scorpio and the South Node both rule excretion and release. This may be one reason why the South Node is considered exalted in Scorpio! However, this point is far more unconscious then the North Node. For example: We could say that abortion is a North Node in Scorpio action, while miscarriage is a South Node event.

Pisces: *Vital force is draining from the feet, weakening them.*

Lymphatic action could either weaken or speed up (because the South Node encourages excretion, and Pisces co-rules the lymph system). Foot fatigue, hot or cold feet, lymphatic toxicity, engorged lymph nodes, weird or engrossing dreams, psychic invasion (entities or magical attack), hypnosis, onset of psychical problems, suicidal ideology, astral porousness, supernatural problems, or mental illness.

This transit also corresponds with blood chemistry issues, blood toxicity, heated blood, boils, problems from mixing drugs and alcohol, drug overdoses; STDs.

Plastic poisoning, waterborne pathogens, hormone poisoning, seafood poisoning, inability to process alcohol, bloodworm, increases or decreases lymphatic action—good unless other toxin-clearing systems are down! Sexual addictions, seductions, boils, carbuncles, hot-wet rashes, dye allergies, watery cysts.

Note: Many of these items listed are shared with the North Node in Pisces, but for opposite reasons! Thus, the great usefulness of medical astrology.

The South Node and sign Pisces both enhance excretions, (as do the other excreters, Mars and Scorpio). The Lunar South Node when transiting Pisces can weaken the immune system and blood, producing an invitation to problems in these areas.

Conversely, the North Node's passage through Pisces would act to invade, engorge, obstruct or attack these regions—and Pisces, as a delicate sign, offers small resistance.

SOUTH NODE TRANSITS OF NATAL PLANETS
Health Potentials for Predisposed Nativities
Transits do not always manifest as health concerns or benefits.

Applicable to both natal and transit charts, these partial lists of expressed symptoms apply only to predisposed nativities. These conditions are obviously uncommon and require multiple testimonies beyond the presence of the Nodes.

Manifestation of symptoms may be enhanced by lifestyle choices, and taking preemptive measures can reduce, remove or prevent potential issues from manifesting. It is not possible to list all potential expressions.

SOUTH NODE CONJUNCTIONS
Transit South Node Conjunct Natal Sun

This transit is one of the most fatiguing of all transits. The vital force drains away more readily than usual. Weak, elderly or convalescing people should avoid strain.

The heart muscle may weaken, eyes may weaken, some experience brain fatigue. This is a good time to strengthen the heart, eyes and brain. Do all you can to bring more vital force into the system, or prevent leakage, unless your physician advises otherwise. Some interesting methods are detailed in *Astrology & Your Vital Force*.

Surgical and Medical Tips: Unless the responsible physician advises otherwise, this is generally not the best time for surgery, due to the temporary weakening of the vital force and heart. If you must have surgery, see protection techniques in the above cited book. Strengthen the eyes, brain and heart.

Herbal Note: Cardiac, brain and circulatory tonics are useful: Hawthorne Berry, Rosemary, Linden, Yarrow, Angelica, Gingko etc.

Renaissance doctors would place gold nugget or a bag containing three to five Solar herbs directly over the heart. Turquoise and amber heart amulets are strengthening to the magnetic field of the heart in specific cases. Do not self-treat. A great deal material is available in *Astrology & Your Vital Force*.

Transit South Node Conjunct Natal Moon

This transit is one strong testimony of temporarily lowered fertility. If pregnant, consult your naturopath or doctor for measures to strengthen the womb. The transit reduces edema in most cases; however in rare cases it causes it, by weakening lymphatic action. Female hormones may dramatically lower (especially progesterone): breast shrinkage, poor milk production, onset of perimenopause and menopause is possible if occurring for age-appropriate women.

Amenorrhea, or conversely, menorrhagia. Weakens digestion; appetite may lower; malnourishment, poor absorption, nutritional deficiency, starvation, anorexia; dehydration (especially in Fire signs). Lung action may weaken (this is dangerous for COPD,

TB, etc.), brain fatigue, weakened eyesight, emotional difficulties, severe depressions, sorrow, grief, loss, extreme sensitivity. Past-life memories may impinge on waking consciousness.

Mother issues may influence the health. Your mother's health may be important at this time. Memory loss or onset of dementia (only in the predisposed). Potassium deficiency. The lymphatic drainage of the brain may slow, requiring assistance.

This is a cataract-prone transit. Psychic protection is essential at this time! Often, a sense of overpowering loss.

Surgical and Medical Tips: Never take psychotropics under this transit! Avoid channeling, chanting, hypnosis. Be sure to drink enough pure water. This is NOT the best time to become pregnant because the uterus needs to rest.

Herbal Note:: If pregnant, consult with your doctor about Red Raspberry Leaf tea. This notorious herb is successfully used by midwives to strengthen the placenta's attachment to the uterus. Do not self-treat.

For confusion, brain fog, depression or psychic porousness, see *The Earthwise Herbal Repertory,* by Matthew Wood. St. John's Wort is famous for allaying moderate depression. Vervain is useful for preventing nightmares. Juniper berries and leaves worn about the neck will help close off astral porousness (hearing voices, etc.).

Bilberry, and red, orange and yellow foods may offset eye weakness. Bach Flower Essences might assist in depressed cases (Mustard, etc.). Psychic strengthening is a must. For prolapsed uterus or bladder, Horsetail, Bayberry. For poor lactation in nursing mothers: Borage. Do not self-treat.

Transit South Node Conjunct Natal Mercury

Weakens normal mental powers and function. Weakens communication or removes desire to speak, weakens sensory nerves or hearing, weakens hands or fingers, provokes carpal tunnel syndrome and repetitive-use hand injury, shoulder or arm issues; stuttering. Insufficient lung action or inspiration, poor oxygenation, bronchial or lung infections due to reduced strength of these organs.

Brain issues involving the speech or conscious mind, cerebrum. Nervous breakdown, nervous sensitivity, deficient nutrients to nerves, onset of mental illness, dementia or perceptual problem (rare), memory loss, acuity, coordination may be "off;" clumsy; astral impingement on sensory faculties, such as hearing voices, etc; increased psychism.

Herbal Note: Nutritive nervines are useful: Oat Straw, Milky Oat Tops, Parsely, Nettles, Alfalfa, et al. Cold pressed oils. Do not self-treat.

Medical Tip: Those with mental illnesses that interfere with rational processes or the interpretation of sensory input should be watched carefully under this transit.

Field Note: An excessively talkative high school friend requested my company on a particular weekend. However, I noticed that the transit South Node would be exactly conjunct his natal Mercury at that time. Knowing this would be challenging for someone so loquacious, I suggested that we move my visit off to another week. He said no, it must be that week. When I arrived, he had contracted laryngitis, and couldn't utter a word. We spent the visit in silence.

Transit South Node Conjunct Natal Venus

Potential lowering of blood sugar, estrogens and/or copper. Decreases libido and attractiveness; provokes onset of hair loss; infertility, kidney weakness, issues with ovaries or testes, venous insufficiency, varicosities. Influences the health of sisters and aunts.

Herbal Note: Wild Yam, Sarsaparilla, Saw Palmetto (males), Maca Root, Ginseng (both white and red, varying by your gender), and Licorice are a few of the many herbs with properties useful for managing female hormones. Nettle Seed is a specific for kidney disease. Sage, Mullein, Rosemary and Rue are excellent for veins. This is very general information. Do not self-treat!

Surgical Tip: Unless your responsible physician advises otherwise, it is best at this time to avoid cosmetic surgery of any kind; or surgery to ovaries, breasts or kidneys. However, this aspect may demand their removal, and in this context suits the symbology.

Removal works better than addition! For best results, it might be wise to delay that voluntary breast enhancement procedure to a more appropriate time.

Field Note: When a sister leaves, is ill, or even dies, it is amazing how often a recent South Node eclipse has occurred in close orb to natal Venus.

Traditionally, the wearing of a diamond and/or the taking of tincture of white diamond can offset the deficiency of Venus' Indigo Ray, indicated by this transit. A Jyotish astrologer trained in *Upaye* (remedies) should be consulted.

Transit South Node Conjunct Natal Mars

This transit potentially weakens the muscles, and decreases testosterone, adrenalin and iron. Available energy lowers. This transit presents the practitioner with a conundrum. Typically, the transit (or natal) South Node fatigues any planet it conjoins. However, we have a special case with Mars because both Mars and the South Node stimulate excretion. So, I've made it a point to watch this transit closely in available cases. It appears that often the native will indeed experience the expected lowered energy and reduced libido. However, others experience increased sexuality, or unmanageable surges of temper, energy or aggression.

Potential internal or external hemorrhage. Excretion may increase, due to both Mars and South Node governing excretion. However, that would be more typical of the reverse aspect, transit Mars conjunct the natal South Node. It is more likely that normal excretions (Mars) are weakened during a transit South Node passage, producing more circulating toxins in the lymphatic system and bloodstream.

Mars is the fighter. Mars' temporary disablement could signal an open door in the immune system. Digestive fires and metabolism may also be temporarily lowered. Acid-Alkaline balance may lurch to one side. This aspect sometimes coincides with poisoning, boils and rashes.

Field Note: One yogi born with the natal South Node conjunct her natal Mars in Scorpio suffered a mysterious, undiagnosed flow of blood from her colon for several years.

Field Note 2: As the transit South Node, plus transit Uranus (with an eclipse at same point), occurred simultaneously in Aquarius (sign of the ankles), exactly conjunct a client's natal Mars in Aquarius, he broke his ankle in a skiing accident. This was an astrological "no-brainer" skiing avoid, but alas, he was unaware.

Surgical and Medical Tips: Unless the physician insists on immediate surgery, it is wise to let the exact conjunction of the South Node over Mars clear a few weeks or months. Mars rules the surgeon's knife. Should professional opinion agree, this may be a time to assist natural excretion, sweating and blood cleansing. Avoid transfusions, transplants or hormonal treatments unless your physician advises otherwise. The doctor's opinion rules.

Herbal Notes: For anemia, Nettles, soaked Black Raisins, Beets. For sagging libido, Maca Root, Gingseng, Saw Palmetto, Sarsaparilla. Exhausted adrenals respond well to combined Oat Straw and Borage (Wood). For hemorrhage or internal bleeding: Yarrow, Cayenne, Sage, Storks Bill, Yellow Dock, et al. Do not self treat.

Transit South Node Conjunct Natal Jupiter

This transit is weakening to the arterial circulation and de-celerates both blood pressure and liver function. Invigorating and athletic. This transit is useful for fat loss and the clearing of cholesterol from the blood and vessels. Influences pituitary gland function, with odd results caused by hormone decrease. Generally warming to the body. If convalescing, don't overdo it too soon! Internal hemorrhage prone.

Can increase tendency toward thoughtless liver damage or the entry of liver flukes or pathogens. Liver function may weaken or conversely, the liver may dump something excessively into the blood (cholesterol, glycogen, etc.). Possible blood sugar level changes.

With three or more testimonies, either Lunar Node transiting natal Jupiter can coincide with the onset of diabetes in predisposed persons. Expected medical insurance can fail to come through. Physicians may be neglectful or careless.

Herbal Note: This aspect is highly miscarriage prone. Traditionally, herbalists used Raspberry Leaf tea to strengthen the bond of the placenta with the uterus. This transit lowers fertility in both genders, but not so much as when the South Node crosses the Moon (for women).

Transit South Node Conjunct Natal Saturn

Decreased bone density. This transit is the biggest single warning that calcium and/or other minerals are leaching more rapidly from the bones. Extremely weakening for elderly persons, and increases proneness to falls and bone breakage. May relate to onset of some skin cancers, moles, warts, and a wide array of skin diseases.

Dental decay, teeth loss, teeth weakening, hearing loss, deafness, weak joints, cartilage degeneration, weakened ligaments and tendons, brittle nails. The nervous system is affected, especially in Air signs. If natal Saturn is severely afflicted, this transit threatens nervous exhaustion. The general strength and integrity of the whole physical vehicle is potentially lowered.

The gallbladder may fail to excrete enough bile, or conversely, too much. Cornell associates Saturn with the white blood cells. This seems counterintuitive, but if he is correct then this transit could signal a lack of or change of white cells for predisposed nativities.

Hypothetically, bone spurs, toxic accretions and/or heavy metals might more readily release from the body. While so doing, be wary as to not leech out your minerals too!

Field Note for Physicians: When noting this aspect, always test for bone density. All too often you will discover that your patient has been rapidly losing calcium "for unknown reasons."

A friend was soon to experience a "doubling" of this aspect: transit South Node conjunct natal Saturn while simultaneously transit Saturn was moving to conjunct the natal South Node!

She was already suffering a mysterious muscle-wasting disease and was gradually losing the use of her limbs. If nothing was done, she would be in a wheelchair by the time the doubled aspect came due in one year.

Armed with this knowledge, she set to work on her mineral nutrition. Seaweed, mineral rich herbs, and better food choices. She also found the best osteopath and Rolfer in her area. This was the perfect therapy choice, because Saturn governs bodily structure! By the time the aspect came through, she was much improved (instead of worse) and kept on improving! It took a few years, but now she enjoys good muscular health.

Herbal Notes: For mineral loss or weakening bones: Oat Straw, Alfalfa, Red Clover, Nettles, Maca Root, Pumpkin Seeds, Dandelion, Parsley, etc. To facilitate heavy metal cleansing: Cilantro, et al. Bile moving herbs: Dandelion, Agrimony, Yarrow, Butternut, Burdock, etc. Do not self-treat.

Transit South Node Conjunct Uranus

Hypothetically, this transit decreases electrical activity in the body, often suddenly and without warning. Predisposed persons may experience inexplicable problems of an electrical origin.

Strange chakra disorders, strange shooting pains, numbness, tingling, psychic experiences, hormonal imbalances, spasm, paralysis, electrical malfunction in the heart or brain, seizure, and peculiar "undiagnosable" conditions. Possible association with the onset of some types of mental illness in predisposed persons (rare).

Theoretically, this aspect could be useful in cases of hyper-electrical activity in the body, heart or brain. Uranus is never dependable, and results in any direction can reverse suddenly.

One never knows what responses might occur for any treatment under this aspect. EMF fields are especially disturbing to the body at this time. We bathe in these now, oblivious to their widely proven influence on many physical and cellular functions.

The reader can readily find scores of references and research studies from India, Japan, Scandinavia, Germany, and others, available on the Internet. *The Secret of Life: Electricity, Radiation and Your Body*, by scientist Georges Lakhovsky, is a worthy read.

Field Note: One barefoot man I encountered at the sacred headwaters of Shasta, California had fallen deathly ill (for years) immediately after a teacher encouraged him to drink his specially prepared eclipse water. It is interesting that some ancient traditions instruct to cover all water that must be left outdoors during eclipses!

Medical Tips: Theoretically, vibrational oscillation and/or electrical treatments of all kinds would be dangerous during this transit, or give unexpected results. The physician must be consulted on decisions regarding these treatments. Pacemakers and other electrical monitoring devices should be carefully watched, lest they malfunction or "go down."

Those suffering "undiagnosable" problems at this time might take an accounting of the EMF levels of their daily environment especially the bedroom. Excellent meters are available online; search "EMF protection, meters, products" etc.

Salt influences electricity, and so do crystals (salt is a crystal). Ancient Europeans had diverse treatments for epilepsy involving the drinking of water, either poured over crystals, or water in copper bowls under Lunar eclipses.

It appears that some sort of electrical-charge reversal is involved, transferred to the sufferer via the charged water. Normally however, one should never drink water left out under any type of eclipse! However, this does seem to be an ancient technology for healing epilepsy, a condition thought to be caused by little understood electrical brainstorms.

Transit South Node Conjunct Natal Neptune

Because Neptune and the South Node are quite similar in action, the client's natal Neptune, and all its personal meaning, is doubled under this transit! This is similar to the transit of the North Node over natal Neptune, although considerably more vulnerable.

One's normal psychic boundaries are weakened, requiring vigilance. The veil thins now between the physical plane and the astral plane producing greater vulnerability and sometimes clairvoyance/clairaudience.

This aspect warns against hypnotherapy, as unpleasant packages from the deep subconscious could leak upward into the conscious at this time. Some rare psychiatric conditions or depression may commence (only for predisposed charts).

One is also more easily victimized by other people or entities with powerful minds. Beware mental suggestion and strengthen conscious resolve! Become conscious of your musical, social and media environment, choosing these selectively. Tune your psychic radio to only high vibrations, and request spiritual protections. Some people are more susceptible at this time to their vital force being drained by stronger persons or even nefarious beings.

One's sleep and dream life are profoundly influenced. Fatigue is symptomatic. The bodily regions governed by the sign of natal Neptune may leak vital force, thus weakening. This transit can sometimes signal the onset of cellular change, or suggest the presence of a hidden virus, fungus, or mold. Avoid adopting voluntary implants that may leak or poison in the future. Neptune has a gift for leaking and slow, secret poisoning!

Possibly tumor prone, usually hidden. When symptoms arise under Neptune-Node contacts, keep looking. The transit North Node to natal Neptune is more inclined to tumors, though sometimes this reverses.

Hidden viruses or poisoning are very typical, but far more so if the transit itself is reversed, i.e. with transit Neptune conjunct the natal South Node. This transit increases the tendency to be seduced into drugs, or to become addicted, or enslaved.

Be wary of deception and seduction related to the sign and house position in the natal chart (and in general). This is obviously not the time to take the "eye off the ball" with teenagers!

Neptune has some governance over all opiates, alcohol and relaxing substances. Theoretically, these would be insidiously harmful at this time. Neptune is never obvious in action, allowing one to "go to hell in a handbasket, singing all the way." Vibrational-based and intuitive therapies of diverse kinds are potentially risky or misapplied at this time (homeopathy, shamanism, trance, seeking information from spirit guides, hypno-suggestion. This is no time to allow oneself to be placed into a trance state, and thus vulnerable to powerful people or entities.

The potential for drowning is heightened in some charts, with added testimony.

If your physician agrees, strengthen the function of any weak body part governed by the sign of natal Neptune. If contemplating a voluntary medical procedure or new medication, this transit warns to obtain a few opinions first.

Herbal and Medical Tips: Many of this transit's proclivities can be counteracted with improved psychic boundaries. Consciously tune the inner vibrational radio to a good station. Vervain is a traditional herb for preventing bad dreams. Avoid Mugwort and other dreaming herbs at this time! Juniper leaves and berries, worn about the neck are traditional for closing an astral door (hearing voices, etc.). Don't self-treat.

Transit South Node Conjunct Natal Pluto

In rare cases for predisposed charts, this transit may signal the onset of a genetically inherited disease, or a disease of karmic origin. Always note the bodily regions governed by the sign of natal Pluto. May suggest the entry of dangerous bacteria into the bloodstream. Inclines to damage of a significant nature through radiation-therapy, lasers, chemotherapy.

Could hypothetically be useful for a thorough removal of diseased tissue or cancer—Pluto rules destruction and regeneration. The South Node aids removal, and Pluto does too! Although not necessarily preferred for any surgery, this time is certainly superior for removing parts, rather than adding-on.

Because both South Node and Pluto govern poisoning (along with Mars, Neptune, Saturn, North Node and signs: Scorpio, Aquarius, Pisces), this conjunction can testify to poisoning as much as does Mars-Neptune. Check for parasites in the colon, organs or bloodstream. Radiation poisoning is also a candidate.

This conjunction might warn of danger incurred through hormone therapies, stem cell transplants, organ transplants, blood transfusions, chemotherapy etc. Danger of drug overdose.

Potential sepsis or gangrene. This transit could signal the reception of HIV, STDs, etc. Be extra careful of parasite infestation, especially if natal Pluto is in an Earth or Water sign.

It is not impossible that symptoms presenting may be due to hexing activity. This is equally true of the North Node's passage of Pluto. However, the reverse is far more potent in this regard: transit Pluto conjoin either natal Node!

Transit South Node Conjunct Natal Ascendant

The focus of this book is more upon planet interaction and less upon houses. However, the passage of the Dragon's Tail over the natal Ascendant is so impactful to health that it must be discussed.

In my experience with scores of cases over many decades now, the arrival of the transit South Node to the sign of the Ascendant produces a nearly immediate sensation of malaise, all the more so if nearing the precise degree.

Sometimes this effect commences the very day the transit South Node enters the sign of the natal Ascendant. What is happening here is that a receding celestial tide is dragging vital force away from the bodily field. Fatigue and heightened sensitivity result. Many sleep more and eschew crowds.

Ambition recedes with the tide too, replaced by a period of spiritual inquiry or more negatively, depression. The bodily region governed by the natal Ascendant sign is weakened unless provided with extra support. To *know the transit* gives the ability to counteract it. The native needs to pull more vital force back into the bodily field. There are many ways of doing this, some detailed in my book *Astrology & Your Vital Force*.

Utilizing the methods of the Ascendant sign's element is helpful: pranayama (for Air signs); high nutrient raw foods and mineral baths (Earth signs); swimming in/or drinking natural water (Water signs); color and gem therapy for Fire signs (gems refract color).

Realistically, most methods work for all elements. Additionally, certain opaque stones worn over the heart help prevent the leakage of vital force.

NODAL SQUARES AND THEIR HEALTH IMPACT
Health Potentials for Predisposed Nativities
Transits do not always manifest as health concerns or benefits.

Refer to this same section in previous *Chapter 8, The Lunar North Node.*

THE NODAL QUINCUNX
Health Potentials for Predisposed Nativities
Transits do not always manifest as health concerns or benefits.

Refer to this same section in previous *Chapter 8, The Lunar North Node.*

THE PLANETS

Chapter 10
MERCURY
SENSE RECEPTION,
NERVES, CONNECTIONS

Properties, Rulerships and Actions

Rules: Gemini and Virgo

Exalted: Virgo *(Jyotish)*; Aquarius *(West)*

Detriment: Sagittarius and Pisces

Fall: Pisces, Leo

Metal: Mercury

Minerals: None cited. This is curious, because as a nerve conductor, one would think he shares rulership of sodium, table salt, normally assigned to Saturn and the electrical sign Aquarius.

Vitamins: B1 *(Jansky, Nauman)*

Gem & Cosmic Ray: Green Emerald, Green

Herbal Categories: Nutritive nervines, including all herbs that act to specifically assist and strengthen the function of the sensory nerves and the smooth conduction of neural signals, from the sense organs through the afferent nerves to the central nervous system.

Sedative nervines and antispasmodics are commonly listed as belonging to Mercury. While these are calming to nervous complaints, they are certainly not in themselves Mercurial by nature, i.e., nervous! Similarly, many soporifics (sleeping herbs) and psychotropics are also placed on Mercury's traditional lists; these relax the mind while functionally resembling sleepy Neptune, sweet Venus or the nurturing Moon

Body Rulership & Organ Affinity: Mercury governs hands, fingers, speech, and the afferent nerves, which transmit signals from the sensory organs to the central nervous system (CNS). Mercury also has a considerable influence over the sense of hearing and is almost always natally co-implicated in cases of deafness. He holds general rulership over the peripheral nerves (with Gemini) and governs the speed of synapses.

The Jyotishi state that Saturn also has a strong governance of "the nerves." The electricity-ruling Uranus is strongly involved. Both Mercury and Uranus strongly influence the electrical conduction of the nerves.

Gemini and its opposite sign Sagittarius govern the voluntary nervous system: Sagittarius reigning over the CNS and lower spinal nerves with Gemini ruling the peripheral nerves. Aquarius is also considered to strongly influence the spinal nerves. In contrast, Virgo and Pisces appear to rule the sympathetic and parasympathetic nervous systems.

Obviously, the four "mutable" signs have the greatest influence over the nerves (Gemini, Sagittarius, Virgo, Pisces). Mercury rules two of this group: Gemini and Virgo.

The great prophet and medical psychic Edgar Cayce states that Mercury governs the pineal gland. He is unique in this viewpoint, but considering his venerable reputation, not to be scoffed at.

Mercury influences the bronchial tubes (with Gemini), the lungs (with Gemini, Cancer and the Moon), and hearing (with Aries, Taurus, Mars, Saturn). His governance of speech implies rulership over the speech centers of the brain.

General Action: Mercury's primary action is nervous. Mercury stimulates the nerves of the bodily regions governed by the zodiac sign he tenants, either natally or by transit. He is indicated wherever one finds neural pain, malfunction, or itch. This planet is also implicated, with Mars, in cases of bedbugs, lice, fleas, flies, mice and various infestation of insects and small vermin!

All manner of sensory and communication disorders are under

Mercury's auspices, as his direct influence is over the peripheral sensory nerves. His natal placement indicates the efficiency and speed of neural synapses and the transmission of sensory data to the brain through the afferent nerves.

Mercury-Mars equals pain. Neurological pain is most evident when Mercury is in hard aspect to transit or natal Mars, and secondarily Uranus. His negative transit expresses as nervousness and/or neuralgia in the bodily region ruled by that sign.

Conversely, in certain conditions the neural flow is reduced. For example, when natal Mercury is blocked by Saturn, confounded by Neptune, weakened by the Lunar South Node, or when in Pisces.

Mercury, the "celestial messenger," is the fastest moving of the true planets. While his natal aspects, (occurring at birth) can be quite strong, his transits are brief affairs excepting for his many yearly "stations," when he appears to stand still from Earth's point of view.

Even though his transit influence is brief, never underestimate him! The ray of this tiny lightweight often functions as the proverbial "straw that broke the camel's back." So often one sees the heavier planets delay a pending crisis awaiting the day that Mercury adds his weight.

The transits of Mercury can be useful in the diagnoses of mysterious symptoms. In studying maladies that began during an exact transit of Mercury to a natal planet, consider those nerves in the bodily regions governed by the sign of transit Mercury. Also consider the nerves ruled by the sign of the natal planet that Mercury currently afflicts. For additional clues, observe the element of transit Mercury (Fire, Earth, Air or Water); consider these literally! With pathogens, the element describes their literal source.

Medications and their prescription are very generally Mercurial affairs, but must be further assigned by type (e.g, stimulants are Mars, and opiates are Neptune). It is a good idea to check aspects from transit Mercury (and also to natal Mercury) at onset of a course of medication. At the time of receiving a prescription, a helpful transit of Mercury offers one positive testimony of its efficacy. However, a prescription received during the transit conjunction of Mercury on the natal South Node or Neptune warns of error or hazard.

Positive: Natally, sensory nerves are functioning normally and at good speed. The nervous system can handle normal stress and does not keep one up all night! The peripheral nerves are healthy. Hearing and speech are fine.

Negative: When natal Mercury is seriously afflicted by transits, the nervous system and brain is disturbed, more or less. Afflictions to and from both Mercury and Uranus are implicated in epilepsy, speech impairment, and tremors. Mercury's negative health transits are associated with pain and itch of neurological origin. The optimal function of the hands may be impaired.

Temperature & Moisture Level: Traditionally, both transit and natal Mercury is a chameleon, adopting the temperature, gender and moisture level from the zodiac sign he passes through and the planets he conjoins. Yet, on his own accord, Mercury is cool and dry. He is "friends" with cold Saturn and the gently normalizing Venus. That being said, transit Mercury is quite capable of inflaming the nerves when moving through Fire signs, or when conjunct or quincunx either transit or natal Mars.

Transit Frame & Orb: Strongest effects within one astrological degree by conjunction, square, opposition, quincunx, trine or sextile to any natal planet. Normally, this is a time period of only one to two days. The exception occurs when Mercury "stations," standing still from Earth's viewpoint. At this time, Mercury can sit near just one degree of ecliptic longitude for a several days, making his transit impact far stronger, perhaps even threefold!

Additionally, Mercury's nervous influence pervades the bodily regions of the sign he transits, from his ingress to his exit of that sign.

Field Notes: One client was born with natal Mercury positioned in a stellium of other planets, all in the nerve, arm and speech governing sign, Gemini, in the 6th house of health, conjunct the weakening South Node. She was epileptic, paralyzed in one arm, and bore a speech defect. She was also married to a schizophrenic. She passed away in her thirties.

An acquaintance born absent one hand shows Mercury conjunct the South Node in the third house, Aries. A client with a missing finger was born with Mercury conjunct the South Node in Gemini; it was his pinkie, the Mercury-ruled finger!

MERCURY THROUGH THE ELEMENTS & SIGNS
Health Potentials for Predisposed Nativities

Most of these conditions are obviously uncommon and require multiple testimonies beyond the presence of Mercury. These symptoms may apply to both natal and transit charts.

However, Mercury's **transit** is too brief to indicate any of the chronic conditions listed below. Instead, he can produce brief annoyances as listed, or similar, as he passes through each sign.

Manifestation of symptoms may be enhanced by lifestyle choices; and taking preemptive measures can reduce, remove or prevent potential issues from manifesting. It is not possible to list all potential expressions.

Mercury in Fire Signs

Aries: Eyestrain, neuralgic pains in ears or head, rages, impulsive or rash speech, accidents to arms or hands, bites and stings, dry bronchial tubes or lungs.

Leo: Disturbance to the electrical rhythm of the heart (arrhythmia), heart flutter, spasm in heart vessels, fits of anger, twisted wrist, neuralgia in back. Mercury in this sign influences the nerves of the gallbladder, upper back and wrist.

Sagittarius: Sciatic neuralgia, religious mania, excited and distracted mental states, ADHD, hyperactivity, paralysis, electrocution, verbal exaggeration.

Mercury in Earth Signs

Mercury being a conductor of electrical current through the nerves, is more grounded in Earth signs. This may lessen the impact of his transit.

Taurus: Neurologically caused deafness, neuralgic pains in ears or teeth, tinnitus, problems of cervical nerves, spasm of vocal cord or larynx, spasm of upper esophagus, speech defect caused by malfunction of nerves of tongue and vocal cords, nervous loss of voice; thyroid disturbances, choking, jaw misalignment, bruxism, TMJ.

Virgo: Nervous digestion and all its perturbations, active solar plexus, neurological pains in upper digestive organs; may contribute to autoimmune reactions and allergies; insomnia.

Capricorn: Gallbladder spasm (also seen in Leo), pituitary disturbance, growth extremes due to pituitary malfunction, "trick knee," neural pain in knees; dry skin and dandruff, itchy skin issues, sensitive skin, flea and insect bites; moles and freckles; "nervous" rheumatism, brittle mental state influencing issues of joints, ligaments and tendons; OCD.

Mercury in Air Signs

Gemini: Influences the nerves of the lungs, bronchial tubes and hands; neurological problems of arm and hand function, disturbance of sensory nerves or afferent nerves, some neurological brain disturbances; mental disconnection, attention disturbances, stuttering, speech disturbance. Asthma, whooping cough; frozen shoulder, dislocated shoulder, sprained or twisted arms, hands or fingers, emphasized hands (natal), increases need to communicate.

Libra: Influences the nervous system of the kidneys. Renal spasm; headache and eyestrain by reflex to Aries; shooting pains in lower back, lumbago (with Saturn). May influence ovarian nerves.

Aquarius: Because Aquarius has some rulership of the spinal nerves, this position is associated with an overall heightened neurological sensitivity and an increased need for calm and quiet. Natives with this natal position should avoid loud noise and chaos.

Pathologically, this transit or natal position can signal hyperfunction or disease of spinal nerves, all manner of undiagnosable problems (due to the body's little-understood electrical system), nervous breakdown, nervous exhaustion, odd mental states, sudden bolts of psychic information, sudden lack of oxygen, weird circulatory disturbances, neuralgia of the lower leg.

Should Mars, Saturn or Nodes be simultaneously in Leo, this may indicate demyelination of the spinal sheath. The transit is hypersensitive to electromagnetic fields and devices.

Mercury in Water Signs

Cancer: Nervous stomach, neuralgic pains in breasts, ribs, pericardium or pleura; emotionalism and sensitivity; phobias; extreme noise sensitivity; allergies; effects memory in both directions, eating disorders, noise, hypersensitivity.

Scorpio: Sensitive bladder, bed-wetting; genital pains or itching; neurological causes of impotence; colitis, nervous colon; nasal issues; colorectal parasites, crabs, bedbugs, lice, worms; shooting pains in Scorpio-ruled regions.

Pisces: Neurological problems of feet, sensitive feet, foot neuralgia, restless feet; narcolepsy, sleep walking, lucid dreaming, psychic trance states, extreme sensitivity to noise; increases mental confusion, depression, forgetfulness, dementia. Enhances memory too, but usually of childhood, or from the distant past.

MERCURY'S TRANSITS OF NATAL PLANETS

Most of these conditions are obviously uncommon and require multiple testimonies beyond the presence of Mercury.

These symptoms may apply to both natal and transit charts. However, Mercury's transit is often (but not always) too brief to indicate any of the chronic conditions listed below. More typically,

Mercury manifests these symptoms as brief annoyances as he passes through each sign. Symptomology may be enhanced by lifestyle choices, and taking preemptive measures can reduce, remove or prevent potential issues from manifesting. It is not possible to list all potential expressions.

MERCURY'S CONJUNCTIONS
Health Potentials for Predisposed Nativities
Conjunction does not always manifest as health concerns or benefits.

Mercury's strongest transit is the exact orb conjunction!

Transit Mercury Conjunct Natal Sun
A very brief and typically ineffective transit. Increases alertness and the neurological impulses throughout the bodily regions ruled by the Sun's sign. Potentially stimulating to the nerves governing the heart, eyes or brain, especially in Fire signs.

Transit Mercury Conjunct Natal Moon
This is a brief aspect that is generally not notable. However, it speeds the mental-emotional informational exchange and is thus excellent for psychotherapy, dream work and journaling.

Mercury conjunct the Moon increases neural sensitivity and emotional cognition; stimulates the nerves of the body part ruled by the sign of the natal Moon; and increased enervation of the stomach. Asthmatics and epileptics might take heed as this brief transit may increase neural reactions precipitating events.

Pregnant women should take every caution under this exact conjunction, because it increases the neurological response of the uterus, especially if stationing on the exact degree of the Moon. Therefore, avoid plane flights, EMF stimulus, and the like.

This aspect is either stimulating or irritating to those with mental illness.

Field Note: Pamela Sackett, the genius who coined the term "emotion literacy," and creator of ELA (Emotion Literacy Advocates) was appropriately born in with Mercury and Moon conjunct.

Surgical and Medical Tips: This transit could heighten neural sensitivity, neural pain, and nerve reaction especially for those with natal Moon in Gemini or Aquarius, or for whatever bodily region is governed by the sign that Mercury transits through.

Transit Mercury Conjunct Natal Mercury

Briefly increases nerve function, for good or ill.

Herbs: Both sedative and nutritive nervines are helpful. Do not self-treat.

Transit Mercury Conjunct Natal Venus

Calm Venus is rarely disturbed by slight enervation. Also, Mercury and Venus are "friends," being harmonious together.

Perhaps this conjunction heightens the nervous reactivity of the kidneys, ovaries or veins. May increase female genital sensitivity. The skin may become sensitized. The sign of natal Venus receives a heightened neurological stimulus.

Transit Mercury Conjunct Natal Mars

This conjunction increases alertness and quickens the motor nerves. The adrenal "fight or flight" mechanism speeds up. Insomnia is one typical manifestation. It can be enhancing to hand acuity, hand-eye coordination and athletic finesse (excellent for high focus, small muscle sports (e.g. gymnasts) and sharp shooting (e.g. golf, archery). Increases impatience and tendency for vehicular speeding. Improves ability to use tiny, sharp tools.

Mercury potentizes Mars, creating inflammation, pain and neuralgia/neuritis in the bodily regions ruled by the sign of natal Mars (or the sign opposite, square, or quincunx). Unless stationary, this conjunction is brief but potent. However, the conjunction in reverse is much stronger (transit Mars conjunct natal Mercury).

This conjunction is associated with insect bites, animal bites, bedbugs, lice, beestings, insect infestations, and exposure to plant toxins. If one already has an itching, festering or inflamed bite, boil or wound, then this brief transit requires antipathetic remediation.

Adrenal response is "nervous" and readily triggered. People are more inclined to seek neuromuscular stimulation with coffee, cigarettes, etc. Increases mania and manic tendencies, anger control issues, and bipolar disorders in those prone, especially in Fire signs and sometimes in Air.

People experience bouts of muscular tension. Muscle strains are common. Produces a nervous effect on the male sexual system. Insomnia is a typical manifestation of this transit.

Accident Prone! Avoid playing with venomous creatures, sharp tools, or weapons. Take great care with mechanical equipment and driving. Accidents occur through risk, impatience and poor judgment. Weapons should be removed from the proximity of children and angry persons. Mercury-Mars loves to play with knives in Air (element) and guns in Air and Fire!

Field Note 1: Mercury-Mars-Uranus contacts are typical in electrocution cases according to one fascinating research study conducted by one of my three long-term apprentices, Clayton Cruce, researched three categories of electrocution (lightning strike, mechanical, and death penalty by electrocution) in his *Research Monograph, Electrical Series Volume 1.* Trines are just as common as conjunctions, squares and quincunxes. The orb is typically 1°.

Field Note 2: Mercury-Mars natal conjunctions in Capricorn and Virgo bring itchy skin. In my practice, this has been infallible when natal Jupiter tenants an Earth sign with the natal Sun in Virgo, Capricorn or Aquarius. Today, it presented itself once again, begging my question: "Does your skin itch?"

"Oh yes!" she replied, "My skin always itches."

Surgical and Medical Tips: Take any hint of anaphylaxis (severe allergic reaction) seriously! Delicate surgery can be performed on male areas, adrenals, muscles, provided transit Moon and/or Jupiter are in good aspect and sign. However, this conjunction can temporarily heighten pain and irritable response to medical procedures! A trine from transit Jupiter and/or Venus will assist. Also, an exact sextile or conjunction from Venus will offset the irritation.

Herbs: Should symptoms agree, professional herbalists may consider their nervines, anodynes, muscle relaxants, sedatives, anti-venomous herbs, antibiotics. Blue Vervain, Lemon Balm, Valerian, Wood Betony, and Lycopus are all calming in different ways. For intense neuralgia: Prickly Ash, St. John's Wort (with Scullcap or Lavender). Don't self-treat.

Transit Mercury Conjunct Natal Jupiter

This brief influence is unclear, and rarely negative. Pituitary action may be momentarily disturbed, resulting in a few days of hormonal changes. Brings "luck" for health news and knowledge.

Liver function is stimulated, amping up functions such as bile production, digestion, blood constituents, and cholesterol. This would seem important knowledge for those suffering from hepatitis or liver disease. This conjunction may coincide with an onset of beneficial liver medication. Strongest if stationing.

This conjunction enhances neural response and reactivity in the bodily regions ruled by the sign of natal Jupiter.

Surgical and Medical Tips: Unclear. May influence liver surgery by exciting liver and gallbladder function. May testify to either a "good" diagnosis or a correct one!

Transit Mercury Conjunct Natal Saturn

This conjunction can bring a firm diagnosis or bad medical news. Often, something essential must be considered or decided at this time, related to either Saturn's generic rulerships or the bodily parts governed by the sign of natal Saturn, or any planet he squares, opposes, or quincunxes. Sometimes a surgical decision or treatment mode is pondered.

Potential nervous sensitization of the skin or joints, more attention drawn to the bones, ligaments, tendons, nails, cuticles. Possible dental issues or dental decisions of import.

Field Note: While writing this section, a friend asked me to check prospective dates for elective prostate surgery. All dates looked horrible, so I suggested obtaining more selections. As I delivered this news, transit Mercury was exactly conjunct his natal Saturn. Saturn rules both his 7th house of consultants, and his 8th house of surgery. It is also closely square to his natal Mercury-conjunct-South Node in Scorpio (the specific sign-ruler of the prostate).

Transit Mercury Conjunct Natal Uranus

This transit is far more remarkable in the reverse. (See *Transit Uranus Conjunct Natal Mercury*.) Any pairing of these two planets heightens electrical activity! Both planets conduct current, and Uranus is fond of reversing a current state of being! This lends itself to extremes.

If negative, there is some increased potential for spasm (in the body zone ruled by the sign of natal Uranus), various neurological issues, increased tremor, mental disturbances or even seizure, but only in individuals so prone.

Positively, this brief transit is conducive to the general alertness, reversing spasm, or reawakening of nerves following damage.

Transit Mercury Conjunct Natal Neptune

Mercury's brief conjunction with Neptune clouds diagnosis and predisposes to faulty prescription. If you receive a diagnosis or new medications at this time, ask more questions. There is also a tendency to misunderstand medical directions or misapply them.

Conversely, this conjunction can bring intuitive revelations on the source of a complaint, or a long-standing mystery might be solved (e.g. they finally find the bug in the microscope).

This transit briefly heightens any tendency to self-diagnose, self-medicate or engage in substance abuse.

This conjunction can bring too much or too little sleep and enhance dreams; encourages drug experimentation or purchase; can signal drug overdoses or, conversely, sudden release from addictions.

This transit awakens the astral senses, enhancing clairvoyance or clairaudience. However, this tendency could make it a difficult time for schizophrenics. Those suffering from dementia or Alzheimer's will be extra confused.

For investigating mysterious symptoms that begin on this conjunction, consider the entry of an insect, food or microbe-borne pathogen, or secret chemical. For clues, consider the Element of the transit Mercury.

Surgical and Medical Tips: Hypothetically, one should be careful of unpredictable effects from anesthesia.

Transit Mercury conjunct natal Neptune can result in a few days of fuzzy thinking, whereas the reverse scenario (the conjunction of transit Neptune over natal Mercury) is so often seen at the onset of dementia. The same goes for Mercury-South Node conjunctions.

Transit Mercury Conjunct Natal Pluto

This brief aspect corresponds to Pluto-type medical procedures, such as colonoscopy, sinus exploration, radiation therapy, or chemotherapy. We often see a Mercury-Pluto contact at these times.

Negatively, this transit can increase suicidal ideology or criminal thoughts. One cogitates upon death, "Should we purchase a grave plot or go for cremation?"

This aspect may correspond to the testing and diagnoses of various plagues, such as Lyme disease, HIV, bacterial infection, or genetic issues. Insect or animal bites incurred during these few days may go septic. Nurses need to be more careful when handling needles and fluids. Assists diagnosis.

Surgical Tip: This transit can be one testimony of a diligent surgeon, but it also heightens the chance of post-operative bacterial invasion.

Transit Mercury Conjunct Natal South Node

Intellectual and communication functions are temporarily weakened at this time. This conjunction reliably warns of potential error in medical prescription and diagnoses; faulty hearing and misunderstood communication; or the advice nurse gets it wrong. People feel disinclined to speak. Medical orders are misunderstood. This is an excellent time to rest the voice or go on silent retreat!

This aspect may contribute to brain or neurological complaints. This transit briefly emphasizes a weakness in the bodily region of the sign of the natal South Node. Trouble through insects. Plant allergies kick up. Hands, fingers, thinking or breathing may be slightly compromised (unnoticed in healthy individuals).

The bronchial tubes and upper lungs can temporarily weaken. Asthmatics might take extra cautions. Stuttering may occur or be a natal condition related to this placement. "Mental health day." This aspect disinters old memories. PTSD prone. Profoundly depressing.

Surgical and Medical Tips: Be on red alert for medical misinformation or prescription error! Medical records and paperwork can go missing, not arrive on time or contain serious errors. Watch for that missed call.

Unless the responsible physician disagrees, this period is a time to avoid medical procedures of all kinds. Use an orb of a few days on either side of the exact conjunction to both the "mean" and "true" South Lunar Node.

Transit Mercury Conjunct Natal North Node

Mercury's transit of the North Node signifies an increase of nerve force entering one's bodily field. Neural function improves for those convalescing from a wide array of complaints. Strengthens hearing and speaking. Hand acuity improves.

Heightens alertness. Medical advice and prescription are helpful, unless countered by stronger more negative aspects. Herbal medicines are potentized. Brings helpful news!

Negatively, may briefly increase neurological pressure, tension, drying or hardening in the bodily region ruled by the sign of the natal North Node. If occurring in Fire or Air signs, there can occur an excess inflow of nervous energy; nervousness (Air) and irritability or temper (Fire) can result. Insomnia prone.

Surgical and Medical Tips: Brings helpful healers, nurses, advice, herbs and medications, provided no reverse testimonies coincide. This is an excellent time for speech therapy and stroke recovery.

This conjunction is a positive, but minor, testimony for medical procedure and surgery; not reliable if used alone, without wholistically studying the entire chart. Use an orb of a few days on either side of the exact conjunction to both the "mean" and "true" North Lunar Node.

Transit Mercury Conjunct Natal Ascendant

First, be certain the Ascendant degree is really true. This aspect is generally neurologically quickening to the body, for good or ill, most especially to the regions governed by the Ascendant's sign. Effects last for the duration of Mercury's transit through the Ascendant sign, though are more pronounced within 3° of the true Ascendant degree.

MERCURY'S SQUARES
Health Potentials for Predisposed Nativities
The square does not always manifest as health concerns or benefits.

Mercury's square aspects (90°) behave similarly to his conjunctions, but at perhaps 60% strength. Normally, they don't have much clout unless occurring within an orb of 1°.

Mercury's transit squares bring minor irritations, generally lasting 1 to 3 days, or they go entirely unnoticed. However, should Mercury station near an exact square, his normally slight, brief influence is compounded and lasts continuously from his first contact of the natal planet (while he is in direct motion) until his last contact recurs again during direct motion (after his retrograde period). In this case, the aspect can last as long as five weeks, greatly increasing the importance of the square.

Always check and make sure Mercury is not going to back up and revisit the square, then turn around and do it a third time!

The same rule holds for all planets. Our point here is that this scenario turns a negligible transit into a major one!

Use the previous text for Mercury's conjunctions to each planet for squares. However, there is an important difference.

In considering the square, we have the electrical stimulus of Mercury coming from his current sign and applying to the sign of the natal planet he squares by transit. The signs and quadruplicity of the planets involved would seem of paramount importance.

See *Chapter 3: Aspect Mechanics*, for further explication on the different types of squares and their medical interpretation. Here is a helpful formula.

Square Delineation Formula

Transit Mercury delivers neurological tension or increased neural stimulus from the bodily zone ruled by his current sign position _____ *(give sign and body parts)*, to the planet he squares _____*(give the planet, and the body parts and functions ruled)*, and the sign of that natal planet _____ *(give the sign and body parts it rules)*.

As discussed above, Mercury's square can bring minor irritations generally lasting only 1 to 3 days. However, **Mercury-Mars and Mercury-Uranus squares** are exceptions to this rule. These amp up neuro-electric response! In both examples that follow, the square from transit Mercury can heighten tendencies toward insomnia.

Transit Mercury's Square of Natal Mars

This transit produces that sudden "minor" event that can be a real doozie; e.g. the backyard bee sting that wrecks the summer. This tiny brief aspect can add just that extra touch of pressure needed to produce a motorcycle or skateboard accident. Never underestimate Mercury's square of Mars!

Transit Mercury's Square of Natal Uranus

A transit that heightens electrical current and is implicated in associated maladies, e.g. seizures, spasms, mental extremes, intestinal gripes or painful gas.

TRANSIT MERCURY OPPOSITION TO NATAL PLANETS
Health Potentials for Predisposed Nativities
Opposition does not always manifest as health concerns or benefits.

Many authors describe all 'hard' aspects (conjunction, square and opposition) as behaving in the same manner. However, the opposition has distinct properties. Foremost, an opposing transit confronts and pulls upon the vital force of the natal planet opposed. The exact outcome is hard to define.

What we do know is that the pull is exerted from the opposite sign, not the same sign, as with the conjunction. Also, the pull is weakening to the planet opposed because it comes from the opposite side of the circle of ecliptic longitude. It is essential to note the houses and signs in the polarity concerned. This is discussed in *Chapter 3: Aspect Mechanics.*

It is beyond the scope of this text to discuss all sign and polarity combinations. Here is a formula.

Opposition Delineation Formula:
Transit Mercury in sign _____ *(give sign),* and the bodily regions ruled by this sign _____ *(give sign's body regions)*, will pull upon the planet he opposes _____ *(name planet)*, and its bodily functions _____ *(describe bodily functions)*, in the bodily regions ruled by sign of the natal planet _____ *(list body regions).*

The nature of this pull will be Mercurial: fast changes or neurological attenuation of the natal planet so opposed. Mercury oppositions present the natal planet opposed with "news." Therefore, this transit can signal the arrival of medical news, test results, exams, or a consultation with a medical professional.

An opposition from Mercury could provoke an insightful diagnosis or review of a medical problem related to the planet and sign opposed.

MERCURY'S QUINCUNX
Health Potentials for Predisposed Nativities
A quincunx does not always manifest as health concerns or benefits.

All quincunxes are sneaky and hard to diagnose. However, they are not mild aspects. They are, in fact, the preeminent health aspect. This is because a quincunx (150°) replicates the directional angle ("house") to the natal Ascendant of the malefic 6th house (of health) and 8th house (of chronic health problems, surgery and death.)

The planet quincunxed by Mercury cannot "digest" or receive Mercury's ray. A transit quincunx from Mercury signals a brief neurological insufficiency or malfunction related to the functions of the quincunxed natal planet. Sometimes this is no small matter!

General Surgical Tip: Mercury governs a surgeon's skill and Mars the surgeon's knife. Surgery is unwise should the planet representing the topic of surgery be receiving an exact quincunx of Mercury, especially if either sign involved coincides with the bodily region concerned.

Field Note: A ten-year-old boy had facial surgery on the precise date of an exact quincunx of transit Mercury to his natal planets in the indicated facial region. Most transits that day were fair-to-middling. The surgeon accidentally nicked a facial nerve, resulting in a mild paralysis of a facial muscle.

This impressed me so much that to this day, I strictly avoid suggesting surgery dates on exact Mercury quincunxes to **any** natal planet, but especially those governing the region under the knife.

Transit Mercury Quincunx Natal Sun
The heart, eye or brain is briefly not receiving the normal supply of electrical current, and/or is neurologically disturbed in a manner difficult to diagnose. In other cases, the brain suddenly receives too much current. The life force is suddenly affected.

This brief transit could be relevant for epileptics or those with unpredictable neurological disorders of the heart, brain or eyes. It can also indicate small matters, such as an eye twitch. This transit lasts only 1 to 3 days, unless stationing.

Transit Mercury Quincunx Natal Moon

This transit lasts only 1 to 3 days, unless stationing. It can affect brain chemistry in ways hard to diagnose, but for clues look to the signs of both transit Mercury and the natal Moon. It can also bring about strange moods or disturb the timing of menstrual cycles and most monthly bodily rhythms.

The neurological flow to the whole body is disturbed. This transit may relate to cellular moisture levels, implying a disharmony between the matrix and the nervous system. Mental health and stability may be temporarily destabilized in those so prone.

For most people, this transit is insignificant. However, it is quite important if occurring at birth (natal Mercury quincunx natal Moon).

Learning disorders abound for the natal quincunx of Mercury to Moon. Sometimes this natal aspect produces disassociation between the conscious mind and the subconscious feeling reactions: "I can't explain to you what I feel…," or, "I can't remember my dreams…."

Folks born with this natal quincunx sometimes cannot verbally define precisely what they are feeling, or conversely have times of unconscious emotionality, disassociated from rational thought.

Some manifestations might be sleep walking or inability to remember emotionally-based reactions (e.g. "What are you talking about, I didn't say that!") To close friends, they may appear as if they are two people, one side being extremely rational (without feeling), and one side being all emotional (and illogical).

Transit Mercury Quincunx Natal Mercury

The flow of neural current and information through the nerves may be briefly "off." Sensory information may be addled. This may cause clumsiness, lack of hand coordination, or momentarily exacerbate a neurological condition. Nerves may be strained. This transit lasts only 1 to 3 days, unless stationing.

Transit Mercury Quincunx Natal Venus

For most people, this transit is nil. For a few, the ovaries, kidneys and veins may not receive enough nerve force. Kidney hormones may release erratically, producing electrolyte imbalance. Estrogen release may be slightly erratic. There could be odd sexual interests or changes of inclination or tastes. This aspect can produce a minor irritation to skin or female organs.

Transit Mercury Quincunx Natal Mars

These two planets are not friends! All aspects between Mercury and Mars possess a first-rate health potential. Nerve conduction to muscles and motor nerves is briefly lowered. Timing and muscular coordination and contraction may be slightly "off."

For most people this aspect is insignificant and goes unnoticed. For athletes, it could impair timing just enough to lose that race! This is that loose shoelace that bedevils the professional skater.

Alternatively, this aspect can produce a significant neuromuscular inflammation, especially if the pulling of a muscle occurs during Mercury's station. Effects last typically 1 to 7 days (unless stationing), although, if unattended, can set off a longer-term inflammation process.

This brief aspect can produce first-rate accidents! Be careful with equipment, driving and risky sports. Be careful with electricity, knives, needles, and sharp tools.

If you are camping under this transit, bring your bug net! This transit is associated with unforeseen stings, insect or reptile bites, animal bites, plant toxins, poison sumac and the like. This aspect is like that unsuspected miniature poodle that flies out of nowhere and bites the postman!

This transit creates a nervous incoordination between the thyroid and adrenals, essential information to sufferers of Graves' disease and hyperthyroid. Strange neurological sexual effects, genital inflammation or male performance issues may ensue.

For clues, study the signs of both transit Mercury and natal Mars carefully, and remember the words "nervous irritation."

This aspect can coincide with a surprise, but brief, bout of acute neuralgia, itch, shingles, herpes eruption, or pain.

Field Note: Mars rules peristalsis and Mercury enervates. This week, a neighbor experienced a frozen bowel, unresponsive to a surprising array of laxatives—even the two pints of ripe berries produced nothing! The chart revealed that transit Mercury (neural enervation) was exactly quincunxing her natal Mars (peristalsis).

This was compounded by the fact that her natal Mars was itself in quincunx to her natal Saturn-in-Scorpio, the sign governing the colon, and expulsion from same.

Surgery Tips: This tiny transit, when in exact orb, constitutes first-rate surgical danger. If the responsible physician agrees, avoid all surgical procedures when this aspect is within at least a 1° orb. Also see the reverse: *Transit Mars Quincunx Natal Mercury.*

Transit Mercury Quincunx Natal Jupiter:

Unclear to this author; for most people the effects are insignificant. Indigestion can occur, with the cause baffling to doctors. There is possibly some problematic effect upon the ducts, vessels and/or valves of the gallbladder, duodenum, pancreas, liver, cecum, etc. For clues, consider the signs involved.

May briefly disturb nerve signals to/from the pituitary, liver or gallbladder. The liver and gallbladder may be more sensitive to fats during these dates. Transit lasts 1 to 3 days, unless stationing. Station is always strong!

Surgical Tip: If the responsible physician agrees, avoid liver, gallbladder or pituitary surgery at this time. Clear the exact transit by at least 1 day.

Transit Mercury Quincunx Natal Saturn:

For most people the effects of this transit are insignificant, though it is strong if found between natal Mercury and natal Saturn.

Nerve signals to the skeletal system are momentarily deficient; electrical charge is not reaching the bones. Sudden instability, "trick knee," falls or spinal subluxations; teeth pains, surprise dental issues, earache, joint pains of unclear origin. Check sign of transit Mercury and natal Saturn for clues.

Regulation and timing of bodily processes may be "off" for 1 to 3 days (longer when stationing).

Be alert for symptoms caused by secret heavy metal poisoning, or the ingesting of heavy metals. Potentially a good time to test for heavy metals (Saturn). This quincunx influences the ears and hearing.

Surgical Tip: If the responsible physician agrees, avoid bone, skin, ear or teeth work at this time. Beware that the metal Mercury is not in amalgams to fill new dental cavities. This time period is a poor choice for removing Mercury amalgams or for leeching out heavy metals from the liver, etc. Clear the exact aspect by at least 1 degree, more if possible.

NOTE: There is limited information available for the quincunx of transit Mercury to the trans-Saturnian planets.

Transit Mercury's Quincunx of Natal Uranus

For most, this transit goes unnoticed unless stationing. It lasts 1to 3 days, unless stationing. It influences the electrical current of the nerves. Those with unstable or scrambled brain signals, seizure disorders, spasm, and other neurological diseases, may find this transit challenging.

Strange spasms may occur. Should natal or transit Mars be configured with Mercury and Uranus, there can be neural pain, sometimes severe. Electrocution-prone.

If you are dependent for breath on an electrical oxygen producing device, have it checked, or have a backup. All electrically-based medical devices should be checked for malfunction as this aspect approaches. Take care with pacemakers!

Surgical Tip: In rare cases, unforeseen electrical problems occur with medical equipment or with the electrical functioning of the heart, brain, spinal nerves, or peripheral nerves. Odd and unforeseen things can go suddenly wrong. If possible, surgery should clear this transit by a few days.

Because this brief transit excites electrical reactions, it is wise to have strong sedative and antispasmodic herbs on hand. Lobelia, Catnip, Prickly Ash, Vervain, St. John's Wort, et al. Select for herbal temperature by using the elemental antithetical to the sign of natal Uranus (hot to cold, cold to hot, etc.) Do not self-treat.

Transit Mercury's Quincunx of Natal Neptune

Neptune can indicate a health mystery, hidden virus, and so forth. Mercury is news, and the quincunx means something around the corner at an odd angle, unseen. Therefore, look for something hidden, overlooked or unseen, or, conversely, being exposed, as in something long-hidden appearing in a microscope, psychic vision, or dream!

Watch for secret poisons (for example a small carbon dioxide leak). Check the signs of transit Mercury and natal Neptune for clues. Potentially, a time one could contract a virus, especially from birds, small animals, children, or people in Mercurial professions (secretaries, porters, waiters, mail person et. al.).

Be careful of small, darting vehicles or animals while driving; they may be in your blind spot!

This transit is also prone to misinformation, faulty advice and misdiagnosis, such as tuberculosis diagnosed as a minor virus. It is prone to all manner of drug mistakes: mixing drugs, wrong prescriptions, overdoses, and taking alcohol with drugs.

This transit signals a high alert for asthmatics and anyone else with impaired oxygen reception. If you use a CPAP machine, make sure it is clean.

Surgical tip: There is a heightened potential for electrical malfunctions, machine and equipment failure, surgeon distraction, or misinformation. If the responsible physician agrees, allow the aspect to clear by 3°.

Transit Mercury's Quincunx of Natal Pluto

This aspect may be indicated in snake bites, bee stings, animal bites, plant venoms, secret radiation exposure, poisons and deliberate poisoning. Watch for Mercury poisoning!

This is the time when the dentist insists yet again on those "low radiation" X-rays. There may be hidden but potent dangers inherent in medical treatment, or in herbal regimes commenced at this time.

Medical or genetic tests may be required. Family DNA secrets may be revealed by accident; "You're my Dad?"

Surgical Tip: Because Pluto governs transplants, transfusion, and cadavers, it appears that this transit would be antithetical to transplants because sufficient nervous force (Mercury) is lacking for the transplant or transfusion (Pluto). If the responsible physician agrees, allow the exact quincunx to clear by a few days.

Transit Mercury Quincunx the Lunar Nodes

Generally not observed, except in Horary astrology. However, this does not mean there is no effect! Personally, I would avoid surgery on the date of an exact quincunx from transit Mercury to the Nodes, and definitely so if the surgery involved nerves, brain, ears, bronchial tubes, lungs, arms, hands, or fingers.

Chapter 11

VENUS
Relief

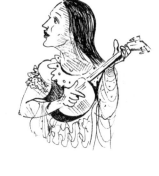

Properties, Rulerships and Actions

Rules: Taurus, Libra

Exalted: Pisces

Detriment: Scorpio, Aries

Fall: Virgo

Metal: Copper. Strangely, baby girls are born with 30% more copper in their bodies then infant males! Adult females also retain more copper than males. Traditionally, Venus rules female sexuality, and copper too!

Minerals: Molybdenum *(Jansky)*

Vitamins: Niacin, E *(Nauman, Jansky)*, P, Rutin, Niacinamide *(Jansky)*

Gem & Cosmic Ray: White Diamond is said to refract the Venus' Indigo Ray and is therefore the traditional gem of Venus *(Jyotish)*.

Body Rulership & Organ Affinities: Venus influences blood sugar, female hormones (with Moon), the veins (with Aquarius), the ovaries and kidneys (with Libra), and the skin (with Saturn and Capricorn). She influences the "thick lymphs" of the body and holds some co-influence with the Moon over mucus. Female genitalia. Venus has a definite influence with Mars and Scorpio over testes, prostate and seminal fluid (but not the sperm).

Temperature: Normalizing: gently cooling if hot and pleasantly warming if cold. Contrary to this designation, traditional texts list Venus as "cold in the first degree," (i.e., cool). Ancient, Medieval and Renaissance physicians assigned both temperature and moisture to the known planets. With few exceptions (Blagrave), medical astrologers became habituated to binary thinking, listing signs and planets as "hot or cold" with seemingly no "warm" nor "cool."

Gender too became static, with most planets being male and all female planets "cold." The simplest of astro-medical observations forces the practitioner to rethink some assignments, particularly that of Venus. The below discussion supports my firm opinion that the traditional assignment of "cold" to Venus cannot be correct.

The pop-rock group, *Shocking Blue,* aptly recounted Venus' charms in their 1969 mega-hit, "Venus:"

> *"A goddess on a mountain top… Was burning like a silver flame…*
> *The summit of beauty and love… And Venus was her name."*

Nothing cold about that!

Venus presides over mid-spring, and beauteous sign Taurus, a season when the sexy magnetic forces of Earth are the most concentrated. She governs love and physical attraction, molecular action that cannot be described as cold. Indeed, May-born Taurus folks are notorious for their warm hands, attractively magnetic natures and huge appetites. Cold? C'mon, this ain't right!

Venus also governs Libra, the most temperate sign of all. The warm and lovely metal copper is Venus' personal metal, and female her traditional gender. Out of respect for astrologers who disagree with gender-assigned planets, I'll include that persons of all genders can be born with strongly "Venusian" traits, and furthermore, that these traits do not exclusively "belong" to females. Additionally, all genders have some degree of the Venus-ruled female hormones and copper in their physical makeup.

Medicinally, Venus' ray is a wound-healing vulnerary and soothing demulcent, active in relieving pain. Her effect on the body is primarily relaxing. She also increases the romantic libido (as opposed to Martian lust). She rules sugar, too, and her general properties sweeten our lives in so many ways. Furthermore, the physical planet Venus is a greenhouse and very warm indeed!

So, we may now ask, how can Venus be "cold?" Well, she can't be! There is just nothing cold about her. How about pleasantly cool then? If you lived in the Sahara, yes, you might very well experience Venus that way. Conversely, if you lived in snowy Norway, Venus' action would be sensed as pleasantly warming !

How can Venus be both pleasantly cooling and warming? Because Venus' ray produces that one action the early medicine didn't always envision: normalizing! Venus, the peacekeeper, is ever seeking to produce the happiest mean between any two extremes. Think of the function of her home sign Libra, the scales!

Overall, Venus' influence upon the physical body is gently warming and moist (whereas Luna, the Moon is always cool-cold and moist). However, lady Venus can present as happily cooling and moist, as circumstance demands!

Her temperature-normalizing actions explain why some tradions list her as cold! However, she is never cold, but gently cooling as needed. In sum, it would seem appropriate to re-designate Venus' traditional temperature assignment from "cold" to "warm/cool as needed!"

General Action: Demulcent (relieving inflammation or irritation), vulnerary (wound healing), anodyne (relieving pain), hemostatic (arrests flow of blood), relaxing, calmative, antispasmodic, normalizing, softening, soothing, magnetic, a female aphrodisiac.

Special Note: Venus' pain-allaying properties are so strong by transit that one can readily witness an immediate pain reduction within a bodily region the day that Venus enters the sign decan ruling that zone.

Positive: Venus is the planet that normalizes extremes. She is experienced as pleasure. Neither hot nor cold, she refreshes when hot and, conversely, pleasantly warms when chilled. When we are parched, Venus brings moisture. Never drying, she is however slightly hemostatic, staying the hemorrhage of wounds. Her influence is anodyne and vulnerary.

Note: Designated as the "Minor Benefic," sweet Venus' transit, trine, or sextile cannot be relied upon to rescue an afflicted natal planet. The conjunction is her miracle moment! An exact conjunction of transit Venus to any natal planet in trouble is a sure helpmate and safeguard.

Negative: Being lazy and indulgent, Venus transits can bring the excesses of Venus. Envision the contented, languid person, of soft flesh, reclining in an easy chair, sampling chocolates (illustrator Duff's depiction of Venus ruled Libra). Now, think of this same characterization directed at any other natal planet. Naturally, that planet's function loses tone or suffers from excess sugar consumption, leading to candida. Venus builds cysts (usually benign) and is substance-addictive.

She governs venereal diseases, an honor shared with Mars and perhaps the Nodes. Her conjunction relaxes the organ or bodily sign she is transiting through or natally tenanting. In rare cases, Venus can kill. Imagine a slow, lazy heart, barely beating, and along comes Venus. True, she could help if the weak heart were due to an internal tension or stiffness (Saturn). However, if the heart is just plain lazy, Venus would increase that direction! The heart stops.

Excess: Productive of cysts in the bodily region ruled by the sign of natal Venus. Also inclines to bacterial and yeast inviting sugary conditions in the body zone where natally indicated. All the proof one needs of this fact is the astonishing frequency of correlation between genital yeast and colon candida with natal Venus in Scorpio!

Venus also tends to prolapse of bladder, uterus, rectum, etc., and lazy tissue tone. She inclines toward sugar and wine indulgence and excess blood sugar.

Deficient: Low copper, low female libido, low female hormones, dry skin and/or hair, baldness, weak kidneys (with related acne due to resultant toxins in blood), lack of sparkle or attractiveness, low blood sugar (or too high!). Low copper can be implicated in iron deficiency anemia, thyroid dysfunction and heart palpitations.

Transit Frame & Orb: One to three days by transit conjunction, square, opposition, or quincunx to a natal planet, longer for stations. However, Venus influences the bodily regions of the sign she transits from ingress to exit.

VENUS THROUGH THE ELEMENTS & SIGNS

These partial lists of symptoms apply only to predisposed charts. Most of these conditions are obviously uncommon and require multiple testimonies beyond the presence of Venus.

Although my emphasis is on Venus' transit influence on the body, these symptoms may apply to both natal and transit charts. Venus' transit is typically too brief to "cause" many of the chronic conditions listed below. Instead, she can exhibit brief annoyances along the lines described, as she passes through each sign. Typically, the transit of Venus relieves pain in the body, and is a general assist.

Manifestation of symptoms may be enhanced by lifestyle choices, taking preemptive measures can reduce, remove or prevent potential issues from manifesting. It is not possible to list all potential expressions.

Venus in Fire Signs

Aries: In this case, Venus is experienced as "cooling." She allays inflammation of brain and eyes, cools overheating of arteries and the cardiovascular system, refreshes. Gently relaxing to the heart, circulation, arterial circulation, brain and eyes. Gives "sparkle" to eyes and face.

Leo: Relaxes and cools heart; relaxes thoracic region and spine. Venus' effect on the gallbladder in gall-ruling signs Leo, Virgo and Capricorn is of interest. Her transit can either loosen existing gravel and allay pain or, conversely, increase the thick sludge obstructing the gall ducts.

Sagittarius: Relieves sciatica and hip pain; improves synovial fluids and relaxes tense muscles and nerves in this region that may press on the sciatic nerve. It is astonishing to observe how fast sciatic pain diminishes when transit Venus ingresses into Sagittarius!

Field Note: A friend suffered sciatic inflammation for weeks as Mars made his way through Sagittarius in the 6th house of health. However, the day of Venus' ingress into Sagittarius brought instant, lasting relief. This was compounded by Mars exiting the sign around the same time! This effect has been witnessed multiple times.

Venus in Air Signs

Gemini: Calms the brain and nerves, relaxes the veins and capillaries (warming), sweetens speech.

Libra: Relaxes kidneys and is mildly diuretic, relaxes lumbar region, balances hormones and alkalizes blood, increases mucus production in the urinary tract. Increases sugar cravings.

Aquarius: Increases oxygen to heart, enhances tendency towards social drinking; encourages socializing, comforts the distraught, allays extreme mental states. Improves oxygenation of blood as copper assists the work of Mars, the governor of the oxygen-carrying blood hemoglobin. Aquarius greatly influences the quality of the blood cells.

Venus in Earth Signs

Taurus: Increases food cravings, gluttony, and sugar cravings. Increases mucus in ear-nose-throat. Relaxing and mellifluous effect on vocal chords, but can build vocal polyps. Relaxes neck and may slow thyroid or thymus glands.

Venus' brief transit through Taurus for individuals with fat-choked neck vessels may be problematic as increased blood sugar/alcohol/food indulgence could threaten an infarction (tissue death).

Virgo: Relaxes anxiety, increases vessel flexibility, softens intestinal lining, and improves gut absorption. Moistens, lubricates, and is mucus producing; moistens dryness of skin, hair and mucous membrane (especially needed for both Virgo and Capricorn). Significant influence on blood sugar, either up or down!

Capricorn: Softens hard tissue, beautifies and nourishes skin, assists in muscle building, reduces tendency to self-starvation. Venus' effect on the gallbladder in gall-associated signs Capricorn, Virgo and Leo is of interest. Her transit can either loosen existing gravel and allay pain or, conversely, increase the thick sludge obstructing the gall ducts.

Note: There is a big difference between a natal position of Venus in Capricorn or Virgo and the transit of Venus through these signs. By transit, she softens their innate dryness. Natally, she can sometimes indicate dry skin and hair because Venus, governing the beautifying hormones, is at detriment in these drying signs!

Venus in Water Signs

When transit Venus is conjunct the natal Sun in Water signs, the weak or cool heart is gently warmed and personal magnetism increased. Water signs are sexy, and Venus increases magnetism and fertility when transiting through them. However, if the heart or brain are too moist, she may increase this moisture!

If positive, the transit action of Venus will either gently warm or pleasantly cool the lymphatic system (Water signs Pisces and Cancer), as needed. She alkalizes the stomach (Water sign Cancer) and the blood (the blood is approximately 80% water; and allows for the improved absorption of copper). Estrogen is better assimilated in Water signs. It is notable that the feminine Water signs and Venus-ruled Taurus are more common in aging males who keep their hair.

For those with Sun, Moon or Ascendant in Water signs, transit Venus is fertility enhancing and sexy. She moistens and softens the colon, rectum and vagina, thus assisting evacuation. However, she can also suggest sugar-induced candida, yeast, excess mucus and low peristalsis.

Cancer: Fertile. Relaxes, softens and alkalizes the stomach. Grows breast tissue, improves lactation, and is breast softening.

Negatively can be productive of breast cysts, clogged milk ducts, or swollen breasts.

Scorpio: Candida prone, vaginal and colon infection, increased sexual desire, and STD prone. Vaginal, uterine and bladder prolapse; vaginal polyps.

Sugary or stagnant, mucous-engorged colon; nose mucous, chronic nose infection (due to excess sugar), "smoker's" voice.

Pisces: Cools or warms lymphatics as needed, but can produce lymphatic stagnation. Fertile, sexy, increases libido; in rare cases is prone to bouts of nymphomania. Eases mental distress, depression and mental illness. Allays foot pain or, conversely, can weaken the foot muscles. Natally, Venus in Pisces can bring good or pretty feet, and/or delight in foot decoration or shoes.

VENUS TRANSIT OF NATAL PLANETS

Most of these conditions are obviously uncommon and require multiple testimonies beyond the presence of Venus.

Although my emphasis is on Venus' transit influence on the body, these symptoms may apply to both natal and transit charts. Venus' transit is typically too brief to "cause" many of the chronic conditions listed below. Instead, she can exhibit brief annoyances along the lines described below as she passes through each sign. Typically, the transit of Venus relieves pain in the body and is a general assist.

Manifestation of symptoms may be enhanced by lifestyle choices; and taking preemptive measures can reduce, remove or prevent potential issues from manifesting. It is not possible to list all potential expressions.

VENUS' CONJUNCTIONS
Health Potentials for Predisposed Nativities
Transits do not always manifest as health concerns or benefits.

Transit Venus Conjunct Natal Sun

This transit is relaxing, magnetic and generally supportive to the Vital Force, brain, eyes and heart. However, if one suffers a lethargic heart muscle, it can increase this tendency. Should natal Venus be conjunct the Sun at birth, the magnetic effects are lifelong, unless temporarily reversed by transits. Venus' transit conjunction can also increase fluidic pressure to the eyes or brain.

Surgery Tip: This conjunction within 1° is one helpful testimony for surgery to the heart, eyes, or brain, provided the tissue is not swelling. **Remember, electing safe surgery dates is the province of your doctor (first) and a highly skilled medical astrologer (second).**

Transit Venus Conjunct Natal Moon

Enhances female hormones, fertility, milk production and libido. Sensitizes skin and touch-pleasure. Increases receptivity and relaxation and is warming to emotions (never cooling in this regard, though acts as a balance to reduce the "hot" emotions of anger or mania).

Can stimulate cyst growth in breasts and uterus, or in the body regions of the sign she is transiting. Increases water retention and moisture, softens, hydrates; alkalinizing to stomach and improves appetite. Decreases eye pain, but can increase headaches related to fluidic pressure, or hormone imbalance. This conjunction is soporific, easing sleep. People feel affectionate!

Surgery and Medical Tips: This conjunction within 1° is one helpful testimony for surgery to the stomach, breast, womb, eyes, brain, and lung. Enhances efficacy of mucilages and demulcents. Remember, selecting safe surgery dates is the province of your doctor (first) and a highly skilled medical astrologer (second).

Field Note: Use this conjunction, if you need to help get a client pregnant! I'm now the proud "father" of many. Of course, it is important to combine with additional fertility heightening aspects.

Herbal Note: Licensed health practitioners may find this aspect to be one of the best times to treat a dry mucus membrane or an unhappy, acid stomach with Venus and Luna's demulcent herbs. Peach Leaf is a specific Venusian herb for the chronically upset, hot stomach attendant with a pointed, red tongue (Wood).

This aspect is excellent for fertility-enhancing herbal treatments (see above *Field Note*). Herbal treatment for insomnia, depression and PTSD are more successful at this time.

Transit Venus Conjunct Natal Mercury

Very soothing to neuralgia. Relaxes the nerves; enhances love of beauty in word and music. A significant testimony of good health for those born on this conjunction because it eases the mind.

Surgery Tip: This conjunction within 1° is one helpful testimony for surgery to peripheral and afferent nerves, hands, fingers, arms, bronchial tubes, lungs, brain, and ears. Remember, selecting safe surgery dates is the province of your doctor (first) and a highly skilled medical astrologer (second).

Herbal Note: Licensed health practitioners will discover this to be an effective time to introduce needed neural sedatives, mental calmatives and soporific herbs (Lemon Balm, Hops, Blue Vervain, Wood Betony, Scullcap, etc.), and anesthetic herbs specific to neural pain (e.g. Hypericum, Lavender, Vervain, etc.).

This transit allays seizures and is useful for seizure preventative treatments. Edgar Cayce stated that a tea made from Passiflora fruits and flowers was specific to epilepsy. His methods are very specific and worth looking into.

Transit Venus Conjunct Natal Mars

Stimulates the libido; influences copper-iron balance and female-male hormone balance, resolves excretion issues due to dryness and calms excretion issues due to excess heat or inflammation (e.g., assists cystitis). Greatly comforts wounds, and can reduce hemorrhage, and vomiting (emesis).

Venus "holds onto" fluids when needed, and relaxes tension as required. Temporarily calming to any inflammatory issues indicated by the natal Mars, including male issues. Male libido is enhanced at this time. For males, sperm count and virility may significantly increase the few days around this transit. For women, this transit is sexy too!

Surgery and Medical Tips: This conjunction within 1° is one helpful testimony for medical procedures involving the male organs, prostate, adrenal glands, blood or marrow transfusions and gallbladder. This brief time is useful for the onset of libido enhancing treatments. Remember, selecting safe surgery or treatment dates is the province of your doctor (first) and a highly skilled medical astrologer (second).

Herbal Note: Licensed medical practitioners may find this aspect to be effective for staunching internal or external bleeding, allaying raw irritation, burns, pain, and inflammation with appropriate herbs, (Yarrow, Aloe, Calendula, etc.). Venus' magnetic energy is calming to Mars' complaints. One does not need to use the specific herbs of Venus, because the aspect is enough to enhance any herbs of choice for these above purposes.

This conjunction potentizes herbal treatments designed to assist male virility, sperm quantity and motility.

Transit Venus Conjunct Natal Jupiter

Increases all of Jupiter's extremes. This is a prime tumor and cyst building combination. However, since this transit typically only lasts a few days, the reverse (transit Jupiter conjoining natal Venus) is far more important or if occurring in the natal chart.

Softening to liver, relaxing to tense arteries. The portal circulation can become sluggish under this transit, and veins can excessively relax causing varicosities. Sugar levels in the bloodstream may spike up or down. Both benefics together are definitely nutritive and somewhat fattening.

This brief transit can also act to calm a "hysterical" Jupiter—remember how the Greek God Zeus (Jupiter to the Romans) could behave? This could be useful in cases where the liver was processing nutrients too rapidly or dumping excessive cholesterol or bile.

Because of Venus' relaxing qualities, it is doubtful that she would help with arterial engorgement or plethora of blood (both Jupiterian ailments), unless due to hard blockage or inflammation. Normally, she increases Jupiter's tendency for engorgement.

Venus calms Jupiterian mental conditions, such as religious mania, excessive elation, megalomania, and egotism. However, she contributes to his natural narcissism!

Field Note: This combination is super-fertile, producing growths of all kinds. Natally, it is common to see cysts, polyps, some cancers and obesity with Jupiter and Venus conjunct, sextile or trine, especially in Water and Earth signs.

Surgery Tips: This conjunction within 1° is one helpful testimony for surgery to the liver or arteries.

Remember, selecting safe surgery dates is the province of your doctor (first) and a highly skilled medical astrologer (second).

Transit Venus Conjunct Natal Saturn

Venus is softening to Saturn's hardness and gently warming to Saturn's frigidity; pleasantly warming to all cold states.

This transit helps smooth rough skin and allay all skin diseases (except those due to sugary blood). Brings nutrients to bones, assists hair growth, strengthens nail, improves circulation, opens the gall.

If occurring at birth, this conjunction produces some personal sexual issues, i.e., shyness, fear, or frigidity. Also, kidney or venous function may become impaired, if neglected.

Surgical and Medical Tips: This conjunction within 1° is one helpful testimony for surgery to teeth, knees, bones, skin, right ear, gallbladder. Excellent for skin treatment. A perfect few days for onset of treatments to reduce emotional and physical rigidity, especially in the body part that natal Saturn tenants.

This is a good time for skin treatments, to soften gall or kidney stones, and reduce bone spurs. Remember, selecting safe surgery dates is the province of your doctor (first) and a highly skilled medical astrologer (second).

Field Note: One friend was born with Venus conjunct Saturn in close orb in Cancer, the sign of the breasts, in her 12th house (late life). She developed breast cancer at 70. If she had only known, she could have remediated this tendency! See *Herbal Note.*

Herbal Note: Licensed health practitioners should note that this aspect provides an effective time for the introduction of skin assisting herbs for softening, smoothing, mending or moistening (Linum, Plaintain, Chickweed, Rose, Comfrey, et al.).

Dandelion Root, Red Clover and Poke Root are specifics for the cleansing of breast tissue. This conjunction instructs those so born to keep the entire female system free from toxic buildups. For males, attend to the testes and prostate gland. Do not self-treat.

Transit Venus Conjunct Natal Uranus

Effects of transit Venus conjunct natal Uranus are often minimal or unfelt and far briefer than the reverse (transit Uranus conjunct natal Venus). However, this transit can minimize a natal Uranus' tendency for extremes, provided it is so doing.

Conversely, this conjunction can produce unexpected shifts for Venus issues, or the items ruled by the astrological houses governed by Venus in the natal chart. Watch for sudden blood sugar or hormonal shifts.

Surgical and Medical Tips: This conjunction within 1° is one testimony to avoid surgery to the kidneys, ovaries, vagina, face or skin. The current-reversing nature of Uranus would be baleful for onset of hormonal therapies, haircuts (unless you want weird), and beauty treatments. Remember, selecting safe surgery dates is the province of your doctor (first) and a highly skilled medical astrologer (second).

Field Notes: This conjunction, when occurring natally, is frequent in sexual extremists and pioneers. In Aries, Leo, or the 8th or 10th houses, a strong Venus-Uranus conjunction is commonly noted in sexual exhibitionists.

The last time this turned up, I asked my client if she enjoyed displaying her wares in a radical way. "Oh yes! I'm a belly dancer...."

Transit Venus Conjunct Natal Neptune

This conjunction is extremely magnetic and sweetening. This brief period enhances pleasure, seduction, sleeping and all manner of escapist indulgence. A remarkably sexy aspect, prone to hypnotic attraction. One could not find a better conjunction for applying anodynes and demulcents. Be wary of opiates and painkillers, as addictions can be formed.

Sleep inducing herbs are potentized! All vibrational therapies that work through the unseen (Neptune) are given a boost. An excellent time for magnetic healing, music therapy, homeopathy, flower essences, aromatherapy and prayer. Also, a prime time for a relaxing massage.

Surgical and Medical Tips: This conjunction within 1° increases the efficacy of narcotics and painkillers, so be careful with dosages. Remember, selecting safe surgery dates is the province of your doctor (first) and a highly skilled medical astrologer (second).

Field Note: It is common for natives born with Venus conjunct Neptune to fall prey to the lure of social wine drinking, then gradually morphing into addiction without realizing it. "Mom thinks I'm an alcoholic, do you?"

Herbal Note: This is a relaxing influence, and opening. Licensed herbalists can find few better aspects for commencing specific herbal treatments for insomnia, tension, or female frigidity.

Transit Venus Conjunct Natal Pluto

Venus conjunct Pluto is very brief but intense. However, you won't see the long term physical manifestation you might with the reverse (transit Pluto conjunct natal Venus). Often, something happens in the emotional or social life, or occurs in the life of a beloved relative, most likely, but not invariably, a female.

This is a good aspect to finally receive a diagnosis of a long-term pestering issue. This conjunction is inviting to parasites and STDs. Sexual desire may be unusually intense, as can surfacing sexual-psychological issues. This is a good time for women to avoid strangers.

Surgical and Medical Tips: This conjunction within 1° inclines those predisposed to drastic facial reconstruction surgery, tattoos, Botox injections, piercings or sexual reassignment decisions. This conjunction is useful for allaying wounds because it reduces sepsis and is preventative to bacterial attack. Hormone therapies or synthetic chemicals may have drastic results. Remember, selecting safe surgery dates is the province of your doctor (first) and a highly skilled medical astrologer (second).

Transit Venus Conjunct Natal North Node

A surplus of Venus energy enters the physical system at this time. This brief period, seldom lasting longer than one week unless at station, places Venus' significations at the great celestial entry portal. Opportunity presents itself for overindulgence in pleasure. Produces sugar craving. Blood sugar and alcohol levels may rise. Be safe! Check transits to natal Venus. This can be a nice time for a haircut!

Surgical and Medical Tips: This conjunction within 1° is one helpful testimony for surgery in general, bringing plenty of loving care and attentive nurses. Excellent for skin care and all demulcent and softening treatments. Female hormone treatments can present unexpectedly excessive response. Note: Selecting safe surgery dates is the province of your doctor (first) and a highly skilled medical astrologer (second).

Field Notes: Venus conjunct the North Node at birth can produce a nearly supernatural level of personal sexual magnetism; the native can get whomever he or she wants! Venus normally collects women, while Mars on North Node collects men.

Elvis Presley had Venus conjunct the North Node and was followed by screaming mobs of girls. TV's recent famous Bachelorette "Becca" was born with natal Venus and Mars on the North Node. She readily managed to win the hearts of all 16 bachelors on the show! However, a warning comes with Venus-North Node conjunctions—beware how you use the attractive powers afforded you.… There are karmic penalties for its misuse.

One gorgeous client born with Venus conjunct North Node collected women too, but was substance addicted to almost everything including sugar, destroying her life. Another case was so beautiful that she stopped traffic. However, her genetic portrait led her to undergo a preemptive radical mastectomy to avoid her family plague, breast cancer. This malady is linked in many cases to excess estrogen (Venus). This conjunction suggested she was correct in her decision.

Transit Venus Conjunct Natal South Node

Venus is not "lucky" here. All things ruled by Venus in the natal chart are temporarily on the great celestial "exit door." Venus' traditional significations are briefly lowered: sugar, copper, kidney function, estrogen, magnetism. This is a good time to refrain from sex, sugar and alcohol because they may have an exhaustive or deleterious effect during these few days.

This aspect is quite significant if occurring natally in the birth chart. Potentials include inefficient kidneys, diabetes, weak skin clearance (I've seen multiple cases of severe acne), psychological-sexual confidence issues (usually related to appearance), dietary obsessions, low estrogen, low libido, low copper related anemia (copper supports iron) and thyroid issues (low copper connection).

Surgical and Medical Tips: This conjunction within 1° is one testimony for surgical avoidance, especially for body parts and procedures ruled by Venus, such as kidneys, ovaries, female genitalia, buttocks, skin, and lips; facial cosmetic procedures, breast enhancement or reconstruction. It is best to avoid commencing voluntary hormonal replacement therapy or hair augmentation (for baldness) at these times.

Remember, selecting safe surgery dates is the province of your doctor (first) and a highly skilled medical astrologer (second).

Field Note: Some cases born with this conjunction in Virgo appear to have low estrogen.

Venus influences the shine and abundance of the hair. One male client was born with natal Venus ruling his Libra Ascendant. His Venus was natally positioned in Aries (Venus' detriment and the sign of the head), closely conjunct the natal South Node. He was quite bald by his mid-twenties but corrected this with hair plugs.

Transit Venus Conjunct Natal Ascendant

First, be certain the Ascendant degree is really true. This aspect is soothing and magnetizing to the body, most especially to the regions governed by the Ascendant's sign. Effects last for the duration of Venus' transit through the Ascendant sign, though are more pronounced within 3° of the true Ascendant degree.

The native appears sexier and more attractive to others for a few days around exactitude!

VENUS' SQUARE, OPPOSITION & QUINCUNX
Health Potentials for Predisposed Nativities
Transits do not always manifest as health concerns

These transits are fast moving and of small orb. Normally the "hard aspects" of transit Venus are not powerful unless one suffers Venus-related issues, such as difficulties with kidney, blood sugar, hair loss, ovaries and hormones. Venus hard aspects can also "add to the load" of more powerful planets.

The Square encourages the excesses of Venus and can soften or overly relax the squared natal planet for a few days. Venus loves pleasure; and her squares can produce a passive loss of discipline with food, sex, drugs, chocolate, wine, sugar, and the like. See *Chapter 3, The Square,* for squares by sign combination.

A Venus Opposition slightly pulls off the vital force of any planet she opposes. This typically goes unnoticed unless the native is very weak. In that case, a Venus opposition within 1° can be the proverbial straw that breaks the camel's back! However, her opposition is often good, bringing balance, help and sweetness (the very functions of Venus) to the natal planet she opposes. See *Chapter 3, The Opposition,* and *The Six Polarities,* for polarity delineation.

The Venus quincunx is especially brief, lasting only two days or so, unless stationing. The natal planet quincunxed may not receive enough sugar, copper or estrogen during this transit. One might say metaphorically that the natal planet does not receive enough love at this time! See *Chapter 4 "The Quincunx!"*

The Venus quincunx can produce a hidden hormonal swing or deficiency related to the signs and planet involved. Transit Venus quincunxes to the natal Sun, Moon or Ascendant are not good times for beauty treatments or haircuts!

VENUS' SEXTILE & TRINE
Health Potentials for Predisposed Nativities
Transits do not always manifest as health concerns or benefits

The sextile (60°) and trine (120°) are considered "good" aspects. However, never expect a sextile or trine from transit Venus to rescue anyone, or save the day in surgery. Her close-orb sextiles and trines are mildly helpful towards offsetting sepsis, bleeding or pain. The exact conjunction of transit Venus is the only Venusian aspect reliably "benefic" enough to save a life.

Transit Venus' soft aspects often represent a helpful nurse, sister, lover or wife, who sneaks in the craved hamburger or provides needed caresses. Venus sextiles and trines saves lives through love!

Of course, the stronger the transit and natal Venus, the greater the impact. For example, an exalted transit Venus in exact trine to the natal planet in trouble can do wonders for anyone with a strong, positive, natal Venus.

Chapter 12

MARS
HEAT, ENERGY, EXCRETION

Properties, Rulerships and Actions
Rules: Aries, Scorpio

Exalted: Capricorn

Detriment: Libra, Taurus

Fall: Cancer

Metal: Iron (traditional)

Minerals: Cobalt, phosphorus *(Jansky, Nauman)*, molybdenum, selenium, and sodium *(Nauman)*. However, sodium is traditionally allotted to Saturn due to its tightening and drying nature. Also, sodium is an electrically conductive crystal and Saturn is one of the governors of the nervous system.

Vitamins: B12 *(Jansky, Nauman)*, F, Folic Acid *(Nauman)*

Gem & Cosmic Ray: Red coral *(traditional Jyotish)*, Yellow.

Body Rulership & Organ Affinities: Muscles, adrenalin, adrenal gland (with the Aries-Libra axis), cortisol, red blood cells, "the marrows" *(Jyotish)*, thumb *(Hill)*, with Mercury, Gemini and Virgo; the motor nerves (with Aries, Sagittarius), nose (with Scorpio), sense of smell, vision (with Aries), the left ear, gallbladder, and gall (with Saturn, Leo, Virgo, Capricorn), stomach acids and digestive fire, pancreatic and duodenal enzymes, testosterone, spermatozoa (with Sun), spermatic cord and male genitalia (with Scorpio).

General Action: Acute, acidic, heating, stimulating, inflaming, irritating, invading, infecting, pungent, penetrating and excreting (with Scorpio). Physical invasions of pathogens, fevers, hemorrhage, eruptions, redness of skin. Mars with Mercury gives insects, itch, hot neuralgia and pain.

Mars governs catabolic processes. The penetrating action of Mars works in both directions! Ruling penetration of skin barriers from the outside-in, Mars works through outside entities to produce bacterial entry, bites, stings, cuts, wounds, and stabs; and Mars governs the surgeon's knife. Mars also works from the inside-out pushing waste, semen and fluids out of the body. Thus, Mars is ever active in diaphoresis, catharsis, emesis, urination, defecation, sweating, nosebleed, mucous release, boils, rashes, all "red" skin reactions, abortion, miscarriage, and the like.

Mars Retrograde: Mars retrograde is pathologically worse, as his excreting actions are turned inward, with potential for autoimmune disorders and various types of auto-toxicity.

Positive: Mars, the Lesser Malefic, is also our great friend and indispensable ally. For example, a happy Mars gives strong muscles, excellent athletic prowess, courage, "nerves of steel", ambition, good blood, excellent excretion release, strong immunity, strong libido, and virility.

He provides our available surface energy, whereas our deep battery of vital force is the Sun. These two work together to indicate our natal energy level and metabolic burn-rate.

Negative: Inflammation and injury, with the body location and manner depending on the sign and element.

Mars overheats and dries when in Fire and Earth signs. He irritates the nerves in Air signs, causing neuralgia. In Water, Mars is both hot and wet, producing all manner of boils, fungus infections, itch, pus, sepsis, and the like. A blocked Mars overheats the interior, resulting in GERD, skin conditions, itch, colitis, diverticulitis, and similar maladies. This tendency is furthered if retrograde, and especially strong in Earth signs.

Excess Mars: Strong Mars heightens testosterone, adrenalin and iron, producing sex addiction, hyperactivity and mania. When excess Mars is obstructed or blocked, the same types of maladies occur as described above.

Deficient Mars: Deficient Mars gives fatigue, lassitude, poor sense of smell, timidity, anemia, depression, asthenia, impotence, muscle atrophy, general weakness, addictions; contributes to deprivation. The normal excretion of toxins is impeded and turns inward producing boils, rashes, skin disease, sweat disorders, constipation, parasites, and so forth, depending on the sign and element.

The tendency to overheat the interior also occurs when Mars is deficient and blocked! This is because Mars always heats. When obstructed, the trapped heat builds, causing inflammatory conditions as described above!

Transit Frame & Orb: Mars transits are most obvious within an orb of 10°, and very potent at 1°. So often the degree following exactitude is productive of surprise events, so don't take your "eye off the ball" as soon as exactitude clears. Mars' station is extremely strong, doubling his impact for 1 to 3 days.

Temperature & Moisture Levels: Hot and dry when in Fire, Air and Earth. Hot and moist in Water.

You will not see this "moist" designation in traditional texts. This is odd because: a) Mars rules the Water sign Scorpio; b) Mars was assigned as the ruler of the Water triplicity (both by day and night in some texts); c) Mars in Water signs produces a wide array of obviously hot and wet eruptive conditions. (See *Mars Through the Elements & Signs* below.) These are strong testimonies for allotting Mars as hot and moist in the three Watery signs.

I cannot entirely agree with tradition's assignment of governance of the dark, cold-moist Water triplicity to hot Mars because common "horse sense" would assign this honor to Luna! The cold-moist Moon rules the water in our bodies and the tides in the sea.

MARS THROUGH THE ELEMENTS & SIGNS

Applicable to both natal and transit charts, these partial lists of expressed symptoms apply only to predisposed nativities. These conditions are obviously uncommon and require multiple testimonies beyond the presence of Mars.

Manifestation of symptoms may be enhanced by lifestyle choices, and taking preemptive measures can reduce, remove or prevent potential issues from manifesting. It is not possible to list all potential expressions.

Mars in Fire Signs

Fire signs and Mars speed the burn-rate and the metabolism. Thus, the ingress of Mars into a fire sign increases the caloric burn-rate, especially in Aries and Sagittarius. Also, digestive enzymes and appetite are typically strong.

Aries: This transit is prone to accidents to the head and eyes, premature ejaculation, mania, rages, high fever, brain fever, meningitis, conjunctivitis, shooting pains in head, eyes or upper teeth.

Especially natally, there is a predisposition to dry, itchy eyes, dry hair, strong scull, strong jaw, good muscular action, strong metabolism, hyperactive motor nerves, strong or excessive adrenal response, and aerobic action. Stroke-inducing.

Leo: Accelerated heartbeat, carditis (heart inflammation), heart attack, stroke, injury to heart or spine, spinal cord inflammation, overheating, sunstroke, spinal cord injury, meningitis, temper fits. Natally, a positively placed Mars in Leo provides a strong heart muscle, strong back, dry spinal sheaths, muscular sclerosis.

Sagittarius: Hyperactivity, mania, panic, paralysis, dry lung (reflex to Gemini). Pain in or injury to lower spinal nerves, hips, thighs, femurs, and other Sagittarian parts. Injuries incurred from horses, dogs, driving, sports, risky behavior, firearms, or arrows. Stimulates the neuromuscular system.

Natally, can be associated with strong hips and thighs, athleticism, good runners, overactive motor nerves, addiction to "uppers," satyriasis (excessive male sexual desire), sciatica, hyperthyroid, Graves' disease. Insomnia is classic. Davidson says, "Too full of life."

Mars in Earth Signs

When in Earth signs, Mars obstructs poisons from fast exit. This manifests in skin conditions and arthritis, especially with Mars in Capricorn; throat infections for Taurus in reflex to a stuffy colon;

and diverticulitis, colitis and appendicitis for Mars in Virgo. Earth-sign Mars is one testimony of internal dryness. The Earth metabolism is slowest of all the elements. The calorie burn-rate is slowest in Capricorn and Taurus. Gives great stamina!

Taurus: Neck injury, throat inflammation or infection, ear infections, ear injury, eating disorders and addictions, malnourishment, heavy metal poisoning, infected teeth or salivary glands, overeating, excessive masturbation, vocal cord inflammation or infection, tongue inflammation, tonsillitis.

Virgo: Abdominal hernia, duodenitis, pancreatitis, colitis, diverticulitis, dry intestine, intestinal worms or parasites, liver flukes, liver diseases, liver injury, hepatitis, appendicitis, jaundice, splenitis, splenectomy, injury to upper digestive organs or intestines. Health exercises, yoga, diet extremes, orthorexia, anorexia.

Capricorn: Skin changes or skin cancer, itchy skin, excessive release of toxins through skin, excessively oily or dry skin, eczema, psoriasis, pituitary excitation, excess bile production (jaundice); knee injury, tendonitis at knee.

Stomach issues and nausea (by reflex to Cancer causing acidic stomach), vomiting; iron poisoning, bone infections, dental carries; may briefly contribute to cellular changes in skin or bone, influences kidney function, stimulates anterior pituitary, especially near 4° Capricorn. If natally positive, strong knees. Increased excretion of toxins into joints, precluding arthritis, rheumatism or gout.

Mars in Air Signs

Mars excites the nerves and speech when transiting the Air Element, more so in Gemini, and less in Libra.

Gemini: Dislocated shoulder, bronchitis, neuralgia anywhere but especially to shoulders, arms, hands, fingers, scapula, or clavicle. Dry bronchial tubes, dry asthma, dry upper lung, tuberculosis, nervous stimulation or burnout, insomnia, accelerated speech and gesticulation. Natally, fast reflexes and hand-eye coordination, fast fingers, fast metabolism, alertness due to heightened nervous and mental activity.

Libra: Kidney infection or inflammation, blood in urine, ovarian infection, dizziness, vertigo, hormonal imbalance, acidic blood, heated blood, injury or removal of kidney or testes, lumbar injury, lumbago. Sex and love addiction, excess sodium or potassium excretion (because one of the adrenal hormones is in excess or deficiency), hormonal caused acne, insufficient excretion of uric acids, electrolyte imbalance.

Aquarius: Anemia, leukemia, mysterious blood disorders, blood poisoning, carbon monoxide poisoning, auto-intoxication, mal-formed cells, phlebitis (inflammation of veins), lower leg throm-bosis, circulatory disorders, excitation to spinal nerves, heightened electrical impulses through spinal nerves, ankle or calf injury, neural pain in lower leg, blood clots in calves. This position exacerbates all manner of inherent venous and blood related problems.

Dr. Davidson reported that persons born with their natal Mars in Aquarius should not receive intravenous procedures. One might think then, that this transit might hold similar potential for persons whose charts suggest venous vulnerability.

Mars in Water Signs

Mars' natural excreting function is greatly enhanced in Water, especially Scorpio and secondly, Pisces. **Important!** The normal hot, dry nature of Mars is hot, wet in Water signs. See this discussion, earlier in this chapter, under *Temperature*.

Cancer: Breast pain, trouble nursing, leaking breast implants, breast injury or surgery, plastic poisoning, excess hidden estrogen or progesterone, acidic stomach, "hot" stomach, irritable or inflamed mucous membrane, itchy armpits, elbow injury, stomach ulcers, dry stomach, nausea due to inflammation, GERD, waterborne parasites.

Eating disorder, bulimia, vomiting, stomach surgery, tendency to abortion and miscarriage; injury to ribs, breastbone, breasts, stomach, diaphragm; pericarditis, pleuritis, emotional bitterness, waterborne parasites, alcoholism and drug addictions, family pattern issues, strong allergic response, rashes pleuritis, infection of lower lung, tuberculosis, inflammation of marrow. Stimulates posterior pituitary, especially near 4° Cancer.

Scorpio: Sex addiction, nymphomania, peculiar sexual obsessions, STDs (especially of spirochete origin), HIV, genital fungus, jock itch, vaginal infection, genital yeast, infected penis or testes; enuresis, bladder infection, colorectal bacterial imbalance, colorectal parasites, waterborne diseases (cholera, etc.), candida, diarrhea, rectal bleeding, hemorrhoid, excess excretion (sweat, urine, stool, nose mucous).

Worms, blood worm, parasites, vermin caused disease, stings of all kinds, snakebite, Lyme disease, bedbugs (with Mercury), plant venoms, dirty water, fecal or urine contamination, contaminated water and waterborne parasites. Chronic nasal infection, acne, plastic poisoning, hormone poisoning, smell problems, nose bleed, broken nose, inguinal hernia, "dirty blood." Intense body odor, excess sweating, copious foul smelling sweat, extreme genital odor, reaction to dyes, cystitis, colectomy, injury to anus, rectum, colon, bladder, genitals; and appendicitis (with Virgo, especially 15-18°).

Pisces: Foot pain, strong feet, injury to feet or toes, hot feet, excessive foot sweat; strong lymphatic action (which is good unless other toxin clearing systems are down), lymphatic toxicity, engorged lymph nodes.

Onset of psychic interference related mental illness, weird or engrossing dreams, psychic invasion (entities or magical attack); problems from mixing drugs and alcohol, inability to process alcohol, drug overdoses; blood chemistry issues, blood toxicity, heated blood, plastic poisoning, water pathogens (cholera, et al.), hormone poisoning, copious foul smelling sweat, blood worm; STDs, sexual addictions, seductions; wet excretions, boils, carbuncles, hot-wet rashes, reaction to dyes, the flu.

MARS TRANSIT OF NATAL PLANETS

Applicable to both natal and transit charts, these partial lists of expressed symptoms apply only to predisposed nativities. These conditions are obviously uncommon and require multiple testimonies beyond the presence of Mars.

Manifestation of symptoms may be enhanced by lifestyle choices, and taking preemptive measures can reduce, remove or prevent potential issues from manifesting. It is not possible to list all potential expressions.

TRANSIT MARS' CONJUNCTIONS

Health Potentials for Predisposed Nativities
Transits do not always manifest as health concerns or benefits.

Transit Mars Conjunct Natal Sun

Energizing; metabolism increases, pulse rises. Increases heat throughout the system, including the muscles, nerves and spinal cord. If the natal Sun is strong, this heightens energy and some people feel fantastic. In weak or convalescing individuals, available energy may rise with danger of excessive heart stimulation resulting in future exhaustion. Elderly or weak persons should be careful of sunstroke and excessive stress or aerobic activity under this transit.

Danger of heart attack stroke, most particularly in Fire signs. Can coincide with accidents to head, brain or eye. In very rare incidences, meningitis. In Earth signs, watch for conditions caused by trapped heat, oppressing the natural release of toxins. The expulsive force increases in all signs, producing high fevers, rashes, and powerful histamine response. Avoid caffeine.

Surgical and Medical Tips: Postpone surgery to the heart, eyes or brain, unless the responsible physician feels it is necessary to move ahead.

Herbal Note: Circulatory balancing herbs: Rosemary, Hawthorne, Yarrow. Stress induced blood pressure reduction: Motherwort, Yarrow, Garlic, et al. Threat of stroke or aneurism: Yarrow, Cayenne. Cooling, moist herbs may be required to reduce internal heat: Cucumber water, Watermelon, Chickweed and pure water.

Do not self-treat. For muscle injury: Peppermint (a rare, cooling stimulant), Rosemary, Myrrh, Camphor. See the *Earthwise Repertory of Herbal Medicine,* by Matthew Wood.

Transit Mars Conjunct Natal Moon

Heats the feelings, fluids and mind. Acidifying, acid stomach, nausea, vomiting, stomach flu, ulcer. Increases temper and alcohol cravings. Prone to fever, inflamed eyes, bursting of boils, pimples or cysts, stings, bites, overheated brain tissue, inflamed meninges. Increases circulating testosterone or adrenalin and heightens any tendency towards anaphylaxis. Sensitizes the eyes and brain.

Inflammation of mucous membranes in the body part governed by the sign of the natal Moon (e.g. conjunctivitis for natal Moon in Aries; or colitis, diverticulitis in Virgo). Acidifies the bloodstream, heated blood, toxic blood, menorrhagia, painful period. Tendency to miscarry or abort, violent expectoration, increases and thins all fluid excretion, potentially dehydrating. Enhances drug reactions.

This transit promotes pathogen entry (colds are common) and is infection-prone, especially to infants and small children. In general, it is also wise to create a more alkaline condition in the body just prior to, and during this aspect. Avoid acidic foods!

Heightens risk of miscarriage. Mennoraghic. Stimulates parturition. The exact orb transit (any aspect) of Mars to natal Moon is one testimony of parturition. This aspect is tough on babies, bringing fever, colic, crying fits. (See *Herbal Note* below.)

Field Note 1: My grandmother was born with a natal Mars-Moon conjunction in Virgo. She suffered stomach ulcers so severe that they necessitated surgery; eventually she cured herself with Lunar-ruled cabbage juice.

Field Note 2: A "Lunar-ruled" friend experienced a sudden attack of anaphylaxis today. I noted that transit Mars precisely squared his natal Moon, while simultaneously the transit Sun had just minutes before ingressed into 0° Aries, heralding in the Spring Equinox, exactly now opposing his natal Saturn posited at 0° Libra. And, to boot, we were still within orb of a full Moon. This is an educative example of how multiple, mutually supportive astrological testimonies collude in acute events.

Surgical and Medical Tips: Pregnant women need redoubled vigilance during the exact passage of this transit. Raspberry leaf tea is said to provide folic acid and other nutrients that help the placenta adhere to the womb. Postpone surgery to the stomach, breasts, brain, eyes or womb unless the responsible physician advises otherwise.

Herbal Note: Herbalists use a wide array of carefully selected Lunar herbs to counteract the baleful, hot rays of Mars. These are your bland, cooling, moistening demulcents: Celery Seed, Celery, Cucumber Water, Chickweed, Marshmallow Root, Cleavers, Green Grapes. Peach Leaf is a specific for a hot irritated stomach.

Golden Seal and Cabbage juice has been used to cure stomach ulcers. For internal ulceration or bleeding occurring at this time, it is best to use the cooling astringents like Yellow Dock or Golden Seal, combined with a demulcent.

These herbs all work on different symptoms and must be selected under advice from a licensed herbalist. Also, alkaline foods do wonders in counteracting the acidifying beams of Mars. Avoid caffeine. Do not self-treat. Vulneraries should be on hand: Calendula, Plantain, Dr. Kloss' burn tincture, Aloe.

Transit Mars Conjunct Natal Mercury

Mars and Mercury are traditional "enemies." Together, this disharmonious duet produces neuralgia, itch, bites, stings, cuts, and intense shooting pains in the bodily region ruled by the position of natal Mercury. When within an orb of 3°, this is a very potent effect that can easily "bounce around" by reflex into bodily regions squaring, quincunx or even trine the sign of natal Mercury!

When we think of an "-itis," we think of Mars-Mercury! Watch the body parts governed by sign of natal Mercury. For example, when Mars transits natal Mercury in Aries, there could be eyestrain, dry eye, or conjunctivitis! In any sign, this aspect is exceptionally irritating to the respiratory organs, but especially so, in Gemini.

Repetitive action inflammation is typical of Mars-Mercury, such as carpal tunnel and tennis elbow. Increases stress. The nerves are heated and irritated, especially when in the masculine Air and Fire signs, but far less noticeable in Earth and Water.

This aspect drys and inflames the upper respiratory tract. Transit or natal Mars conjunct natal Mercury can produce the endless dry, painful cough, painful ears, strokes affecting speech or hearing changes; jitters, tremors, panic, mania, insomnia, excessive taking of stimulants, excessive talking, smoking, fidgeting, outbursts of foul language, extreme reactions to drugs or medications. These effects can occur in any sign, but are very noted for Gemini, Virgo and Sagittarius. "He needs something to do with his hands."

This transit excites bowel action and may excite bouts of diarrhea. Caution: Laxatives will be triply potentiated! A hernia, or sudden-onset hemorrhoids are also common expressions.

Highly accident prone! Conjunctions and all other transits of Mars to natal Mercury (and the reverse) warn of being susceptible to accidents. The most common causes are vehicles, knives, machinery, and animal bites. The hands, fingers and arms are a common accident locus (usually cuts), but also look to the body parts ruled by the signs of transit Mars and natal Mercury.

Herbal Note: Professional herbalists can use a wide array of carefully selected cooling and moistening nervine sedatives (for most cases), soporifics, nutritive nervines (for burnout), adaptogens (for heightened neural and adrenal stress); also sedative herbs Lavender, Lemon Balm, Blue Vervain, St. John's Wort, Scullcap, Passion Flower—these all relax different symptoms. For example, St. John's Wort is specific for assuaging Mars-Mercury neural pains, and Lemon Balm serves as a specific for herpes eruptions.

For respiratory affliction, use the cooling, moist and relaxing expectorants (if in Water signs, use the cooling, relaxing and astringent expectorants.) Do not self-treat.

Field Note 1: Herpes zoster virus can erupt out of its hiding place in the nervous system under this transit. I recall multiple instances of checking the transits of a friend or client in the throes of a sudden herpes eruption. There it was, a close aspect from transit Mars to natal Mercury, and sometimes the reverse. Matthew Wood's favorite herpes remedies are ranuculus bulbosis, 6X and other members of the buttercup family, Wild Cherry bark, Melissa, St. John's Wort, Licorice root and lysine. Do not self-treat.

Field Note 2: It is astonishing how often a close orb aspect of any kind from transit Mars to natal Mercury can produce a motor vehicle incident. If you are concerned, avoid major driving during the exact transit conjunction, square, opposition, or quincunx. One builder friend with Mercury rising in Gemini seems to reliably injure his hands or have a vehicular accident when transit Mars comes around to conjoin it!

Medical and Surgical Tips: Do not underestimate that tiny bug bite, thorn prick or trivial wound accrued during the time of this brief transit. Because neurological reactions are greatly heightened at this time, observe extreme caution with new medications! Postpone surgery to nerves, hands, fingers, brain, and ears, unless the responsible physician feels it is necessary to move ahead.

Transit Mars Conjunct Natal Venus

The negative implications of this conjunction are rare, because these two planets are "lovers." However, this aspect could coincide with the infection, dryness or inflammation of kidneys, ovaries, lips, mouth, female genitalia, or veins. Blood sugar or copper levels may rise or fall. Alcohol, caffeine, sugar, or chocolate consumption may increase (or anything else of pleasurable interest).

This sexy transit heightens libido and is quite useful for women seeking pregnancy! Male energy lines up with female, producing a strong hormonal release. Practice safe sex!

Medical and Surgical Tips: If you are diabetic, be vigilant. Avoid excess sugar and alcohol. Tattoos and piercing are more inclined toward infection. Postpone surgery to kidneys, veins, female genitalia, and testes, unless the responsible physician feels it is necessary to move ahead.

Field Note: I've successfully used this transit for conception.

Virile Mars transiting over natal Venus can conceive a pregnancy all on his own, without any further planetary assistance. However, this is an especially strong transit should it occur when either transit Jupiter or Venus are simultaneously in conjunction, sextile or trine with the natal Moon, or conjunct the natal North Node. Additionally, it is ideal to have the day's Moon phase identical with the birth Moon phase *(Jonas)*.

Herbal Note: The professional herbalist can use cooling anti-inflammation herbs, such as Marshmallow root, Uva Ursi and Corn Silk, to offset Mars-related genital-urinary irritations, to be combined with antibacterial herbs if necessary. Cranberry is an old favorite for urinary tract infections, though might well be combined with a demulcent in this case. Chickweed is a specific for itching genital tissue. Ginkgo, Arnica and many cold pressed oils are useful for Phlebitis. Do not self-treat.

Transit Mars Conjunct Natal Mars

Sometimes the intra-Saturnian planets are little felt when aspecting themselves, including Mars-Mars, Venus-Venus, etc. The "Mars Return" would emphasize any Mars-related condition shown by the sign position of the natal Mars. (See: *Mars Through the Elements & Signs,* earlier in this chapter.)

If natal Mars is neither too strong nor deficient, and well placed, this aspect is of little concern, although, as the *I Ching* says (paraphrased), "Even a tiny pig can rage around!" For those so prone, speeding accidents, drinking, and drug excess are implied.

Medical and Surgical Tips: Beware of exceptional reactions to beestings and medications. This transit enhances the adrenal and immune responses, aka anaphylaxis.

Transit Mars Conjunct Natal Jupiter

This aspect stimulates arterial circulation and accelerates liver function. Invigorating and athletic. Muscles receive more oxygen. Adrenalin and testosterone rise. Metabolism increases. Generally warming to the body. Energy rises, and some people feel great! If convalescing, don't overdo it too soon.

Stimulates the pituitary gland, with odd results caused by hormone increase, such as hot flashes, swollen breasts, high libido. Heats, thins and pressurizes the arterial blood. Heightens any inherent tendency to stroke, heart attack, thrombosis, and sunstroke. There is a tendency towards dehydration, especially in Fire signs. If negative, this conjunction is extremely hemorrhage prone!

Hepatic plethora. This transit is a potentially dangerous stimulant for individuals suffering bipolar, mania, panic, anger control issues or ADHD. Conversely, victims of depression may feel like living again!

Field Note: One young client could not stop dangerous uterine bleeding for some days following a uterine surgery undergone on the precise day when transit Mars exactly conjoined her natal Jupiter in Scorpio, 12th house. Scorpio and Cancer govern the uterus.

Medical and Surgical Tips: Excellent for the commencement of aerobic and movement therapies, provided the patient has a good cardiovascular system and strong heart (check with a physician). Assists weight loss. The exact conjunction of Mars is always a bit intense and heightens the chance of hemorrhage. If even minor bleeding occurs under this transit, act fast. Postpone surgery to liver, pituitary gland, heart, arteries, and veins, unless the responsible physician feels it is necessary to move ahead.

Because Jupiter rules fat, drastic fat removal may be quite effective, although a Mars-Jupiter trine or sextile is safer. Alternatively, a transit Mars conjunction of natal Jupiter may be useful for surgical fat removal if simultaneously transit Jupiter closely trines or sextiles natal Mars! This "doubling" would be protective.

Herbal Note: Herbalists can use cooling hepatics (e.g. Dandelion, Centaury, Gentian) should the liver be overly functioning or heating. In cases of trapped heat within the liver turning inward, herbalists can use both heating plus cooling hepatics, bringing in needed moisture while simultaneously assisting Mars in his releasing functions. Yarrow and should be on hand (for bleeding or hemorrhage). Do not self-treat.

Transit Mars Conjunct Natal Saturn

This natal aspect is traditionally a "doozie" for bone breaks and a poor choice for dangerous sports. In ripe candidates, expect the sudden, painful expulsion of gravel and stone.

Positively, this transit is perfect for general strengthening, bone and muscle building, weight loss. Potentially drying, heating and irritating to bones and joints; joint inflammations, tendon and ligament tears, muscle strains, wounds; potentizes skin diseases. Drying, this aspect is productive of itching skin due to bile salts, gout, jaundice, drying ligament and tendons. The body strives at this time to excrete gravel in kidneys or gallbladder. Ouch!

Heats where cold. Increases circulation to area of body governed by natal Saturn—this could be needed, or alternatively produce a dangerous "road jam" in the vessels, organ or body part of natal Saturn, thus producing cramps, thrombosis, clots, blood pressure issues and the like. Blockages of outlet points (e.g. constipation, blocked ureters, blocked ducts), obstructions in body parts governed by natal Saturn. Excessive mineral or salt excretion. Dries where already too dry! Also, pay attention to the body parts ruled by the sign opposed and the two signs quincunxed by natal Saturn.

Medical and Surgical Tips: Postpone surgery to skin, knees, ears, joints, bones, ligaments, tendons, unless the responsible physician feels it is necessary to move ahead.

Herbal Note: Professional herbalists use a wide array of carefully selected herbs for cooling and moistening joints, relieving joint or skin irritation, bringing back elasticity to ligaments and tendons. For gout, Celery Seed and Black Cherry Juice are both favored specifics. For ligament health, Solomon's Seal Root, and Flaxseed are specifics. For setting bones: Mullein, Boneset, and with caution, Comfrey. (See M. Wood's *Earthwise Repertory of Herbal Medicine.*)

For skin, the cooling Lunar-ruled Chickweed is best to counter-act hot Mars. Plantain and Calendula are also useful anti-arthritic herbs may be in order. For muscle strain: Peppermint is a rare, cooling stimulant, whereas Rosemary and Camphor are warming.

In this aspect, where hot meets cold, your temperature choices are paramount. Do not self-treat.

Transit Mars Conjunct Natal Uranus

Many associate this conjunction with sudden accidents. However, slow-moving individuals generally go unscathed by avoiding high-risk behaviors, wild environments and operation of dangerous equipment! This is a good time for extra caution while driving.

Because Uranus governs electricity, Mars excites the bodily electricity, inclining some to sudden, often ill-advised actions. Hormones suddenly rise or fall. This may shift a delicate neural or hormonal balance, disturbing equilibrium, and causing some to lose control. Positively, damaged nerves can reawaken!

The metabolism may rise. Diabetics should be on high alert when this transit is in close orb. Sugar, iron, adrenalin, cortisol and testosterone shifts may occur. This is a good time to be proactive against cramps and spasms of all types. These might occur because Mars "burns up" our electrically conductive salts by excreting them through urine and sweat. Look to the bodily regions ruled by the sign of natal Uranus and the signs in quincunx to natal Uranus.

Nervous signals or bodily electrical functions are hyperstimulated. This could present such symptoms as tinnitus, unexpected paralysis (usually temporary), neuralgia, epileptic seizure, panic attacks, unpredictable behavior or moods. Electrocution is associated with Mars-Uranus-Mercury *(Cruce)*. Sudden heart arrhythmia is a Mars-Uranian issue.

Surgical and Medical Tips: A notably unpredictable transit for surgery. Anything could happen. The electrical system in the body may have unpredictable reactions. Unless the responsible physician feels it is necessary to move ahead, postpone surgery to the body parts governed by the sign of natal Uranus.

Herbal Note: To treat spasmodic symptoms, professional herbalists can use a wide array of carefully selected cooling sedatives, nutritive nervines, and antispasmodics including Catnip, Black Cohosh, Cramp Bark, Lobelia, Red Clover (see Matthew Wood's *Earthwise*

Repertory of Herbal Medicine). Sodium and minerals can be used in some cases, with a physician's agreement. Do not self-treat.

Transit Mars Conjunct Natal Neptune

This transit is potentially one of those medication doozies. These two planets mix about as well as alcohol and ibuprofen! Be very alert for all manner of drug incompatibility, overdose, and faulty prescription. Because it significantly weakens self-control, this aspect is dangerous for drug addicts and alcoholics.

Potential food poisoning, plant poisons, poison in the cerebral spinal fluid, secret poisons, and sneaky things. Heats the blood and excites the lymphatics. Poisoning to the matrix and interstitial fluids. This transit may evince itself in wet, itchy skin eruptions, carbuncles, boils and excess pus. Fungal, yeast and virus infections are also common. Watch for molds, dust and little-noticed carriers of sneaky pathogens. Check for gas leaks and carbon monoxide poisoning, especially if in Air signs.

Possibilities heighten for sudden drug overdoses, or conversely, miraculous release from addictions. A likely time for medical revelations and innovative cures, especially regarding physical motility and independence. Lymphatic and blood clearance need support at this time.

Field Note: This example displays to perfection the sneaky nature of Mars-Neptune aspects. A client was soon to enjoy a transit of Mars exactly over his natal Neptune, in Scorpio in his 6th house of health and work, I vehemently suggested that during this transit he be wary of "poisoning in the workplace."

He called a few weeks later to tell me what transpired. Heeding my warning, he was very careful all that day about the glass factory, where he worked as a skilled blower. Nothing happened.

At the end of the workday, his boss appeared, regaling him with a bottle of nice wine. He drank some of it, and it made him very, very sick. Poisoning in the workplace!

Surgical and Medical Tips: One should be careful of unpredictable effects from anesthesia.

Herbal Note: Professional herbalists can use a wide array of carefully selected alteratives (blood and lymphatic assisting and cleansing herbs), such as Poke Root, Red Root, Dandelion, Burdock, Red Clover, Beets, Rhubarb, Grapes, Sassafras, Sarsaparilla, Oregon Grape Root, Blue Violet. Cooling herbs are best. For staunching blood seepage, consider cooling astringents Cranesbill, Blackberry. Do not self-treat.

Transit Mars Conjunct Natal Pluto

Unclear and may not be felt in all nativities. More dangerous in reverse, with Pluto transiting natal Mars or if transit Mars is stationing in for a long stay.

This transit is potentially dangerous because of drastically potentized effects of drugs, herbs, lasers, and the like. May suggest the entry of dangerous bacteria into the bloodstream. Inclines to damage through radiation-therapy, lasers, and chemotherapy. Danger of drug overdose, sepsis, gangrene. This transit could signal the reception of HIV, and other STDs. Abstain or practice safe sex. A useful transit for parasite clearance!

Because both planets govern poisoning (along with Neptune, Saturn, the Nodes and certain signs), this conjunction can testify to poisoning as much as does, for example, Mars-Neptune. It would be interesting to see if mandatory amputations are typical under close Mars-Pluto aspects to the natal chart.

Surgical and Medical Tips: This conjunction is dangerous through potentization of procedures such as hormone therapies, stem cell transplants, organ transplants, and blood transfusions. Cleansing reactions can be extreme. Therefore, physicians may consider lower doses.

Speedily treat bites of any kind. Take precautions with all high-tech medical equipment. Be extremely proactive against dangerous bacteria when working around rats, hospitals, needles, and the like. Dangerous for surgery due to potential for bacterial contamination.

Healing powers, hormones and vermifuges (a type of anti-parasitic) are potentized.

Chemotherapy would be extra-effective but also more potent in effect on healthy tissue.

Herbal Note: The professional herbalist should have potent antivirals, antibacterial and anti-inflammatory herbs handy at this time. Chaparral, Olive Leaf, Eucalyptus, Thuja, Rosemary, Oregano Oil, Tea Tree, Lomatium, Grapefruit Seed Extract, Lemon, Garlic et al. Do not self-treat!

Transit Mars Conjunct Natal North Node

Mars' transit of the North Node signifies an influx of stimulating heat into bodily systems, either in general or specific to the bodily regions ruled by the sign of natal North Node. This could manifest in a great number of possible ways: tissue inflammation, hyper-function, exhilaration, increased blood flow. This transit can contribute to stroke, aneurism, heart attack and rages in over-heated natal charts predisposed to these conditions.

Muscles receive more energy. This is a strongly positive transit for competitive athletes! Motor nerves receive excess stimulus.

Testosterone and/or adrenalin surges can add to problems with self-medication, drinking binges, gambling, speeding, fighting, anger outbursts, mania, and hyper-sexuality. Avoid excess stimulants and acidic foods. Basking in the sunshine is dangerous, especially if the transit Mars afflicts your Sun, Moon or Ascendant to or from Leo or Aries. Iron levels may rise.

Surgical and Medical Tips: This transit could mean a successful surgery only if augmented by a nice trine from transit Jupiter, or similar help. Otherwise, Mars, ruling the surgeon's knife, can be too aggressive at this time. (This is the time your hairdresser decides to cut your hair too short!) Normally, it is wise to avoid surgery during the close conjunction to the natal North Node, unless your physician says otherwise.

Great care should be taken not to over-medicate or mix drugs/alcohol. Muscle, libido and male hormonal treatments could be either quite successful now, or produce extreme results. One receives a heightened dose of "male energy" at this time anyway!

Should symptoms present, check blood ferritin, adrenalin, cortisone and testosterone levels (because these can rise at this time).

Field Note: One individual born with a close Mars-North Node conjunction in Sagittarius in his 5th house was a great athlete and successful in his military career. He had vicious nosebleeds, and also suffered onsets of wild, violent rages triggered by seemingly minor irritations. He later denied, or could not recall these incidents.

A woman I've met with this same natal conjunction in Leo is a heavy metal guitarist who loves to "shred" the guitar.

Herbal Tips: Licensed professional herbalists can antidote an excessive arrival of Mars' heat by using cooling, moist herbs and the metals of the Moon and Venus (silver, copper). Should a hemostatic effect be desired, combine with Saturn's astringents, being careful of a doubly drying effect should transit Mars be in a Fire, Air or Earth sign.

The receiving point of the excess Mars heat will be in the bodily region governed by the sign of the natal North Node. However, this same aspect can helpfully strengthen and energize those who need it!

This is an excellent time to commence blood-building herbal treatment for anemia (Nettles, soaked black raisins, beets, et al). Do not self-treat.

Transit Mars Conjunct Natal South Node

This transit is the first-rate "avoid" for surgeries. See *Surgical and Medical Tips* below.

Understanding this transit requires delicate interpretive skill. First, the natal South Node symbolizes a weak spot in the anatomy. The South Node drains, dribbles, weakens. It also can represent various addictions, psychological issues, fears, and supernatural issues. It is also the point of self-undoing. The Mars conjunction stimulates whatever an individual's South Node means to them!

Occasionally, I've observed this transit to suddenly produce an excessively acidic condition in the body, with attendant hot, itchy rashes. These have been successfully quelled by reducing all acids, including vinegar from the diet. This acidic action of Mars-South Node well follows the Jyotish idea that Mars' traditional Yellow cosmic ray is hot, while the South Node's Infrared cosmic ray is hotter still, on the astral level. However, be aware that the South Node does not invariably produce obviously hot conditions in the physical body.

Also, be alert to the heightened potential for hidden (or not hidden) bleeding. The South Node is the great anus of the celestial wheel, literally the Dragon's Tail. Therefore, this transit strongly potentizes the release of toxins, but also enhances bleeding, leaching, diarrhea and wasting. Sometimes we see an increase in boils, rashes, acne, vomiting, catharsis, diuresis or diaphoresis.

For drinkers, blood alcohol level may produce unusually disturbing results. For anemics or those with blood diseases, this transit (though typically brief) can signal a dive in red blood cell count or function. Blood constituents are not well understood yet by medical astrology. White blood cells perform some obvious Mars functions too, such as defending and fighting.

There is a bright side of this conjunction. If taking a conscious approach, one can find the courage to "cut off" one's psychological weaknesses and addictions: "I'm quitting cigarettes!" However, this requires choice and willpower. This transit can equally stimulate subconsciously driven cravings as the sword of Mars cuts both ways!

Libido can go either way: excessive or non. Boundaries seem slack with blood-borne contagion, so safe sex is a must at this time. Male virility is temporarily reduced during this transit, and sperm count may plummet.

Associated with active "self-undoing" this transit is dangerous for those with suicidal ideologies or life-threatening behaviors. To counteract, one can use Mars to stimulate courage and awareness of one's self-induced pitfalls. This is one of the worst periods of the year for risky sports, prone to all manner of injury.

Psychological issues can arise suddenly with surprising force. This aspect can woefully exacerbate paranoia and fear. Palliative help, such as flower essences, should be kept on hand.

Field Note 1: It is surprising how many times a male client who has opted for vasectomy was born with a Mars-South Node conjunction. Thus, his Mars-ruled ability to impregnate was sacrificed (a South Node function).

One client born on this natal conjunction in Taurus, his 8th house, lost a testicle in an accident.

Field Note 2: One lady yogi born with a natal Mars-South Node conjunction in Scorpio (ruler of the colon) suffered a mysterious, undiagnosed blood flow from the colon for many years.

Surgical and Medical Tips: It is extremely dangerous to have any kind of surgery when transit Mars is within 15° of the natal South Node, both approaching or departing the conjunction (of course, weaker if in a neighboring sign). The effect is especially strong with-in 10° while approaching conjunction, and within 5° while departing—more so if Mars is about to reverse course and go retrograde back over the Node!

Avoid voluntary blood transfusions or transfer of body fluids, especially if in Water signs. Remember, however, the responsible physician must remain the authority on any urgent medical matter.

If you must have surgery at this time, you can review the "DNA Protection Structure" and other tips in my book *Astrology & Your Vital Force, Chapter 18*; or Aubrey T. Westlake's ideas in his seminal work, *The Pattern of Health.*

Herbal Note: Licensed herbalists can choose to either assist or reduce any excess excretions expressing at this time. Be careful! Typically any medical treatments go awry at this time and are best avoided unless one must act. In most cases it would be wise to avoid use of all hot stimulants at this time; e.g. Cayenne, Black Pepper, Garlic, Mustard, Onions, Ginger, and Coffee.

Transit Mars Conjunct the Natal Ascendant

Effects last for the duration of Mars' transit through the Ascendant sign, though are more pronounced within 3° of the true Ascendant degree. First, be certain the Ascendant is really true.

This aspect is generally heating, stimulating and energizing to the body, for good or ill, most especially to the regions governed by the Ascendant's sign. Infants tend to spring sudden fevers at this time. Some natives become bellicose. This is a provocative aspect for sufferers of mania, anger, hyperactivity. Brings courage to overcome disabilities.

TRANSIT MARS' SQUARE
Health Potentials for Predisposed Nativities
Aspects do not always manifest as health concerns or benefits.

The square aspects from transit Mars behave similarly to his conjunctions at perhaps 75% strength. However, they do produce acute events! The dates of the exact square of Mars to natal Sun or Moon must always be watched with caution in ill persons or elderly.

Use the previous text for Mars' conjunctions to each planet. However, there is an important difference to note between Mars conjunctions and squares. In considering the square aspect we, have the heating influence of Mars coming from his current sign to the sign of the natal planet he squares by transit. See *Chapter 3*, the section on *The Square*.

It would be too lengthy to discuss every possible square and sign combination, although these are of paramount importance. If you know the bodily regions governed by the signs (as all students should) you can do this yourself with the following formula:

Formula For Deciphering Mars Squares
Transit Mars heats and stimulates the functions of the natal planet he squares _____ *(name, and describe the functions and organs of that planet)*, and the body parts governed by the planet's natal sign _____ *(give sign and body parts)*. Mars accomplishes this heating and stimulating action from the bodily region governed by the sign he is currently transiting through. _____
(give sign and bodily regions).

For Square type, see *Chapter 3: Aspect Mechanics: The Square.*

Please note that although common, not everyone responds medically to Mars' squares. Mars transits only sometimes express themselves as distinctly medical issues.

A special note on transit Mars squaring the natal Lunar Nodes: Mars here produces a few stressful days, unless stationing (greatly extending the length of effects). This aspect may not always involve health, but more likely does so if occurring in the 6th/12th, 1st/7th or 2nd/8th house polarities.

TRANSIT MARS' OPPOSITION
Health Potentials for Predisposed Nativities
Aspects do not always manifest as health concerns or benefits.

The opposition of transit Mars works like the conjunction, but not as strong. Additionally, as with most other oppositions, Mars pulls upon the vital force of the natal planet opposed, which is weakening because it pulls from the opposite side of the ecliptic. The opposition of transit Mars also creates heat or irritation in the planet opposed. That pulling and heating effect comes from the opposite sign, not the same sign, as with a conjunction. Mars is confrontive, enjoying a good argument.

He aggressively confronts any planet he opposes, putting its functions on defense, and also waking them up!

It is essential when examining the opposition to note the houses and signs in the polarity concerned. Here is a helpful formula:

Mars Opposition Interpreting Formula:
Transit Mars may produce irritation in _____
_____ (*give the sign of transit Mars and body zone ruled by that sign*),
that influences the energy level and smooth function of
_____ (*name natal planet opposed by Mars*),
and its bodily functions_____ (*describe*);
in those bodily regions ruled by the sign of the natal planet
_____ (*give sign and body parts*).
Thus, the entire sign polarity is emphasized.

Transit Mars Opposes Natal Sun

The vital force is challenged from activities symbolized by the sign and house of transiting Mars. Energy is lowered, potential fatigue. Weakens the heart, brain or eyesight. Most obvious for cardiac effects in the Leo-Aquarius polarity.

Transit Mars Opposes Natal Moon

Outside sources or confrontation bring emotional stress. Domestic or marital stress may be contributors to health issues experienced at this time. Miscarriage prone within a close orb.

Appetite is lower, or stomach absorption disturbed. Pulls from the opposite sign at the brain chemistry and mood. Allergens appear, or allergic responses are heightened. Possible fatigue. This aspect is hard on infants, bringing fever, infection, accident, petulance. Parents argue or are annoyed.

Transit Mars Opposes Natal Mercury

Irritation of the nerves from the opposite sign, neural pain. Significantly increases stress coming from outside oneself. This time period is prone to confrontation, argument, accidents, stings, bites, cuts to hands or fingers.

Allergens appear, or allergic responses are heightened. This allergic effect is similar to Mars' hard aspects to the natal Moon. These aspects heighten the potential of catching a respiratory bug.

Transit Mars Opposes Natal Mars

This period is a low point in the personal Mars cycle and may act to lower testosterone, iron or adrenalin.

Transit Mars Opposes Natal Jupiter

Jupiter functions are stimulated and pulled upon from the opposite sign. This could influence the circulation, pituitary, liver functions, and weight. Hemorrhage and stroke prone.

Field Note: A friend aptly arranged her liposuction (fat removal) procedure upon the precise day that transit Mars opposed her natal

Jupiter (the planet that rules fat.) This may or may not be a good idea because Mars-Jupiter contacts can produce hemorrhage.

To ascertain the safety of this aspect, one must also study same day transits to her natal Mars, and other indications. For selecting safe surgery dates, see *Medical Astrology: A Guide to Planetary Pathology, Chapters 22 - 23.*

Transit Mars Opposes Natal Saturn

This aspect challenges something or someone. This aspect is weakening to bone integrity and behaves similarly as the conjunction, though less strong. Bone integrity is "challenged" from a stimulus in the opposite sign. Heightens accident proneness or falling. This is not the best time to play football or climb mountains.

There can be an "attack" on the skin brought by weather, bugs or tattoo artists. This can mean a doctor or dentist is observing your teeth, bones, or other Saturn ruled parts.

This opposition may set up a temporary mismatch or strain between the bones and ligaments, tendons, or muscles. Hypothetically effective for Rolfing or similar fascia and/or muscle-bone restructuring.

Transit Mars Opposes Natal Uranus

Mars now stands opposite to the native's bodily electrical current (Uranus). This could manifest as peculiar changes in the body's electrical current, electric shock or unexpected physical shifts.

Transit Mars Opposes Natal Neptune

Similar to the conjunction, this transit warns of incompatible drug interaction, with a twist. Oppositions are more likely to come to you from others, e.g. perhaps someone approaches you with a spiked glass of wine, or the anesthesiologist is sloppy.

This time period heightens potential for contracting STDs. Potentials include sexual seduction, bacterial invasion, viral entry, mixed medication danger, and also warns of possible inattention to hygiene in hospital settings.

This aspect is a red alert for surfers, divers and others who enter the sea. Avoid risky swims, hot tubs, beer boats, drinking wine in the bath, etc.

Transit Mars Opposes Natal Pluto

Mars and Pluto both govern killing and poisoning, so Mars-Pluto contacts could signify the discovery or eradication of bacteria, vermin and internal parasites. Sepsis potential, but also can signal those drastic medical interventions that arrive to save the day!

TRANSIT MARS' QUINCUNX
Health Potentials for Predisposed Nativities
Transits do not always manifest as health concerns.

All Quincunxes are sneaky and hard to diagnose. The quincunx of Mars is best observed within an orb of 1°, but is of concern within an orb of 3°. The orb is widened should transit Mars be in the sign governed by the natal planet he quincunxes, or vice versa!

The Jyotishi feel that Mars' quincunx is perhaps his strongest aspect, although certainly the conjunction is supremely potent as well. I've been watching this to see if this idea, so foreign to Western astrology, truly works.

Empirical results have completely satisfied me that the quincunx of both transit and natal Mars is indeed strong and, secondly, behaves quite differently than other planetary quincunxes.

Normally, a quincunx means a disconnection between the two planets placed in an angular relationship of 150° distant from one another. In essence, a quincunx is a conspicuous non-aspect, the very meaning of another term for this aspect: the "inconjunct."

In practice, however, this singular Mars quincunx does not disconnect. Rather, the natal and transit quincunx of Mars somehow magnifies his heat as thrown upon the natal planet involved, to the point of endangering its function! The connection is super strong (instead of a non-connection), perhaps as potent as an exact conjunction. But unlike the conjunction, the Mars quincunx occurs out of left field, bringing unexpected incidents, so often baffling to physicians.

All you need to do in these cases is study the bodily parts and functions of the sign of transit Mars and, then, note how it relates to the sign of the quincunxed natal planet. See *Chapter 4: Quincunx!*

For instance, you might find a transit Mars in Virgo quincunx the natal Sun in Aries. Out of the sheer blue, an intense eyestrain appears for this person. The sign Virgo then, is your clue for the cause and means of treatment. Chinese tradition notes that liver problems (Virgo) outlet in the eyes (Aries).

View the transit Mars quincunx in this manner: Increased astral heat is coming from Mars, through one of the bodily parts ruled by the sign he is currently transiting. This astral heat is then delivered to the sign of the natal planet being quincunxed, and most precisely, to the natal planet too! Thus, we see two signs involved, that of both transit Mars and the natal planet.

Field Note: A friend reported an odd incident today that perfectly demonstrated the weird or shocking effect of the Mars quincunx. Mars rules dogs, amongst other things, and this day transit Mars was stationing and exactly quincunx this man's natal Ascendant.

On his walk, he suddenly encountered an English Bulldog having a seizure. This caused him considerable distress as there appeared no way to help the dog, nor discern his people.

Eventually the seizure cleared, and the dog appeared fine. The unforseen effects, alarm and distressing helplessness, of the transit Mars quincunx is well demonstrated here. One must be on one's toes!

Transit Mars Quincunx Natal Sun

This aspect can produce an unexpected heating of the heart or brain, and/or the bodily region indicated by the sign of the natal Sun. This presents a danger of stroke, seizure or heart issues in the predisposed. Watch for unexpected sunburn, snow blindness or fires. Accident prone! If the physician agrees, delay hospital release.

Surgical Tip: Any type of surgery at this time carries enhanced risk. Unless the responsible physician feels it is necessary to move ahead, it is generally unwise to commence surgery under this aspect, especially to heart, brain, eyes, or spinal cord.

Transit Mars Quincunx Natal Moon

Mars can suddenly overheat the lunar functions and the body regions indicated by her natal sign when directing his quincunx within 3°. The effect is "out of left field." Can correlate with stomach unrest, nausea, fever, acidic system, miscarriage, irritation of sensitive tissues throughout the body, inflamed mucous membrane, asthma and allergic reactions, sudden panic, PTSD. Be alert for unwanted sexual attention. This aspect hits babies hard: surprise fevers, infection.

Surgical Tip: Any type of surgery at this time carries enhanced risk, even mortal potential, should other testimonies coincide. Unless the responsible physician feels it is necessary to move ahead, it is generally unwise to commence surgery under this aspect, especially to stomach, breast, uterus, womb, eye or brain.

Transit Mars Quincunx Natal Mercury

This transit stimulates and heats the nerves, causing irritation and inflammation, especially to the bodily regions governed by the sign of natal Mercury. Herpes eruptions, bug bites, neuralgia, overstimulated nerves, panic, and accident proneness (watch for small, darting animals and vehicles), violent itch.

Surgical Tip: Any type of surgery at this time carries enhanced risk. Unless the responsible physician feels it is necessary to move ahead, it is generally unwise to commence surgery under this aspect, especially to nerves, brain, hands, fingers, and ears.

Transit Mars Quincunx Natal Venus

Women need to be aware of their surroundings at this time. Males can be sexually aggressive, unexpectedly from an unseen corner. Everyone should be alert to STDs.

Mars can suddenly heat, inflame or infect the kidneys, veins, testes or female genitalia. Don't neglect minor infections in these areas. An unexpected kidney stone expulsion could be prompted.

Surgical Tip: Any type of surgery at this time carries enhanced risk. Unless the responsible physician feels it is necessary to move ahead, it is generally unwise to commence surgery under this transit, especially to kidneys, veins, ovaries, testes, and vagina.

Transit Mars Quincunx Natal Mars

The author is unclear on the effects of this quincunx. Hypothetically, Mars' own functions would be temporarily diminished (testosterone, adrenalin, iron, excretion, muscles, libido, male genitalia.) However, the bodily region governed by the sign of natal Mars may heat up or come under attack (possible wounds, bacteria, boils, rash, bites, and the like).

Transit Mars Quincunx Natal Jupiter

Mars may suddenly heat or infect the arterial circulation or liver. Parasitical attack upon the liver is sometimes observed, associated in the Medieval mindset as "choleric" symptoms and "overheated blood." There is danger for those predisposed toward heightened arterial pressure, aneurism, stroke and heart attack. The liver may dump an excess of some nutrient or fat into the blood.

Natally, this aspect can prevent the native from gaining weight, because Jupiter rules fat.

Surgical Tip: Any type of surgery at this time carries enhanced risk. Unless the responsible physician feels it is necessary to move ahead, it is generally unwise to commence surgery under this transit, especially to liver, blood vessels, and pituitary; or for body fat removal and/or transference.

Transit Mars Quincunx Natal Saturn

Mars acts to suddenly dry and heat the bones, ligaments or tendons. Strains, tears, ligament or tendon injury, muscle cramps, bone fractures are common. The mismatch of sudden heat applied to a cold, tense area of body (as indicated by natal Saturn's sign) can throw the body out of alignment.

Sudden skin irritations or hot eruptions are common. However, in rare cases this aspect can be significantly useful in heating or drying all these same areas above as needed. The heat of Mars can break up the stasis of Saturn.

Surgical Tip: Any type of surgery at this time carries enhanced risk. Unless the responsible physician feels it is necessary to move ahead, it is generally unwise to commence surgery under this transit, especially to bones, ligaments, tendons, skin and nerves.

Field Note: For natal Mars quincunx natal Saturn, I've observed that muscles, (Mars), and ligaments-tendons-bones (Saturn) can misalign. Also, proteins do not seem to assimilate correctly.

I've observed severe muscle atrophy, slippery ligaments, misaligned shoulder, and hip joints out of socket resulting in severe muscle torsion. Also, severe, ongoing sweats (Mars) causing mineral deficiency (Saturn).

Transit Mars Quincunx Natal Uranus

A Mars backhanded attack on Uranus can produce mysterious disturbances to the electrical rhythm of the body, electric shock, electrocution, hyperactive nerves, and seizure. Motor nerves experience a "blip" with odd effects. Sleep disturbance, insomnia.

This quincunx could influence the thyroid gland and the heart rhythm. It is important to consider the bodily region ruled by the sign of natal Uranus. Hormonal treatments may throw unforeseen curves as related especially to male hormones, thyroid, and adrenals.

Surgical Tip: Any type of surgery at this time carries enhanced risk. Unless the responsible physician feels it is necessary to move ahead, it is generally **unwise** to commence surgery under this transit, especially to the nerves, heart, spinal cord, thyroid or adrenal gland, and brain; or for gender reassignment.

Transit Mars Quincunx Natal Neptune

Transit Mars fronts a secret attack on natal Neptune. This quincunx of Mars is heating and strong but never as immediately obvious as the conjunction, square or opposition! In this case, the blood or lymphatic vessels may present puzzling symptoms, or delayed diagnosis. Misdiagnosis may invite viral or bacterial invasion to take hold. A drug interaction may cause symptoms, but nobody figures this out.

Another potential would be that of symptoms arising at this time related to a bite, prick or sexual encounter overlooked in the previous weeks, months or even years. Latent pathogens, STDs or spirochetes such as herpes, streptococcus, syphilis, Lyme Disease, quietly start up. Secret poisonings. Should mysterious symptoms arise under this transit, don your Sherlock Holmes cap.

Transit Mars Quincunx Natal Pluto

Increases danger of unforeseen bacterial entry. This aspect is "needling" and increases the tendency for medical procedures and tests to take place, such as colonoscopy, biopsy, and blood tests. Mysterious ulceration. Note the bodily region governed by the sign of natal Pluto.

Transit Mars Quincunx Either Natal Node

Heightens stress related to the meaning of either Node in the bodily regions governed by at least one, if not both, natal Nodes.

Chapter 13
JUPITER
Fats, Expansion, Growth

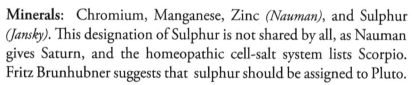

Properties, Rulerships and Actions
Rules: Sagittarius and Pisces

Exalted: Cancer

Detriment: Virgo and Gemini

Fall: Capricorn

Metal: Tin

Minerals: Chromium, Manganese, Zinc *(Nauman)*, and Sulphur *(Jansky)*. This designation of Sulphur is not shared by all, as Nauman gives Saturn, and the homeopathic cell-salt system lists Scorpio. Fritz Brunhubner suggests that sulphur should be assigned to Pluto.

Vitamins: Vitamin B6, Biotin, Inositol Choline *(Jansky, Nauman)*; F, K *(Jansky)*; B15 *(Nauman)*,

Gem & Cosmic Ray: Blue and Yellow Sapphire. This stone is said to produce the Blue Cosmic Ray.

Jupiter's reputation as the "Great Benefic," does not necessarily apply to health! True, Jupiter's cosmic blue ray protects health and nourishes the body. However, Jupiter is equally famous for creating a wide array of liver, blood and fat related maladies. How can this be? Jupiter rules fat and expansion. The pathological expressions of excessive growth include tumors, hypertension and obesity.

Jupiter's association with the pituitary gland *(per Edgar Cayce)* explains why Jupiter is implicated in all manner of hormonally linked growth extremes, including acromegaly, enlarged organs, gigantism and dwarfism. Jupiter is famous for obesity. However, exceptional height is just as Jupiterian as is expansive girth! Whether growth occurs horizontally or vertically depends in part upon

Jupiter's sign and house placement plus the full testimony of the whole natal chart! Diabetes is a malady of Jupiter and Venus.

Body Rulership & Organ Affinities: Liver, pituitary gland *(Edgar Cayce)*, blood *(Cornell)*, arterial circulation. Jupiter governs fats and oils. Fats assist in the protective cushioning of the bones and nerves.

Note: The blood's constituents are not well understood in medical astrology and require revision.

General Action: Expands, grows tissue, fattens, gives plethora, engorges; can promote plethora. Healthy manifestations include bringing fatty protection to nerve and bone, good lipid distribution and adaptogen enhancement. Jupiter also acts to protect and preserve life in the body.

Positive: A healthy Jupiter is one testimony of a happy, healthy, fully-fleshed person of normal to corpulent weight. In medical emergencies, the exact trine from Jupiter can literally "save the day." Jupiter's rays protect life or conversely, endanger it through excess pressure—of a kind determined by the element. Additional chart testimonies help discern if Jupiter will protect or harm. A happy natal Jupiter assists liver function.

Negative: Obesity (or conversely, emaciation). This depends on if we are viewing Jupiter in excess or deficiency *(see below)*. Right now, let's stick to a review of the excesses of his natural functions. Jupiter's excess brings problems caused by a surfeit of circulating cholesterol. Growth disturbances including anything leaning in the direction of too much (height, weight, appetite, and waistline).

Disturbed Jupiter can create gigantism or dwarfism. Jupiter can play a significant role in diabetes; edema, high blood pressure, aneurysm, heart attack, blood engorgement, arterial sclerosis, enlarged organs, liver disease, diabetes.

The "good" trine from Jupiter encourages growth, tumors, edema or blood surplus, especially so if occurring in Earth and Water signs when also trine the natal Venus, Moon or Saturn.

Note: In special cases, Jupiter reverses the growth principal, going small instead of large. See *Field Notes* under *Transit Jupiter's Quincunxes.*

Excess Jupiter: All problems of excess *(see above)*. The natal sign of Jupiter often indicates an enlarged body part (e.g. Jupiter in Sagittarius sometimes produces long femurs or large buttocks)

Possible symptoms include: obesity, excess tissue or bone growth, cysts and tumors, excess bile or cholesterol production, high arterial blood pressure, especially in Fire (flushed face, red palms), edema (in Water).

Deficient Jupiter: There are many conditions that could signify a weak Jupiter. Jupiter's ray will definitely be deficient if in Virgo, Gemini or Capricorn in the 6th, or 8th houses and/or conjunct the South Node or Saturn.

A natally afflicted Jupiter is far more likely to produce liver impairment than any temporary transit of Jupiter. However, if one's liver is already impaired, the transits both to natal Jupiter and from transit Jupiter become important.

Possible symptoms include: skinny, dry, depressed, cheerless, hopeless, lacks oil; nervous due to lack of fatty protection in nerve sheaths; undernourished or small; growth deficiencies; delayed puberty, low libido.

Temperature & Moisture Level: Warm and moist. Jupiter is cooler in Water Signs, explosive in Fire signs, cheerful in Air signs and impaction prone in Earth signs.

Transit Frame & Orb: Jupiter spends approximately one year in each sign, with long retrograde stretches. He enjoys a huge orb, ranging by various opinions as between 7-15°. This means that Jupiter's conjunction, square, trine, or opposition can toggle back and forth for months! The same rule does not apply to Jupiter's quincunx, a singular aspect strongest at 0-3°. This tiny orb can be extended in some cases, especially with reception, or by station, or if obvious symptoms present.

JUPITER THROUGH THE ELEMENTS & SIGNS
Health Potentials for Predisposed Nativities
Not all transits manifest as health concerns or benefits.

Applicable to both natal and transit charts, these partial lists of expressed symptoms apply only to predisposed nativities. These conditions are obviously uncommon and require multiple testimonies beyond the presence of Jupiter. Manifestation of symptoms may be enhanced by lifestyle choices, and taking preemptive measures can reduce, remove or prevent potential issues from manifesting. It is not possible to list all potential expressions.

Jupiter in Fire Signs

Aries: Sudden rushes of blood to brain vessels (migraine), glaucoma, eye pressure, brain or eye tumor, aneurysm, mania, rages; possible increase in oily face or hair, balding.

Surgical Tip: Jupiter in Aries is an excellent assist for surgery to Leo and Sagittarius regions, such as heart, spine, spinal cord, coccyx, hips, femurs, and gall bladder. It could be protective to regions ruled by Aries (e.g. brain, eyes, face, upper jaw), although could bring a surfeit of blood, osmotic pressure, and similar.

Leo: Increases blood pressure, fattens back, increases body heat, increases liver heat. Engorged gall bladder, congested portal circulation, fits of anger. Prone to balding. Dangerous to those with enlarged hearts. Aneurysm alert.

Surgical Tip: Jupiter in Leo is an excellent assist for surgery to bodily regions ruled by Aries and Sagittarius. Influence on Leo body parts is generally protective, although could bring a surfeit of blood, fat or fluidic pressure to those areas.

Sagittarius: Growth spurts, increased weight on thighs or buttocks, increases pressure throughout the arterial circulation, increased mental excitement. Dangerous to those with ADHD, excited mental states, religious mania. Increases energy and urge to be in motion. Balding. Jupiter in Sagittarius in hard aspect to Sun and Mars is strongly associated with hyperthyroid and hyperactive adrenals.

Field Note: Jupiter in Sagittarius, for day births, and especially when simultaneously positioned above the horizon, inclines to height. I saw this in my nephew's chart when he was newly born, and against all common sense, predicted exceptional height. Although both his parents are short, he achieved a height of six feet and two inches!

Surgical Tip: Jupiter in Sagittarius is an excellent testimony for surgery to bodily regions ruled by Aries and Leo. Jupiter is protective to Sagittarius regions, although could also indicate a surfeit of blood pressure or "wild fire" in the system. See a remarkable *Field Note* under the section, *Transit Jupiter conjunct natal Sun.*

Jupiter in Earth Signs

Taurus: Impactions; obstructions; fat deposits in neck arteries; vocal cord polyps; large mouth, teeth or lips; huge appetite leading to heart issues or obesity; excess ear wax; tongue, mouth and esophageal cancer (with Saturn or Nodes); slows liver function; rich blood. Enhances fertility and milk production.

Surgical Tip: Transit Jupiter in Taurus is surgically protective to bodily regions governed by Virgo and Capricorn. In theory, Jupiter should protect Taurus regions, although it is equally likely to produce hemorrhage or fluidic blockage. The transit trine is safer.

Virgo: Slows liver function; "picky" liver; enlarged liver; upper intestinal bloating; enlarged or distended duodenum, increased tendency toward diabetes, imbalance of duodenal, pancreatic and liver enzymes. Bile release is either "dry" or disturbed. Sometimes excessive bile (jaundice), or enlarged spleen. Hernia. If happy, good intestines! Hypothetically, should enhance immunity unless severely afflicted.

Surgical Tip: Transit Jupiter in Virgo is naturally protective to surgery for bodily regions ruled by Taurus and Capricorn. In theory, Jupiter in Virgo would protect Virgo regions too, although this position could equally indicate hemorrhage, fatty or fluidic pressure, or "uncooperative" loose or bulging, prolapsed intestines. The transit trine is safer.

Capricorn: Slows liver; produces too little or too much bile; jaundice; skin growths; oily skin; plugged skin glands; enlarged or swollen knees; growths on knees; slippery ligaments or tendons; obesity disturbs knees; trick knee; weak cartilage; big bones; either strengthens or weakens bone structure (much depends on natal aspects between Jupiter and Saturn). If positive, can improve or heal knee, joint and skin issues.

Surgical Tip: Transit Jupiter in Capricorn is surgically protective to the bodily regions governed by Taurus and Virgo. In theory, Capricorn's body regions should be protected too, although Jupiter could equally signal pressure, impaction or hemorrhage. The transit trine is safer.

Jupiter in Air Signs

Gemini: Scatters thought, increases capillary circulation and pressure in capillary bed. Shoulder dislocation; hyper-mobility of shoulder, arm, or hand ligaments. Speech disturbance, lung tumor (possibly benign), cysts, excess fluids or blood in respiratory tract, blood clots in lungs, strong arms, large hands, enlarged lungs, fatty growths in Gemini regions.

Surgical Tip: Transit Jupiter in Gemini is quite helpful for surgery to bodily regions ruled by Libra and Aquarius. Jupiter is, in theory, protective to Gemini body parts although could equally bring excess fluidic pressure, swelling, or displacement to Gemini parts. The transit trine is safer.

Libra: Fatty or enlarged kidneys, excessive urination, ovarian tumors or cysts, slipped lumbar discs, excess release of one of the adrenal hormones and resultant problems, lumbar fat gain "love handles."

Surgical Tip: Transit Jupiter in Libra assists surgery for bodily regions ruled by Gemini and Aquarius. In theory, Jupiter in Libra is protective to Libra regions, although it could equally signal, swelling, hemorrhage, circulatory obstruction or, lumbar pressure. The transit trine is safer.

Aquarius: Varicose veins are a hallmark, when occurring natally! Large shins; excess fluid in lower leg; dislocated ankle; lower leg thrombosis, slippery tendons or ligaments in ankle and shin; shin bones either too long or short; odd blood issues; if positive: good legs; improves circulation and oxygenation of blood, plethora, circulatory disturbances.

Field Note: For decades, when viewing a prominent and/or afflicted Jupiter in Aquarius in adults of all ages, I inquire, "Do you have varicose veins?" An affirmative (and surprised!) response is so typical that I would rate this effect at 80%.

Surgical Tip: Transit Jupiter in Aquarius is beneficial for surgery in bodily regions governed by Gemini and Libra. While in theory it is protective to Aquarian regions, Jupiter's placement in Aquarius could also warn of hemorrhage, traveling clots from lower leg, and/or swelling, or fatty blockages of vessels in legs. The transit trine is safer.

Jupiter in Water Signs

Cancer: Jupiter is exalted in Cancer; produces huge appetites, and "beer belly." Water and gas bloating is common. Fertile! Jupiter in this sign exerts a strong influence on pituitary function.

Jupiter in Cancer influences breast growth in either direction. It would be interesting to note if Jupiter in Cancer natives have statistically more or less breast cancer. (Jupiter protects but also grows!) In my clientele it is rare.

Field Note: Jupiter is hirsute in Water, and bald in Fire! It is common for men born with Jupiter in Cancer (and sometimes Pisces, Scorpio and Taurus) to maintain full heads of thick hair well into their advanced years. Obviously, this cannot be true in all cases, but it is conspicuous. What could be the connection between Jupiter's element and hair?

Jupiter governs fat; the sex hormones require fats. Jupiter rules the pituitary gland *(Edgar Cayce)*, with the help of Cancer and Capricorn *(Cornell)*. Both pituitary rulerships work well in practice. This gland plays a strong role in many aspects of sexual development.

Water sign Scorpio governs the genitalia, whereas, sexual pleasure is ruled by Pisces. The most fertile signs are Taurus, Cancer and Pisces, followed by Scorpio. Taurus is the "exaltation of the Moon," the bringer of moisture.

Hypothesis: The female sex hormones best receive the oils they require when Jupiter moves through either the Water signs or the home of the Moon's exaltation, Taurus. The hormones linked to male hair retention may benefit from this connection!

Field Note 2: Cancer rules the stomach. One slender friend, born with Jupiter in Cancer, is always mistaken for being pregnant, even though she's not—to the continual embarrassment of all.

Surgical Tip: Transit Jupiter in Cancer is protective for surgery to bodily regions ruled by Scorpio and Pisces. Jupiter in Cancer in theory is protective to Cancer regions but could equally produce fluidic profusion, hemorrhage and swelling. The transit trine is safer.

Scorpio: Transit Jupiter in Scorpio is associated with profuse urination or bowel movements, excess sexual activity, size extremes of sex organs, large bladder, prolapsed bladder or uterus, uncontrolled urination, bed wetting, uterine or bladder tumors, colon polyps or tumors; large nose, excess sweating, hemorrhoids, boils, groin hernia, prolapsed rectum or vagina, testicular swelling, enlarged prostate.

Surgical Tip: Jupiter's transit of Scorpio is protective to surgery in bodily regions ruled by Cancer and Pisces. In theory, Jupiter would also protect Scorpio regions. However, it is equally possible that Jupiter signals hemorrhage; prolapsed vessels, or excessive fatty or fluidic pressure to Scorpio body parts. The transit trine is safer.

Field Note 1: One friend was born with natal Jupiter conjunct both Neptune and the North Node in Scorpio on her Nadir. Her bladder would come under so much sudden pressure that when she had to urinate, there had better be a toilet immediately nearby!

Field Note 2: Jupiter in Water, for night or sunset births, and especially so when simultaneously positioned under the horizon inclines to breadth and obesity.

Pisces: Excessive blood cholesterol (liver makes too much); liver functions are sloppy or excessive; lymphatic pressure, engorged lymph nodes, glandular swellings, pituitary related growth extremes, large feet, mega-obesity, fluidic build up; increases phlegmatic conditions; glandular extremes; excess sleep; excess sex.

Pisces lacks boundaries, so Jupiter in this sign goes to extremes. Pisces is also a bit sloppy, so Jupiter brings disorganization of glandular coordination. Because Pisces rules the lymph system, Jupiter here is possibly an immune system protector! Increases fertility.

Surgical Tip: Jupiter's transit of Pisces is protective to surgery in bodily regions ruled by Cancer and Scorpio (with other testimonies). In theory, Jupiter would also protect Pisces regions. However, it is equally possible that Jupiter signals hemorrhage and profusion of blood or fluidic pressure to the feet. Because Pisces and Cancer govern the lymph system, Jupiter's transit in Water signs may offer extra protection for surgery to the lymph nodes. Good for prayer and all manner of spiritual protection!

JUPITER'S TRANSITS TO NATAL PLANETS

Applicable to both natal and transit charts, these partial lists of expressed symptoms apply only to predisposed nativities. These conditions are obviously uncommon and require multiple testimonies beyond the presence of Jupiter. Manifestation of symptoms may be enhanced by lifestyle choices, and taking preemptive measures can reduce, remove or prevent potential issues from manifesting. It is not possible to list all potential expressions.

JUPITER'S CONJUNCTIONS
Health Potentials for Predisposed Nativities
Not all transits manifest as health concerns or benefits.

Transit Jupiter Conjunct Natal Sun
Significantly raises the vital force. Energizing, hopeful, and expansive. Arterial circulation increases, warms, dilates, giving the heart more oxygen. However, more fat can travel to heart vessels. This transit may warn of migraine, high blood pressure, aneurism or stroke, especially if in Air or Fire signs. Strongly associated in Fire with and hyperadrenalism, especially with involvement from Mars.

Positive: A healthy time all around! Often signals a reprieve or miraculous cure.

Surgical Tip: Normally, Jupiter protects the life, the brain, heart and eyes. If negative, this could signal a surfeit of blood or hemorrhage to these same regions. One would need to assess the whole natal chart and all existing transits.

Herbal Note: Professional herbalists use a wide array of carefully selected cardiac herbs to control hypertension, blood plethora, migraine, etc. Hawthorne, Garlic, Rosemary, Angelica, Motherwort and Linden are cardiac favorites. Feverfew, Rosemary, and Cayenne for migraine. Do not self-treat.

Field Note: Three startlingly similar cases of hyperthyroid. Two cases of natal Sun conjunct Jupiter in Sagittarius in the 6th house (Cancer Ascendant) in hard aspect from Mars to Sun-Jupiter. A third case, also with Sun conjunct Jupiter in Sagittarius in hard aspect to Mars, but in the natal 4th house.

The first two folks almost died of hyperthyroid. One was saved through sipping gold solution through a straw (1950s), the other had the thyroid gland nuked out of all usefulness (1990s). The third individual had self-induced hyperthyroid from eating too many iodine-laced chocolates in Catholic school (following the nun with the candy tray around). He had the thyroid removed.

This is one prime example of how medical astrology can solve medical puzzles and also bring to light neglected connections. Hyperthyroid and hyper-adrenalin are both complaints common to the "Mutable Fire" sign Sagittarius. "Mutable" means transitioning moving. Thus, Sagittarius governs wild fire-type energy. Both above conditions produce accelerating heat with a marked fight/ flight response and resultant hyper-vigilant nervousness. Sagittarius governs the lower spinal nerves and sciatic nerves, and influences the entire central nervous system.

Sagittarius is curiously positioned at the exact pinnacle of two quincunxes with signs Taurus and Cancer. A quincunx is the preeminent health-watch angle of 150°, indicating a disconnection between the functions of the two signs involved.

In this case, Taurus rules the region of the thyroid, and Cancer rules the posterior pituitary. It is my personal conjecture that Cancer may also govern the emotional and memory processing systems of the amygdala, hypothalamus, and hippocampus.

Jupiter-in-Sagittarius, configured with Mars and/or the Sun, seems uniquely prone to "hyper" conditions, panic, manias, hyperactivity, ADHD and the "flight" end of the fight/flight polarity. To reason out why this is so, one must research the neural-hormonal links between Jupiter, Mars and Sun as related to the Taurus-Cancer double quincunx to the spinal-nerve sign, Sagittarius.

Transit Jupiter Conjunct Natal Moon

Fertile! If a woman is wanting a baby, this transit can help. Increases estrogenic hormones, enhances milk production, grows breast tissue; increases menstrual flow and therefore not welcome for sufferers of menorrhagia. Increases appetite and water retention, weight gain, pleasantly warms stomach, though can signify bloating. Produces emotional strain—one would think this a cheering aspect, but when in Water and Earth signs, it seems to produce considerable emotional pressure and floods of tears.

When positive, this transit antidotes Saturn's natal ray upon the Moon and therefore quite welcome for sufferers of atrophy; emaciation; weakness; infertility; fear; tension; depression; dryness.

Field Note: I've observed several cases of natal Jupiter-Moon conjunctions in Water and Earth signs corresponding with menorrhagia so severe that the uterus was removed. This combination is prone to endometriosis and fibroids, every bit as much as is the Saturn-Moon conjunction. Jupiter's transit conjunction of Moon can "hatch" this predisposition in a natal chart. Watery tumors are also common, usually benign, but not always.

Surgical and Medical Tip: In theory, Jupiter's conjunction of the Moon is protective to childbirth, breast and stomach surgery and some forms of brain and eye surgery.

However, the trine is preferable because Jupiter by conjunction can also produce excessive fluidic pressure, hemorrhage, uncooperative or slippery vessels and excessive swelling.

Much depends on the condition of natal Jupiter and his aspects to the natal Moon. Transit Jupiter conjunct the natal Moon in Earth signs (especially Taurus and Capricorn) can be obstructive and slowing in childbirth, especially if retrograding back over the Moon. Be alert that the cord does not wrap around the neck.

Herbal Note: Professional herbalists relieve excessive fluidic pressure with diuretic herbs including watermelon seeds, Burdock, and Cornsilk.

For clearing the breast lymphatics: Dandelion Root. Edgar Cayce discusses the homeopathic remedy Cimex for edema. Mullein is a specific for reducing glandular swellings. Do not self-treat.

Transit Jupiter Conjunct Natal Mercury

Jupiter's expansive nature is naturally discombobulating to Mercury. This is not particularly good for the naturally forgetful, or if one suffers any number of neurologically disorganizing conditions. However, Jupiter can also be healing to the mind and nerves! Much depends on the condition of natal Jupiter and its interaction with natal Mercury in the birth chart. If they are in a harmonious trine or sextile aspect, the negative impact of this transit is lessened.

The positivity of the interaction also depends on the natal condition of Jupiter, and the current aspects it is receiving. If natal Jupiter rules malefic houses (6, 8, 12), and/or is badly aspected in the natal chart, or debilitated by sign placement, or is currently receiving difficult aspects, then his transit conjunction of natal Mercury is troubling.

Conversely, if one has a brilliantly placed natal Jupiter, and/or it is currently receiving nice transits too, then the transit conjunction of Jupiter to natal Mercury can be healing and helpful to Mercury-type complaints (neural, perceptive, sensory or mental issues). Cheering. This transit is quite useful should one need to rebuild the fatty protection of the nerves, and/or "oil the brain."

Surgical Tip: In theory, transit Jupiter conjunct natal Mercury would be surgically protective to Mercury's bodily regions (peripheral nerves, hands, fingers, arms, speech and hearing centers of brain). However, Jupiter's trine is preferred because the conjunction can sometimes signal fluidic pressure, engorgement or hemorrhage. This might obfuscate a surgeon's attempt to work with or around delicate nerves or capillaries (both Mercury-ruled). Much depends on the relationship between natal Jupiter and Mercury, as well as natal Jupiter's relationship to the birth Ascendant.

Herbal Note: Saturn's grounding, mineral-rich herbs are good choices for professional herbalists in need of counteracting overly expansive Mercurial states. Oat Straw, Alfalfa, Parsley and Nettles are favorites. This is a perfect aspect for nourishing exhausted nerves! Fenugreek is a wonderful oily tonic for the exhausted. Borage with Oatstraw is a specific remedy from Matthew Wood for recovery from extreme nervous strain, or protracted stress exhaustion. Do not self treat.

Transit Jupiter Conjunct Natal Venus

This transit can produce fatty buildups, tumors, cysts and tissue growth anywhere, but typically in bodily regions ruled by the sign, or by Venus herself, such as the ovaries, breasts or kidneys. Increases female fertility. Raises libido in both sexes and increases sperm production. More oil is available to skin and hair. Productive of polyp growth for some signs, (e.g. colon polyps for Venus in Scorpio or vocal polyps for Venus in Taurus). This transit works for, or against those with arterial or venous issues, because it increases blood flow to relaxed conditions.

Field Note: Sagittarius and Jupiter both govern arteries, whereas Venus, with Aquarius, rules the veins. The Sun and Leo govern the heart. A client suffered an aortic dissection on the precise day that transit Jupiter conjoined her natal Venus (in Sagittarius, 5th house of the heart), as transit Venus simultaneously conjoined her natal South Node (also in Sagittarius).

This happened ten days following a total eclipse precisely conjunct her natal Mars in early Leo, on the degrees ruling the aorta!

She also had natal Leo Moon and Ascendant, both under multiple stressors. Too many dominoes on the stack!

Surgical Tip: Theoretically, Jupiter's transit conjunction of natal Venus would protect surgery to the bodily regions ruled by Venus including breasts, ovaries, kidneys, veins, and vagina. However, Jupiter can also produce prolapse, hemorrhage and fluidic pressure. One must first judge the natal condition of Jupiter and its relationship to natal Venus. The transit trine of Jupiter to natal Venus is safest.

Herbal Note: Professional herbalists use many herbs for reducing hormonal cysts of the reproductive system including Red Clover, Poke Root, Dandelion and Cleavers. There are also excellent herbs for treating fatty kidney, excess urination, etc. Consult a professional herbalist and do not self-treat.

Transit Jupiter Conjunct Natal Mars

Jupiter's transit arouses high energy, strong libido. This is a spirited conjunction—think of a horse released from his stall! In Fire signs, hyperactive, hot tempered, impulsive, and rash. Heightens male hormones and virility, muscles enlarge; this is a lucky aspect for athletes! Increases adrenalin response; raises blood pressure, especially in Fire signs, but works for all.

Excessive drinking and partying is a common manifestation. This transit can stimulate the thyroid into overdrive, especially if occurring in Sagittarius, although some other signs are also prone. I've seen Jupiter-Mars hard aspects so frequently in the birth charts of those afflicted with Grave's Disease, hyperthyroid, etc., that I consider it a rule. This is odd, because neither planet governs the thyroid, yet it supports the notion that adrenal hormones and/or "internal fire" running wild can prompt hyperthyroid maladies.

Surgical Tip: Theoretically, Jupiter's transit of natal Mars supports and protects surgery to nose, male genitalia and muscles in general, although the sign ruling the body zone of the muscle must be consulted. However, Jupiter's transit can cause bleeding or spurting of arteries.

Generally, a lucky time for surgery because Mars rules the surgeon's knife. This time is quite effective for testosterone treatment or adrenalin support. Iron increases, so this is an excellent time for anemia treatment. Rejuvenation!

Field Note: One of my students reported on his recent experience with transit Jupiter conjoining his natal Mars-Sun conjunction in Sagittarius: "I feel like I'm lit on fire from within. Its amazing! My energy is astonishing, endless!" I recall Davidson reporting that natal Mars in Sagittarius had "too much life."

Herbal Note: Bugleweed, Ashwaganda, Lemon Balm and Motherwort are traditional herbs for symptoms of hyperthyroid. Chaste Tea Berry is noted to inhibit excess libido. Yarrow is indispensable for internal or external hemorrhage or bleeding. Do not self-treat.

Transit Jupiter Conjunct Natal Jupiter

Unclear. May emphasize or increase any meanings or issues of natal Jupiter. The bodily regions ruled by the sign of natal Jupiter are highlighted. Hypothetically, this "Jupiter Return" could be an important pivot point for the liver or pituitary gland, or their cycles. Jupiter's 11.8 year cycle ends as another commences.

Transit Jupiter Conjunct Natal Saturn

Typically, this is a strengthening to the entire constitution, although one also must examine the natal Jupiter-Saturn interrelationship. The transit trine aspect of Jupiter to natal Saturn is safer. This conjunction produces expansion and fluidic pressure (Jupiter) upon hardened or stuck areas (as suggested by natal Saturn), usually in the sign regions of natal Saturn.

Increased blood flow can loosen up tight regions; potentially brings better nutrition for bones; halts atrophy; brings oil to dry skin, nails, hair or the bodily regions ruled by the sign of natal Saturn; skin emollient.

Being fatty, this conjunction is welcome to those who wish to gain weight. This transit can also clog the gallbladder, or be productive of gallstones due to a sudden increase in bile. This aspect may bring overweight, causing more pressure to bones and cartilage.

However, it nourishes bones, ligaments and tendons; warms where cold, oils where stiff.

Field Note: One friend sprang an anal thrombosis (clot) during the exact conjunction of transit Jupiter to his natal Saturn-in-Scorpio, sign ruler of the anus!

Surgical and Medical Tips: In theory, Jupiter's transit of natal Saturn would be perfect for bone and skin surgeries and knee replacements. Jupiter can cause physician miscalculations, dis-organization, bleeding, swelling.

Herbal Note: Specific herbs exist for relieving plethoric con-gestion in any area of the body (to be indicated by the sign of this conjunction). Consult a professional herbalist—do not attempt to self-treat. Yarrow and Rosemary are reputed to equalize circulation.

Danger: This aspect can bring about cellular proliferation, cell-ular changes and potential cancer if Saturn's position in the horo-scope is not addressed prior and during. Worse, when transit Jupiter retrogrades over natal Saturn. Knowing this, one can act to preempt.

Transit Jupiter Conjunct Natal Uranus

This long-term aspect is unclear. Jupiter's somewhat chaotic influence could amp up electrical charges, which are ruled by Uranus, with a possibility of spasm, epilepsy, tremor or heart palpitation and electrolyte imbalance. It may also have unpredictable effects upon electrical discharges. Potentially some influence upon thyroid function, or potential growth of thyroid nodules. Positively, assists in cases of paralysis or seizure, bringing welcome reprieve.

Surgical and Medical Tips: This combination produces and encourages extremes (Uranus). May be miracle prone! It might reverse paralysis or awaken blocked electrical current, thus return-ing function.

Transit Jupiter Conjunct Natal Neptune

This transit increases psychic states in those so prone and opens the door to astral influence. Those divorced from Earth plane reality may drift even farther from the shore. Tempts self-medication, and addiction, helping little to regulate behavior. Neptune governs opiates and alcohol, so one might expect an increase of drinking or marijuana use.

Avoid mixing alcohol and drugs together or with swimming, hot tubs or boating. This is that careless "beer and boating" trip without life vests. Problems arise from foolish inattentiveness. A time to review the dose and type of chemical combinations ingested. Produces an engorging influence upon the lymph system, requiring lymph moving herbs or therapies.

Surgical and Medical Tips: Should clotting be a problem, this aspect could produce leaky-bleeding episodes. Be wary of mixed combinations of chemical drugs or drugs plus alcohol, wine plus ibuprofen, etc.

This conjunction can also produce miracles through prayer and angelic intervention. It is sometimes called the "thank the Lord" aspect! Positive for vibrational healing, homeopathy, Bach Flower Essences, music therapy. Great for shamanic practitioners!

Herbal Note: Lymphatic assisting herbs include Poke Root, Red Root, Dandelion Root, Burdock Root, Cleavers, Beets, Violet, Fenugreek (oily). The excess laxity produced by this aspect can be counteracted with Saturnian astringents specific to the bodily regions ruled by the sign of the conjunction. Mars-ruled stimulants may also assist. Do not self-treat.

Transit Jupiter Conjunct Natal Pluto

Unclear. We do not yet know enough about Pluto to truly designate his medical properties. To date astrologers have not observed him through the entire zodiac.

If there is sepsis or bacterial invasion, Jupiter could either protect the body or increase the bacterial proliferation! Why? Because Jupiter is protective but is also a warm and generous planet who increases anything he touches!

Jupiter might prove lucky or protective for radiation therapy of the body part ruled by the sign of this conjunction, and also to the body regions ruled by the two signs of same element that trine this sign. This aspect could suggest "success with radical measures."

Conversely, this conjunction could encourage a rapid proliferation of parasites, especially if occurring in Scorpio, Virgo or Pisces.

Surgical and Medical Tips: Unclear. One testimony of success for dangerous, radical therapies, radiation treatment, laser, organ transplants etc. More testimonies must simultaneously apply. However, should a staph or strep infection proliferate within the body part of the sign ruled by a transit Jupiter in hard aspect to natal Pluto, this could be a real doozie because Jupiter increases growth.

Transit Jupiter Conjunct Natal North Node

One receives a generous dollop of Jupiter's cosmic blue ray when Jupiter transits the natal North Node. A very fertile aspect!

If positive, this stimulates growth and weight gain as needed. This signals the long-awaited growth spurt for the growth-retarded teenager! Weight gain likely in the bodily regions ruled by this sign, or those trined. In Water signs gives water retention or cysts. Tumors are also more likely in all elements, especially in Earth signs. This transit is an excellent counteractive to atrophy, malnutrition and restricted circulation.

Field Note: Multiple times a yearning couple approaches me, anxious as to when they might conceive a baby. Should transit Jupiter be soon approaching either's Lunar North Node (especially that of the intended mother), I confidently state that conception is soon likely, provided the body is viable, and the rest of the chart agrees. The vast majority of these cases are rewarded with happy conception and parents asking, "How did you do that?"

Surgical and Medical Tips: A prime aspect for increasing weight and strength. Be careful of fertility drugs unless you prefer triplets. Miracle surgeries can occur because one strongly receives the protective incoming rays of Jupiter.

Herbal Note: Mullein is a specific herb for relieving glandular congestion and swelling. Do not self treat.

Jupiter's Versus Saturn's Role in Toxicity and Cancer: If at the time of Jupiter's transit to the natal North Node, one already suffers from any excessive condition in the body part governed by the sign of the natal North Node (or perhaps anywhere), Jupiter increases it unless antidoted!

Fatty arterial build ups, venous clots, vessel blockages, high blood pressure. Bloat, edema, diabetes, tumors, or worms—all receive growth potential and must be efficiently counteracted throughout this transit! Jupiter will not stop the growth of brain or other tumors. In fact, he can promote them! However, Jupiter will protect any bodily zone he passes through or trines. This protective function renders him less dangerous when conjunct the natal North Node than natal Saturn or the outer planets.

Both Jupiter and Saturn can trap toxins but for very different reasons! Saturn traps toxins through impaired circulation and/or condensing, hardening and walling off wastes. Conversely, Jupiter creates heightened blood flow, obesity, excess lipids and engorgement. If blood and lymphatic circulation and excretion are impaired, then the portal circulation (under Jupiter) backs up, clots form, etc. In this manner, one sees Jupiter involved in various cancers as much as is Saturn! Traditionally, Jupiterian caused tumors tend to be more benign, but I cannot vouch for this.

Herbal Note: This is a good transit to preempt. There are many herbs available to cleanse toxic matter that is building up in various organs. Note the bodily region ruled by the sign of the natal North Node. Consult a professional herbalist and do not self-treat.

Transit Jupiter Conjunct Natal South Node

This aspect is not the reverse of the transit South Node's conjunction of natal Jupiter, as one might suppose. Here, transit Jupiter is triggering off the natal meanings of the South Node in the natal chart. Many interpretations are possible, depending on what houses natal Jupiter rules, because all things signified by Jupiter in the natal chart will also be crossing this celestial exit point (the South Node). Medically, the South Node represents leaks, weakness, deficiency or loss. Jupiter's arrival here can either activate the leak, or conversely offer a life raft by revealing or protecting you from the leak!

Positively, Jupiter's passage of the South Node much assists in ridding the body of unwanted matter or weight. The Lunar South Node is famous for its deep psychological effects and past life recall, genuine or otherwise. This seems very apt once you witness enough clients heading off for the Zen Monastery under this aspect. Therefore, watch for doors opening to obscure memories and all that may imply. Schizophrenics, dysthymics (persistent depressive disorder), and paranoid persons must be carefully monitored at this time!

Because Jupiter is the general significator of offspring, this transit is notably infertile, and miscarriage prone. Neither is it a good time to put on weight. However, it is excellent for weight loss and for relieving excess water retention—although not as reliable as its reverse aspect, the transit South Node crossing natal Jupiter.

This aspect so often relates more to psychological than physical health. However, if occurring in the "whole sign" 1st, 6th, or 8th houses, first define the precise physical weakness or deficiency suggested by that sign! You can safely assume that this weakness will be pointed out at this time. Perhaps Jupiter can bring a lucky, remarkable, or spiritual cure at this time. Keep in mind that both Nodes can indicate genetically inherited disease.

Jupiter's passage over this point, or any major planet or eclipse, can hatch a problem, especially if the problem is related to Jupiter's train of diseases: diabetes, obesity, high blood pressure, liver disease, pituitary issues, etc. The sign of the natal South Node is essential to note during this transit.

Field Note: As a youth, I visited a venerable old astrologer, Virginia Dayan, who after drawing my chart in white chalk upon her black board, pointed through a dense cloud of cigarette smoke, and casually pronounced: "Loss through foolishness." This simple truth has remained a part of my consulting arsenal for decades.

So often, it is literal. One client experienced Jupiter's transit to her South Node in Aries in the 11th house. She partied for three days, until she fell off a second story balcony and hit her head! (Aries rules the head). Voila!

Surgical Tip: Unless the responsible physician recommends

otherwise, surgery of any kind is not advisable at this time, nor until transit Jupiter is well past the natal South Node and not going to retrograde back over it. If surgery is imperative, refer to *Astrology & Your Vital Force, Chapter 18.*

Transit Jupiter Conjunct Natal Ascendant

First, be certain the Ascendant is really true. This long-term aspect signifies growth and expansion, for good or ill, most especially to the regions governed by the Ascendant's sign. Effects last for the duration of Jupiter's transit through the Ascendant sign, though are more pronounced within 3° of the true Ascendant degree. Some natives gain weight. Expect a growth spurt for young persons.

Generally health-giving. However, if the Ascendant is Capricorn, Virgo, or Gemini, this transit can present major Jupiterian maladies. This tip from Jyotish has proven itself out in practice multiple times. *(See following Field Note.)*

Field Note: A friend who was naturally of great weight, nearly died when Jupiter transited his Ascendant in Virgo. He topped 400 pounds at this time, and nearly suffocated himself in his sleep, forcing him to slumber in a sitting position.

JUPITER'S SQUARE
Health Potentials for Predisposed Nativities
Not all transits manifest as health concerns or benefits.

Jupiter's transit square (90°) brings excess to any natal planet squared. This is observed to be somewhat chaotic, discombobulating, and wild for that planet's natural functions, not dissimilar to effects observed from Uranus or Neptune!

Jupiter's square is similar to his conjunction, yet perhaps more event prone. Jupiter's square packs a punch that his conjunction does not, often forcing an increase of functions governed by the natal planet so squared. Read the conjunctions and add the concept of **excess in action**. Squares always bring action in the physical plane! A square's stimulus comes from the sign that Jupiter transits through, and is felt by the natal planet and sign receiving the square.

Transit Jupiter Square Natal Sun

Disperses, over-taxes or diffuses the native's vital force. Usually manifests as too much to do or being pulled in multiple directions (especially if in the mutable signs). The heart is overtaxed. The brain may experience a surfeit of blood or overheat. Can increase pressure to the eyes. Counteract with reduced activities and slowing down. Avoid significant travel.

Transit Jupiter Square Natal Moon

Noted for discombobulating the general health and throwing off habitual rhythms. Diet and routine are disturbed. Emotionally and hormonally chaotic at close orb. This is a good time to embrace temperance, avoid overindulging on rich foods, regulate the diet, and support hormonal and circulatory balances. According to the old books, "A poor time to begin anything new, move or travel."

Transit Jupiter Square Natal Mercury

This transit confuses the mental focus. Jupiter's expansive nature is not so good for tax accounting and other mentally exacting Mercurial tasks! Students are distracted—"I don't feel like studying." The mind is pulled away into multifarious interests. This square can exacerbate mania, schizophrenia, epilepsy and many neurological conditions.

Transit Jupiter Square Natal Venus

The blood sugar may suddenly raise or lower. Blood copper levels shift. This transit is somewhat disorganizing to female hormones, with an obvious wide range of possible results. This is a good time to have an overall check of breasts, ovaries, testes and hormonal balances.

This square potentially increases either venous pressure or relaxation, enhancing varicosities or hemorrhoids, (especially if between Aquarius and Scorpio). In those prone, kidney function may increase, or one may experience a congestion of the renal circulation. There is a tendency for undisciplined indulgence in wine, sex, song, and sugar.

Transit Jupiter Square Natal Mars

Jupiter's transit square of Mars produces passionate extremes, influencing the instincts and lust for life. Excites temper, anger, libido and action; accident prone; increases tendency to alcohol consumption, and foolish actions. May incite excessive release of adrenal hormones, testosterone.

This aspect heats the blood, increases arterial blood flow, and incites a need for greater aerobic exercise. Iron, Mars' metal, may become excessive or deficient. The energy level is strongly influenced, either up or down! This square increases blood flow to the muscles.

Transit Jupiter Square Natal Jupiter

This square influences Jupiterian functions: hormonal coordination, weight, growth, the liver processes. Being in square to its own natal position would indicate a pivot point in Jupiter's cycle.

Transit Jupiter Square Natal Saturn

Challenges Saturn to open up and stop being so rigid! Because Jupiter increases a warming blood-flow, this aspect improves some types of cold, rigid conditions.

This combination influences growth. Jupiter (growth) creates friction with natal Saturn (regulation of growth, and limitation to growth). Saturn is, after all "Father Time." Jupiter's transit could throw off the body's timing, producing unexpected menopause or puberty; growth or aging spurts; cessation of growth; excess hair or body growth. Jupiter's square can also awaken latent genetic or karmic disease.

Hypothetically, a strong square from transit Jupiter could stir the release of trapped toxins by improving the blood flow to the sign of the bodily region Saturn tenants. However, cleansing treatments undertaken now may induce sudden excessive or dangerous releases.

For example, Saturn rules heavy metals and has a great deal to do with the teeth. Removing one's old dental fillings at this transit might prove catastrophic (not in all cases). Mineral absorption and calcium metabolism are influenced at this time.

Transit Jupiter Square Natal Uranus

Electrical disturbances increase. Possible stimulation in rare cases of heart palpitations, seizures, spasm, tremors, or colic. Possible manifestation of strange visionary mental states or religious mania (rare). Crazy, stupid or unlucky accidents can occur e.g. sudden storm damage or losing control of the motorcycle. This is not a wise time for thoughtless risk: "Hey, let's go outside and watch the tornado!"

Transit Jupiter Square Natal Neptune

This square can produce a number of interesting effects including: flying in one's sleep, sleep walking, fairy visitations, chronic fantasizing, disorganized life, and addictions. Stimulates grandiosity and visionary states, and trance. Increases imagination, escapism and idealism, and may provoke excessive marijuana or alcohol use "I dunno...I just felt like taking up smoking...."

Significant author Eileen Nauman cites this combination as being involved in blood diseases: leukemia, leukopenia, and anemia.

Possible tumor growth and cellular changes. Watch benign tumors closely at this time. Keep the lymphatic fluids moving by getting enough exercise. This transit has the ability to upset glandular coordination.

Transit Jupiter Square Natal Pluto

Unclear. Wide open to research.

JUPITER'S TRINES AND SEXTILES
Health Potentials for Predisposed Nativities
Not all transits manifest as health concerns or benefits.

This book's focus is pathology. The trine (120°) and sextile (60°) of Jupiter are his "good" aspects, rarely fomenting health issues. In Jyotish tradition, Jupiter's forward trine is his strongest aspect and almost always viewed as protective and helpful!

Jupiter's trines and sextiles both work wonders, and are useful for surgical timing. Therefore, I've devoted this section partially to that usage. His sextile is less reliable, but still helpful, especially within tight orb.

JUPITER'S TRANSIT TRINES

Regarding Trine Orbs: The two entire signs in trine or sextile to one another can be used for timing purposes. However, "the closer the orb, the better!"

In surgery, Jupiter's transit trine offers potent protection to the bodily regions ruled by the both the natal planet and sign he currently trines.

Note: All Jupiter's trines to the trans-Saturnian planets must be supported by multiple testimonies from other planetary transits and natal conditions in order to render a sure effect.

Transit Jupiter Trine Natal Sun

Best transit for surgery to brain, eyes, heart. However, multiple testimonies are required to support this aspect. Raises the vital force. Good for convalescence.

Transit Jupiter Trine Natal Moon

Best transit for surgery to brain, eyes, stomach, womb, breast, lung. However, multiple testimonies are required to support this aspect. Very fertile, especially in Water and Earth signs.

Fattening. This transit encourages growth of tumors and cysts, especially if natal Venus is involved by conjunction, sextile or trine, and more so in Earth and Water signs! Enhances energy, contentment, and the sense of well-being.

Transit Jupiter Trine Natal Mercury

Best transit for surgery or nourishment to nerves, hands, arms, fingers, capillaries, ears, bronchial tubes, lungs, speech centers of brain. However, multiple testimonies are required to support this aspect. Improves mental energy and function.

Transit Jupiter Trine Natal Venus

Best transit for surgery or nourishment of ovaries, kidneys, veins, breasts. However, multiple testimonies are required to support this aspect. Can encourage growth of tumors and cysts, especially if the Moon is involved by conjunction, sextile, or trine, and more so in Earth and Water signs. Fertile.

Transit Jupiter Trine Natal Jupiter

This is a generally helpful period in the 11.8 year Jupiter cycle. Can improve any issues distinct to Jupiter or the sign he natally tenants. Jupiter rules fat, and is the general ruler of the liver (with Virgo), the arteries (with Sagittarius), and the pituitary (with Cancer and Capricorn). However, multiple testimonies are required to support this aspect.

Transit Jupiter Trine Natal Saturn

Best transit for surgery or nourishment to bones, skin, nerves. Strengthening. A fine time for tonifying elderly or frail persons. However, multiple testimonies are required to support this aspect.

Note that all trines to Outer Planets must be supported by multiple testimonies from other planetary transits and supportive natal conditions.

Transit Jupiter Trine Natal Uranus

Best transit for nourishment of or surgery to electrical system of body (little is actually known about this system). May bring miraculous assistance or treatment for paralysis, seizure, spasms, tremor, and puzzling neurological diseases.

Note that all trines to outer planets must be supported by multiple testimonies from other planetary transits and supportive natal conditions.

Transit Jupiter Trine Natal Neptune

A wonderful transit for sleep and meditation assistance. This is one testimony of success for vibrational treatments such as music therapy, homeopathy and flower essences. Supports spiritual treatments: prayer, angelic intervention. Brings miracles! Jupiter-Neptune trines open doors, provide useful psychic information, circumventing of red tape, etc. (Grandma's ghost appears, and hands you a sacred herb.)

Transit Jupiter Trine Natal Pluto

Not much is yet known of Pluto's physical expressions. Theoretically this aspect would be protective for laser and radiation therapy; recovery from all radical treatments including chemotherapy; anti-sepsis (not always, because Jupiter can assist the growth of nearly anything!); transplant surgery (anti-rejection); gender reassignment; cosmetic surgeries for correction of devastating injury.

JUPITER'S TRANSIT SEXTILES
Health Potentials for Predisposed Nativities
Not all transits manifest as health concerns or benefits.

Treat this 60° aspect as a half-strength trine. Although weaker in protective clout, Jupiter's sextiles have more "zing" than trines, and are less potentially stagnating.

Sextiles are thought to be more potent for any two signs in sextile that "hear" or "see" each other (i.e., signs equidistant from the 0° cardinal axis—examples are Taurus-Pisces or Gemini-Leo).

Sextiles are also strongest from signs that share planetary "reception." Example: Scorpio-Capricorn—Mars rules Scorpio and is exalted in Capricorn, one of two signs positioned in sextile to Scorpio. Therefore this specific sextile is a potent one!

JUPITER'S OPPOSITION
Health Potentials for Predisposed Nativities
Not all transits manifest as health concerns or benefits.

Jupiter's transit pulls at the energy of any planet it opposes. This reduces the "prana" of this planet, thus weakening in some cases. However, it can also be quite positive!

The "Great Benefic," Jupiter shines his beneficent ray upon the opposite sign, house and any natal planet located there. Theoretically, this is good for that planet! This principle certainly works for careers: folks born with a dignified natal Jupiter on their Nadir, and thus opposite the Midheaven (that preeminent career point), typically have brilliant careers!

Any large planet in transit opposition pulls upon any natal planet, especially the small ones.

For instance, transit Saturn's opposition can bring the function of the opposed natal planet to a halt! Because Jupiter spends approximately one year in each sign, with long retrograde stretches, Jupiter's opposition can toggle back and forth for months!

This aspect is always a bit chaotic for the opposed planet, bringing wild swings and surprises, and wholesale events. In observation, Jupiter's transit appears to possess some of the traits of Uranus (extremes, surprises), and Neptune (poor boundaries, loose control, sloppy).

Jupiter's opposition can sometimes signify a lucky break coming from a medical or angelic intervention, inspiration, insightful diagnosis or treatment. Protection and/or rescue can arrive through spouses, elders, teachers, grandparents, ministers, priests, and doctors, provided the chart gives more supportive testimonies.

When Jupiter opposes a planet, he brings ups and downs, good and bad, storms and fair weather. Remember, Thor, the old Viking's Jupiter, is a storm God! Jupiter's "great red spot" is. in fact, a giant storm!

Oppositions can produce extremely variant effects. The two opposing planets can either become divorced from each other, or happy partners! Obviously, this makes analysis of possible health effects difficult. Your key is to watch the presenting symptoms and see which way the wind blows.

In all cases, the sign polarity of opposition is emphasized. See *Chapter 3: Aspect Mechanics* for help deciphering the sign polarity involved in any considered opposition.

General Field Note: A purely natal opposition between Jupiter and Saturn is often seen in migraine and bipolar disorder. Here we see medical astrology so perfectly illustrated!

Jupiter expands following Saturn's contraction, and vice versa. *Up and down and away we go!* Jupiter's transit opposition can produce similar effects on a hopefully temporary basis. Astute balance of both principals is required.

Transit Jupiter Opposes Natal Sun

This aspect strongly pulls against the native's vital force, creating fatigue, especially in tight orb. Dangerous for heart patients and the frail elderly. May indicate the arrival of a helpful doctor, healer, teacher, spouse or social worker!

Transit Jupiter Opposes Natal Moon

This transit pulls against the flow of the native's vital force. Disorganizing effects on memory, menses, energy, fluid balance. May reduce the blood's nourishing function or distribute nutrients unevenly. Lymphatic imbalances. This is problematic for those with lung, mental and hormonal complaints. There may be a disorganizing effect on the menses or menorrhagia.

There is some influence on stomach, breasts and womb, though not always negative! For instance, a dry natal Capricorn Moon, (so typical of sensitive stomach, infertility, or uterine fibroids) may receive the needed reprieve from the transit opposition of moist, warming Jupiter acting through opposite sign Cancer (a moist, Water sign governing the stomach and breasts). Because it is an opposition, this reprieve comes from without. For instance, a helpful person may arrive, such as a physician, teacher, social worker, midwife, or spouse; or a miracle of grace.

This transit is not necessarily bad for fertility, because the opposition still shines Jupiter's light on the Moon from the opposite sign. However, it could pull against the Moon in some cases, disorganizing a current pregnancy, or weakening the womb's hold.

Transit Jupiter Opposes Natal Mercury

Confusing and draining to mental function; exacerbates symptoms associated with poor coordination. This transit impacts speech, memory, dementia, Alzheimer's, neural speed, small focus clerical or detail work, reliability.

This opposition can bring medical knowledge and health assistance because Jupiter's ray faces natal Mercury as would a teacher or partner. This might be helpful to people with autism and other significant cognitive disabilities.

Transit Jupiter Opposes Natal Venus

Jupiter now pulls energy away from Venus while simultaneously shining a beneficent ray upon her from the opposite sign. This presents an interpretive puzzle.

Certainly, this is an important transit for diabetics because Venus rules sugar. Blood sugar may become problematic, swinging unpredictably up or down. Jupiter is always a little chaotic in his effects. Recall his namesake god, Thor, hurler of thunder bolts?

The opposition to Venus influences those with kidney, breast or ovarian conditions, although it is difficult to ascertain if the influence is positive or negative! The symptoms will let you know. Jupiter's opposition can bring knowledge, diagnosis, good doctors and helpful assistance for Venus-ruled problems.

Transit Jupiter Opposes Natal Mars

Pulls energy away from Mars while simultaneously shining a beneficent ray upon him from the opposite sign! Therefore, it's hard to know the true influence as outcomes may vary. Important for athletes and those with issues involving iron, muscles, male regions, testosterone and adrenalin. Energy may zoom up or down, or both! One typically observes a great excitement of activity across the sign and house polarity of natal Mars.

Jupiter's opposition can bring knowledge, a needed diagnosis, good doctors and helpful assistance for Mars-ruled problems. By no means as strong as the conjunction.

Transit Jupiter Oppose Natal Jupiter

The low swing of Jupiter's own 11.8 year cycle. Disorganizes liver or pituitary function. Glandular coordination may be either "off" or corrected, depending on the chart's other testimonies.

Transit Jupiter Oppose Natal Saturn

Jupiter's expansive ray opposes Saturn's contractive ray. If negative, this produces go/stop conditions such as migraine or bipolar mental states.

The spiritual urges pull one away from material reality. This is plausibly balancing to Saturn-ruled issues, providing something or someone needed from the opposite sign.

This is an important transit for age-related hormonal changes (puberty, manopause, menopause). Can produce sudden slipping of spinal discs, or other bones related to the bodily regions governed by the sign of natal Saturn.

Transit Jupiter Oppose Natal Uranus

Disorganizes electrical signals and hormones. Prepare for unexpected shifts and quite sudden swings up and down. Produces a sudden imbalance within the circulatory, muscular, portal circulation or electrical systems. Potential reactions are dependent on the natal sign polarity of Uranus.

Reduces "grounding," and consequently produces odd mental states and inattentiveness. Problematic for those with mental health issues, hormonal swings, seizure conditions, spasms, migraine, palpitations, diabetes. Can produce sudden slipping of spinal discs.

Transit Jupiter Oppose Natal Neptune

Uncertain. Strange influences. Disturbs Neptune by:

a) pulling at it from the opposite sign; b) shining a spiritual, euphoric ray on an already highly astral planet; c) disorganizing to anything natal Neptune might suggest in the specific natal chart. This is typically unclear due to the secretive nature of Neptune.

Creates both euphoria and/or extreme depression; emphasizes

fluidic disorganization, plethora, or bleeding related to the sign polarity involved.

Transit Jupiter Oppose Natal Pluto

Unclear to this author.

JUPITER'S QUINCUNX
Health Potentials for Predisposed Nativities
Not all transits manifest as health concerns or benefits.

When transit Jupiter aligns with any natal planet by quincunx (150°), within a tight orb of 1-3°, the said natal planet temporarily cannot receive Jupiter's nourishing Blue Cosmic Ray.

Transit Jupiter Quincunx Natal Sun

Here, the vital force doesn't receive the protective, expansive rays of Jupiter. This inhibits the native's heart strength, brain power, and sometimes vision. This can lead to atrophy or weakening of the heart muscle, weakened brain integrity, or vision changes.

May indicate an increased need for magnesium, iodine, or oil soluble vitamins. In elderly persons, this transit can endanger the vital force (life), should other testimonies agree. An unwise time for hospital release!

These effects might sound similar to those of Saturn's quincunx, and yes, they are! However, there are some important differences. Jupiter rules fat. He also influences arterial and portal circulation and governs the liver (with Virgo, etc.).

Jupiter governs the pituitary gland *(Edgar Cayce)*. Therefore, the sign of the natal Sun may fail to thrive due to lack of needed lipids, oxygenated blood, arterial issues or hormonal delivery. Conversely, heart, brain or eye problems can occur from plethoric blood or excess fats! This is a good time to check for hidden aneurisms, and growths.

Circulatory imbalance can produce engorement within the bodily regions governed by the Sun generically, or to his natal sign— or the sign of transiting Jupiter. Jupiter is also disorganizing, and can produce odd, chaotic symptoms, or hard-to-diagnose fatigue at this time.

Transit Jupiter Quincunx Natal Moon

This transit can signal weight loss or atrophy, reduced fertility, scant milk production; it weakens breast and womb. There can be unforeseen problems with a pregnancy. Study the bodily regions ruled by the signs of both the natal Moon and transit Jupiter.

There may be problems with lymphatic drainage, hormones, fluidic circulation. The native may develop eating disorders *(see Field Note)*. One bodily area may lack hydration or blood while another may be overfed, edemic or engorged. More potassium may be required, or silver.

Field Note: Difficulty holding weight, emaciation, anorexia, orthorexia and genetic muscle atrophy has been noted in cases of natal Jupiter quincunx natal Moon. Three of these cases have Cancer Ascendant. Not all symptoms need apply. Don't expect someone who otherwise has a "fat" birth chart to necessarily be corpulent should natal Jupiter be in a sign at quincunx to the natal Moon! The tighter the orb, the stronger. Nourishment (emotional or food) is somehow denied.

Transit Jupiter Quincunx Natal Mercury

The coating of the nerves or brain may not receive enough protective fats. Indicative of potential neural malnutrition, possibly disturbing to hearing, thought or speech; if unattended can bring on any number of diseases associated with malnourished nerves or inherited neurological disease. In rare cases can suggest a hidden pressure or tumor impinging a nerve. Note the body zones ruled by both the sign of transit Jupiter and natal Mercury.

Transit Jupiter Quincunx Natal Venus

The ovaries, kidneys and veins may not receive enough protective lipids or hormonal distribution. One wonders if this may be good for excessive Jupiter conditions, i.e. varicose veins!

Theoretically, this quincunx would have a slowing effect on

tumor growth, but this has not been researched. However, it might be wise to be on the alert for any hidden development of cysts or tumors in Venus' organs: kidneys, veins, ovaries. The bodily zones ruled by the signs of transit Jupiter and natal Venus are essential in your analysis.

Transit Jupiter Quincunx Natal Mars

Quincunxes to and from Mars seem to work differently than for other planets. *(See the discussion, under Mars' Quincunxes, previous chapter.)* However, here we have transit Jupiter as the current time actor, influencing the natal Mars. Transit Jupiter can deny Mars the activating "go" hormones, inducing impotency, lethargy, or depression (Martial types are rarely depressed).

This quincunx impacts the sense of taste and smell, and the production of male hormones and adrenalin. In practice, I've observed clinically diagnosed excess release of testosterone and adrenalin occur with this aspect, and also one extreme case of loss of smell (hyposomia). See *Field Note.*

This transit provides one testimony of adrenal exhaustion, or iron, or B6 deficiency anemia. Produces disturbances and extremes of anything physically governed by Mars. Some report excessive libido followed by none!

Similar to Uranus, Jupiter can produce extreme swings, up and down. All excretory effects may be extreme or "off," such as ejaculation, urination, defecation, nose, internal or external bleeding. It is possible that this aspect could produce hemorrhage or an unexpected bout of non-stop bleeding.

Field Note: Testosterone and adrenalin are considered as "Mars-ruled" hormones. I've seen four cases of natal Jupiter quincunx natal Mars producing three cases of excess testosterone (one female), and one case of excess adrenalin.

Another natal case is noted for loss of smell occurring with natal Mars in Scorpio on the Ascendant, quincunx both natal Jupiter and Mercury in Aries, the 6th house in this case. Scorpio rules the nose and Aries the head nerves in general, with Mercury chiming in. This affliction was most distressing.

Transit Jupiter Quincunx Natal Jupiter

At this time one's natal Jupiter function, and all that its natal sign placement suggests, is not receiving its own essential "prana" or vital force. Therefore, support natal Jupiter and its sign.

Transit Jupiter Quincunx Natal Saturn

This is a prime time to watch for calcium and mineral leaching. Osteopenia can develop. Jupiter and Saturn work together to keep bones, teeth and cartilage strong. In quincunx, this aspect breaks down the cartilage *(see Field Note, below)*. The bones may not grow or set correctly. Theoretically, the fatty marrow within the bones may be affected. This aspect may also influence blood cell size and development and retard growth of nails, teeth or hair.

The natal quincunx of Jupiter and Saturn could indicate poorly developed cartilage (as ruled by Jupiter and Saturn), leading to an easy grinding down of under-protected bones (Saturn), also, the lack of proper nourishment (Jupiter and Moon) to bone (Saturn).

Field Note: I've collected charts of persons who grind down their cartilage, resulting in the early need for hip or knee replacement. In most cases, natal Jupiter and Saturn are in quincunx (150°) or inconjunct (30°), or square (90°). I presume that the opposition (180°) would work too. Conversely, the few cases of folks over the age of sixty with "the bones of a thirty-year-old" have perfect trines between Jupiter and Saturn, with additional helpful testimonies!

Why should this be? Saturn rules the consolidation of boney structure, whereas Jupiter governs growth and fat, protecting the bones, muscles and neural structures with insulating lipids. Ruling the arterial circulation, Jupiter also delivers the nourishing blood to all organs, carrying the minerals (Saturn) where needed.

Surgery Tip: Jupiter quincunx Saturn is a poor time for elective bone surgery. Potentially, this could be a strange time for gall-bladder procedures. However, ones' physician must be consulted.

Transit Jupiter Quincunx Natal Uranus

Not enough information available. Possibly dis-coordinates some part of the electrical rhythm. Could induce spasm, seizure, tremor, odd mental states, blood pressure swings, or sudden sugar imbalance; Jupiter seems to have as much to do with diabetes as Venus.

Transit Jupiter Quincunx Natal Neptune

Not enough information available on this transit (to this author). This aspect could possibly confuse dopamine and melatonin production and absorption; these being some of the more important pleasure producing and sleeping chemicals (Neptune, Venus). The lymphatic circulation may overload, slow or engorge. This is a good time to assist lymphatic cleansing.

Drug and alcohol users may be quietly developing a hidden liver, blood or lymphatic issue. Potential for unnoticed cell changes in the bodily regions ruled by the signs of transit Jupiter or natal Neptune (but could be anywhere because Neptune leaks).

This aspect, while not obvious, should never be ignored! Cancer survivors should keep up their vigilance and not let down their guard as yet. Use close orb of 1°.

Transit Jupiter Quincunx Natal Pluto

Not enough information available to this author. Astrologers cannot yet, with certainty, know all of Pluto's physical implications. It is established that Pluto governs intense therapies that utilize dangerous substances, rays, and transplants.

Pluto may also govern horrifying diseases (e.g. Ebola), killer bacteria, plagues, AIDS, blood and vermin-born disease, cadavers and poisonous venoms. Jupiter's transit quincunx of Pluto would theoretically not be optimum for that trek through the Amazon jungle! Of course, one needs multiple testimonies.

Surgical and Medical Tips: During this time, Jupiter's protections may not be available to natal Pluto. Therefore, this transit may be dangerous for radiation and laser treatment, organ transplants, fecal transplants, hormonal therapies, or transfusions. Always consult your responsible physician regarding surgical timing.

Chapter 14

SATURN
Cold, Dry, Slow

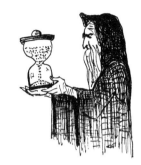

Properties, Rulerships and Actions

Rules: Capricorn, Aquarius

Exalted: Libra

Detriment: Cancer, Leo

Fall: Aries

Metal: Lead (traditional)

Minerals: Calcium

Vitamins: Vitamin C *(Nauman, Jansky)*; Folic Acid *(Jansky)*; P *(Nauman)*

Gem & Cosmic Ray: Blue Sapphire & Violet Ray *(Traditional Jyotish)*

Body Rulership & Organ Affinities: Bones, ligaments, tendons, cuticles, nails, teeth, skin, hair (with Venus), knees, peripheral nerves (Jyotish), gallbladder (with Mars, Leo and Capricorn), the right ear.

General Action: Cold, dry, slow, tense, astringent. Creates restriction, congeals. Reduces circulation and oxygenation. Mineralizes. hemostatic, trapping, congealing, stiffening, hardening, mineralizing, concretizing, and form-organizing.

Saturn delivers cold to both the sign he tenants at birth and transits through. Saturn dries, crystallizes shape and structure, creates tension, reduces circulation and oxygenation.

The larger physiological life cycles are governed by Saturn. He always turns up at the onset of puberty, menopause and manopause. Saturn marches out the stages of life and is the bringer of old age.

Conversely, Luna governs the daily rhythms and monthly cycles. It is fascinating that Saturn and the Moon rule opposite signs Capricorn and Cancer. One might call them "Time Partners."

Saturn's astringency works in two seemingly opposite ways. He can dry tissue, creating atrophy. Conversely, he can trap fluid, creating torpor, and pockets of fluidic stagnation, especially in Water signs.

Because Saturn's rays slow, cool, and stiffening, he can reduce circulation of blood, oxygen and nutrients to the bodily region he tenants at birth and secondarily to the body zone of the sign he currently transits. In this manner, he contributes to chronic conditions and malnourishment. One can preempt these potential maladies by wise health practices with special attention to the bodily region governed by the signs of both natal and transit Saturn.

Conversely, if Saturn's predisposed natal issues are hammered by bad habits, these might "hatch" under Saturn's long, cold transit by conjunction, square, opposition, or quincunx.

It is difficult to comprehend how Saturn builds strength in some cases and osteoporosis in others! Although Saturn rules the strength of the bones, he equally governs osteoporosis and tooth decay when "gone bad." His transits can signal onset of any conditions due to lack of minerals, or poorly absorbed minerals.

When Cold and Dry Precipitates Hot Conditions: Saturn dries synovial fluids, ligaments and tendons. If this occurs within a joint, the unprotected friction results in hot inflammation (Mars). In this manner one often sees Saturn at the base of what one might otherwise assume was a Mars condition! Saturn leads to Mars, as a cart follows a horse.

Positive: Saturn's astringent properties are counteractive to all manner of torpor and prolapse. His transit indicates a good time for strengthening both the heart muscle and the general constitution.

Saturn's concretizing and mineralizing function builds strong bones, good tendons and ligaments, and dense tissue. This occurs when he is enjoys some dignity in the natal chart. Strong men are noted to have "Saturn rising in Leo" *(Cornell)*, although other planets can also display this trait. Cornell's observation is true. The two strongest men I ever knew were both born with Saturn rising in Leo! Of course, one needs at least three testimonies for exceptional muscular strength.

Negative: Saturn, when negative restricts circulation, thus limiting the oxygen and nutrients from nourishing the bodily region he moves through or inhabits at birth. He is also restrictive to the body regions ruled by the signs he opposes and squares.

In this manner, Saturn can signify mineral deficiency and sub oxygenation of cells due to poor circulation. This expresses physically as prolapse of organs, skin and vessels in the sign he natally tenants. And, weak bones and teeth instead of strong ones!

Saturn's beams also constrict the bodily regions governed by the signs he squares and opposes. Body parts governed by the sign that Saturn quincunxes are potentially denied needed minerals. Another of Saturn's manifestation is rheumatic and arthritic complaints due to poorly assimilated nutrients and toxins settling in the joints. Heavy metal poisoning is a specialty of this planet! See next.

Excess Saturn: Saturn dries, stiffens, hardens, and traps. In excess, this can lead to tissue hardening, mineral deposits in joints and kidneys, gallstones, brittle and dry bones, ligaments and tendons or to bone spurs or bone overgrowth. Conversely, excess Saturn's ray can cause poor mineralization if interfering with absorption, processing or circulatory delivery of minerals or vitamins.

Saturn's excess and deficiency are both renowned for all manner of rheumatic and arthritic complaints, but for different reasons. Why? An excess of minerals can settle in joints, causing inflammation and pain. A deficiency of oxygen and minerals creates weak bones or cartilage, promoting joint degeneration.

Saturn governs structural maladies due to organic bone misalignment, malformation or stenosis. In this manner, he contributes to neural pain. Always study Saturn in cases of neuralgia to ascertain if any pressure is due to bones, bone spurs or muscular stricture pressing upon the nerves.

Tumor growth, cancer. Saturn traps toxins! One sees warts and moles for both excess and deficient Saturn, for opposite reasons! An excess Saturn has a predilection to harden and dry skin or block pores. Deficient Saturn deprives the skin of vitamins and minerals necessary for a healthy epidermis.

Deficient Saturn: Osteoporosis, poor teeth, cavities, prolapsed organs due to lack of integrity, weakness, wasting, atrophy, rickets, bent spine, poor hearing, dry skin, skin disease, warts and moles, gall insufficiency, and deafness.

Transit Orb: Saturn's transit moves slowly. Over the course of one year, he typically crosses any planet two or three times before the transit is complete. He is strongest when retrograde and backing up into a natal planet within and orb of 1°, approaching (backwards).

Temperature & Moisture Levels: Saturn is cold, dry and astringent in the extreme, (less cold when tenanting the Fire signs, and less dry in Water signs). He is coldest when placed under the horizon in Earth, and especially Water signs, for night births. This special condition threatens the gradual development of toxicity within the bodily region governed by the sign of natal Saturn.

Cold Saturn is warmest when positioned in Fire signs, above the horizon, in a day birth, and thus least disposed toward causing chronic ailments. Saturn sucks dry and hardens tissue when in the Earth signs.

In Water signs, Saturn acts to either trap moisture in stagnant pockets, disallowing flow, or dries the mucus membrane and other moist coverings.

Although cold, Saturn in Earth signs may trap heat causing the native to feel hot. For a more complete discussion of Saturn in the four elements, see the discussion below in Saturn through the Signs.

SATURN THROUGH THE ELEMENTS & SIGNS
Health Potentials for Predisposed Nativities
Transits do not always manifest as health concerns or benefits.

Applicable to both natal and transit charts, these partial lists of expressed symptoms apply only to predisposed nativities. These conditions are obviously uncommon and require multiple testimonies beyond the presence of Saturn. Manifestation of symptoms may be enhanced by lifestyle choices, and taking preemptive measures can reduce, remove or prevent potential issues from manifesting.

Saturn in Fire Signs

Cold Saturn is warmer in Fire signs in general, and more so if above the horizon in a day birth. These natives rarely suffer the "cold" diseases indicated for Saturn through the other elements. However, he still restricts and tightens the body parts governed by the Fire sign he passes through or tenants natally!

Aries: Restricted blood vessels in head, migraine, aneurism, stroke, blindness, teeth issues, dry eyes, hypopituitarism, blockages to eye or teeth nerves. Contributes to hearing issues and pressures or blockages on the auditory nerves (also see Taurus, Mercury), high blood pressure, heart restriction, heart attack, blindness (rare).

Surgical Tip: Unless the responsible physician feels it is necessary to move ahead, it is traditionally inadvisable to undergo surgery to Aries bodily regions, such as heart, eyes or brain, when Saturn transits through Aries, especially if in hard aspect or quincunx to Ascendant, Sun or Moon. (See sections on these aspects for orbs.)

Leo: Structural back and spine problems, back stiffness, dry or lesioned spinal sheath, insufficient or plugged gallbladder, stiff wrists, high blood pressure, sclerotic heart or heart vessels, small heart, heart problems, sub-oxygenation of heart, heart failure.

Surgical Tip: Unless the responsible physician feels it is necessary to move ahead, it is traditionally inadvisable to undergo voluntary surgery to Leo bodily regions when Saturn transits through Leo, especially if in hard aspect or quincunx to Ascendant, Sun or Moon.

Sagittarius: Rheumatic hips, broken hip or femur, tailbone or spinal cord issues, spinal stenosis, sciatica, arterial inflexibility or blockage, stroke, paralysis to legs, reduced circulation, mental health issues.

Surgical Tip: Unless the responsible physician feels it is necessary to move ahead, it is traditionally inadvisable to undergo surgery to Sagittarius bodily regions when Saturn transits through Sagittarius, especially if in hard aspect or quincunx to Ascendant, Sun or Moon.

Field Note: A colleague once pulled me from a meeting to introduce me to her skeptical friend. True, he openly pronounced his disbelief in astrology. So, I inquired as to the sign of his natal Saturn. My friend relayed "Sagittarius."

Curious, I asked him, "Have you had any trouble with your hip or thigh area?" Stunned, he replied that he had once broken his femur straight through.

Saturn in Earth Signs

Saturn's natural astringency, and bone and muscle building qualities are strongest when positioned in Earth, below the horizon in a night birth (some say day birth). These transits also increase the accretion of toxins within the bodily region governed by the sign of either natal or transit Saturn. Stultifying and slowing to the upper organs of digestion.

Taurus: Predisposed individuals should be proactive against neck issues, hypothyroid, vocal polyps, restriction of neck or ear vessels, hearing reduction, deafness; dental issues, dental root impaction, cracked teeth, cavities, bruxism (teeth grinding); tongue, throat or esophageal cancer, salivary gland blockage, dry mouth, mouth or lip problems; mouth, throat, tongue or esophageal cancer.

Lead poisoning, bad diet, lack of appetite, dietary restriction, dry mouth, blocked salivary glands. This transit is excellent for bone and body building.

Surgical Tip: Unless the responsible physician feels it is necessary to move ahead, it is traditionally inadvisable to undergo surgery to Taurus bodily regions when Saturn transits through Taurus, especially if in hard aspect or quincunx to Ascendant, Sun or Moon.

Virgo: If a chart predisposes to Virgo bodily region issues, it is wise to be proactive during this transit. Duodenal or pancreas insufficiency, spleen insufficiency, white blood cell production issues, poor intestinal absorption, malnutrition due to poor intestinal absorption, intestinal dryness, skin and hair dryness, liver cirrhosis; pancreatic, liver or intestinal tumors; masses or hardening, colitis, appendicitis, Crohn's disease, diabetes, bile insufficiency, immune issues, intestinal stasis, frozen bowel, dry bowel.

Surgical Tip: Unless the responsible physician feels it is necessary to move ahead, it is traditionally inadvisable to undergo voluntary surgery to Virgo bodily regions when Saturn transits through Virgo, especially if in hard aspect or quincunx to Ascendant, Sun or Moon.

Capricorn: If a chart predisposes to Capricornian maladies, it is wise to be proactive regarding these regions throughout this transit or if born with natal Saturn in Capricorn.

Gallbladder insufficiency, gallstones, stomach malabsorption, dry or cold stomach, stomach enzyme insufficiency, uterine and breast thickening, infertility, uterine fibroids, skin tags, vitiligo, dry skin and wrinkling, skin diseases; blemishes and warts need extra watching, plugged sudorific or sebaceous glands, poor subdermal circulation.

Bone loss due to malabsorption of mineral, or conversely an excellent transit for bone building. Special attention should be directed to knees and skin. Dryness and cold of the bodily fluids can lead to knee issues and issues with all joints due to reduced circulation and toxic buildup; dry ligaments and tendons, inflexibility, rheumatism, arthritis, knee stiffening Dryness of synovial fluids, breakdown of cartilage, receding gums, poor cuticles.

Positively, Saturn builds strong bones! Great for weight loss and strengthening!

This transit or natal position accretes toxins in the joints. These then become hot and inflamed. Capricorn is famous for falls, so elderly should take precautions.

Field Note: Saturn entered Capricorn, the sign of the knees, around Christmas 2017. A visitor casually remarked, "My knees have bothered me since Christmas and I can't figure out why." This scenario has played itself out multiple times, as if on a revolving tape loop.

Surgical Tip: Unless the responsible physician feels it is necessary to move ahead, it is traditionally inadvisable to undergo surgery to Capricorn bodily regions when Saturn transits through Capricorn, especially if in hard aspect or quincunx to Ascendant, Sun or Moon.

Saturn in Air Signs

Gemini: Saturn's transit of Gemini tightens the bronchial tubes and upper lungs bringing "cold, dry" style asthma. Therefore, when Saturn transits Gemini, be proactive to prevent drying of bronchial tubes and lungs. This transit or natal position can also bring blood clots in lung, lung tumors and hardening of lung tissue. If you are a smoker, try to stop before Saturn transits through Gemini.

Frozen shoulder. Raynaud's disease. Saturn can encourage arthritis in the shoulders, arms or hands, carpal tunnel syndrome, or indicate bone fracture in any Gemini region. Also, potential speech problems and slowing of mental function.

Surgical Tip: Unless the responsible physician feels it necessary to move ahead, it is traditionally inadvisable to undergo surgery to Gemini bodily regions when Saturn is in Gemini, especially if in hard aspect or quincunx to Ascendant, Sun or Moon.

Libra: This is a good time to be proactive against kidney stones or ovarian tumors. The lumbar spine may need adjustment. The kidneys may require warming. Gravel forming (reflexes as headaches, eye pain).

Surgical Tip: Unless the responsible physician feels it necessary to move ahead, it is traditionally inadvisable to undergo surgery to Libra bodily regions when Saturn is in Libra, especially if in hard aspect or quincunx to Ascendant, Sun or Moon.

Aquarius: Saturn's transit is super cold in the midwinter sign Aquarius, hatching a wide array of cold symptoms in predisposed charts: restricted veins, varicose veins due to insufficient vitamin and mineral absorption, sub oxygenation of cells, chronic depression, cold feet due to circulatory insufficiency, ankle stenosis, weak heart function, spinal nerve conduction insufficiency.

Psychologically, Saturn contributes mightily towards depression in this sign, and loneliness. Light deprivation and social isolation are often factors. Preemption can work miracles.

Surgical Tip: Unless the responsible physician feels it necessary to move ahead, it is traditionally inadvisable to undergo surgery to

Aquarius bodily regions when Saturn is in Aquarius, especially if in hard aspect or quincunx to Ascendant, Sun or Moon.

Saturn in Water Signs

Saturn is coldest and therefore most productive of chronic maladies when positioned at birth in Water signs, in a night birth, under the horizon. For you Greek scholars, this is not the same as the tradition of Hayze, where Saturn would need to be above the horizon.

Cancer: This cold, moist sign increases Saturn's cold nature. However, Saturn is drying and still exerts his drying force upon wet Cancer. This can have two effects: the first being dry mucous membrane and dry, unreceptive stomach. The second being the trapped fluid of lymphatic stagnation. Saturn in this sign is productive of cold, wet conditions or cold dehydration. This is the converse of the more typical hot dehydration of Saturn (or Mars) in Fire. Reduces fertility.

Predisposed charts should be proactive against: chilled stomach, insufficient stomach juices producing ongoing malnutrition, dry mucous membranes, insufficient lactation, breast tumors, thickening or hardening breast tissue or uterus, cold or non-receptive womb, infertility, insufficient female hormones, weakening bones, poor gums, tooth decay, fear, trapped dampness, lung cancer, tuberculosis, cold asthma, fluid stagnation in lower lung, cold lower lung, pancreatic insufficiency, toxic lymphatics, slow lymphatics (the thoracic duct is under Cancer).

Surgical Tip: Unless the responsible physician feels it necessary to move ahead, it is traditionally inadvisable to undergo surgery to Cancer bodily regions when Saturn transits through Cancer, especially if in hard aspect or quincunx to Ascendant, Sun or Moon.

Scorpio: Potential hardening of tissue or tumors of prostate, bladder, testicles, penis, uterus, vagina, nose or colon. Constipation due to fecal impaction, dryness, poor peristalsis or frozen colon. Colitis, Crohn's disease, especially for those with natal Saturn in Scorpio. Keep that colon healthy! Impotence, frigidity, infertility, dry vagina, miscarriage; dry nose, nosebleed (due to malnourished, weakened vessels), plugged sweat glands, anal fissure, hemorrhoids. Nasal impaction, broken nose, chronic nasal congestion or infection, Reflexes to throat and voice. (The sound of the voice reveals the health of the Scorpio regions.)

Field Note: A distraught friend called to relay that her husband was just diagnosed with kidney disease. An ephemeris for his year of birth was handy. His birth date immediately revealed that he was a Libra, the sign ruling the kidneys, and he was also born with many planets crowded into this same sign.

However, my eyes fell upon the real culprit: Saturn in Scorpio on the degree of the urethra, and influencing the general region of the prostate, testes and ureters. I hypothesized that he suffered some long-term obstruction in either the ureters or urethra, and was prone to gravel. She then described how as an infant, he was operated on for an obstruction in one of these tubes, but could not recall which one. Then, she added in all seriousness, "The doctors insist that this has nothing to do with his kidney problem."

Surgical Tip: Unless the responsible physician feels it necessary to move ahead, it is traditionally inadvisable to undergo surgery to Scorpio bodily regions when Saturn transits Scorpio, especially if in hard aspect or quincunx to Ascendant, Sun or Moon.

Pisces: Predisposed folks can preempt this transit's influence: slowed lymphatics leading to toxic buildup, chronic "cold" lung problems, trapped damp in lungs, thickening lung tissue, lung cancer, bone spurs on feet, osteoporosis of feet, osteoporosis in general, chronic depression, past life memory issues, suicidal ideology.

Surgical Tip: Unless the responsible physician feels it is necessary to move ahead, it is traditionally inadvisable to undergo surgery to Pisces bodily regions when Saturn transits through Pisces, especially if in hard aspect or quincunx to Ascendant, Sun or Moon.

SATURN'S TRANSIT OF NATAL PLANETS

Applicable to both natal and transit charts, these partial lists of expressed symptoms apply only to predisposed nativities. These conditions are obviously uncommon and require multiple testimonies beyond the presence of Saturn. Manifestation of symptoms may be enhanced by lifestyle choices, and taking preemptive measures can reduce, remove or prevent potential issues from manifesting. It is not possible to list all potential expressions. Keep well in mind that Saturn is capable of strengthening the body, and is not always a negative influence.

SATURN'S CONJUNCTION
Health Potentials for Predisposed Nativities
Transits do not always manifest as health concerns or benefits.

Transit Saturn Conjunct Natal Sun
Reduces the vital force. If negative, this transit can restrict heart muscle action, raise or lower blood pressure, or reduce blood and oxygen flow to the brain or heart. Conversely, in some natives this same transit strengthens by tightening up the constitution, providing greater stamina and internal integrity. Some of the toughest people I've ever seen are born on an exact Sun-Saturn conjunction!

This aspect is not as reliably dragging upon the internal life battery of vitality as is Saturn's opposition to the Sun. Potential for dehydration of brain, dry eyes; clot, stroke and aneurysm prone in aorta and other cardiac and brain vessels.

The young and healthy may experience less energy at this time, or conversely, increased stamina and personal resolve. However, if someone is dangling near death, Saturn's transit conjunction (or any other hard aspects) to the natal Sun presages a significant lowering of vital force, and possible termination of that physical life.

Surgical Tip: Unless the responsible physician feels it is necessary to move ahead, it is traditionally inadvisable to undergo voluntary surgery to the heart, brain, or eye if this conjunction is in hard aspect or quincunx to Ascendant, Sun, or Moon. Warming and moistening the organ involved, can help counter these poor influences.

Herbal Note: A professional herbalist might use warming, relaxing cardiac herbs, such as Hawthorne, Rosemary, and Linden. If needed, bring more oxygen to the heart, brain or eyes (Gingko, Periwinkle, Yerba Mate, et al.). Do not self-treat.

Transit Saturn Conjunct Natal Moon

This transit is often felt as tiring. The stomach may fail to produce enough digestive acids; cold or dry stomach (drinking ice water is traditionally ill-advised), poor appetite, malnourishment, serious nutritional deficiencies anorexia, starvation, atrophy, GERD (in Fire signs). Drying to mucous membranes and the whole system, dehydration, especially in Fire and Earth signs, lymph fluids may fail to adequately flow allowing toxins to collect; toxins collect in breast, lung or brain tissue.

Typically, progesterone levels plummet and other changes in female hormones occur for both sexes. For women between 48-55, this transit is the harbinger of menopause. Greatly reduces fertility, miscarriage potential, general frigidity, poor lactation, suppressed menses, depression. "How did he get scurvy in this day and age?"

This transit may signal insufficient potassium or silver (Moon), or calcium and Vitamin C (Saturn).

If occurring in an infant's chart, this is no time to leave them with grandma for that week-long break, unless you want a lifelong abandonment issue to set in!

Positive: Promotes tightening of prolapsed womb, bladder, or lung. Counteracts edema. Good for fasting and relinquishing addictions and habits. Confers emotional maturity.

Surgical Tip: Unless the responsible physician feels it is necessary to move ahead, it is traditionally inadvisable to undergo surgery to breast, stomach, uterus, lung, pericardium, brain or eye when Saturn transits over the Moon, especially if they are in hard aspect or quincunx to Ascendant, Sun or Moon. To counteract this influence, warm the constitution, because both Saturn and the Moon are cold.

Herbal Note: Should trapped fluids present, a professional herbalist may use herbs that relieve fluidic congestion. If drying symptoms occur, the warming demulcents are useful, such as Fenugreek and Peach Leaf. Oils and liniments may also be helpful at this time. Undernourishment and atrophy can be remedied with the nutrient herbs, such as Oat Straw, Nettles, Red Clover, Alfalfa, Seaweed. Avoid prolonged use of exclusively drying herbs.

In Earth signs, ease and thin the bile flow and moisturize the intestinal tract. Do not self-treat.

Transit Saturn Conjunct Natal Mercury

Slows neural transmission, which can be good or bad depending on what is needed. Increases any arthritic tendencies in arms, hands and fingers; impairs hearing, interrupts speech. Those unattended repetitive action injuries can go chronic at this time. Drys and plugs upper respiratory organs. This is that endless dry, unproductive cough.

Positive: Focuses and steadies jumpy nerves, steadies a distracted mind, disciplines speech, enhances depth intelligence and scholastic prowess. Good for building nerves, speech therapy, and dedicated and disciplined recovery of skill and neurotransmission after stroke.

Surgical Tip: Unless the responsible physician feels it is necessary to move ahead, it is traditionally inadvisable to undergo surgery to the nerves, brain, ears, arms or hands when Saturn transits over natal Mercury, especially if this conjunction is in hard aspect or quincunx to Ascendant, Sun or Moon.

Herbal Note: For undernourished, stressed nerves, professional herbalists may consider the nutritive herbs, such as Oat Straw, Oat Tops, Parsley, Alfalfa, Nettles, Red Clover, and seaweeds.

For respiratory complaints, use your warming, relaxing demulcent expectoratives. Do not self-treat.

Transit Saturn Conjunct Natal Venus

Cooling to libido, drying to skin and vaginal tissues, influences both puberty and menopause, reduces breast size. Hardening to veins or brings venal prolapse from deficient mineral absorption. Slowed kidney action or kidney stones, skin issues. It is harder to relax at this time. Socializing opportunity and pleasure is decreased. Because the transit can last for months, this increased tension can influence health. However, this aspect assists those who are trying to kick a sugar, wine, or sex addiction.

Field Note: This transit reliably lowers the female libido, and can also obstruct male enthusiasm. It is astonishing how often wives and husbands complain of sexual disinterest as this transit approaches exactitude. Estrogen slumps, with all that this implies. Folks prefer to sleep alone because they are temporarily less cuddly.

When I see this conjunction current in men of a certain age, I inquire, "Are you loosing hair right now?" Answer: "How did you know that?"

Positive: Saturn's astringency can tighten a prolapsed womb. Also, diagnosis of hidden female or kidney issues, tightening of veins, reducing excessive blood sugar, tightening the skin. This transit could equally produce varicosities and wrinkles, due to nutritional deficiencies, poor eliminations and/or oxygenation (depending on the nativity).

Surgical and Medical Tips: Unless the responsible physician feels it is necessary to move ahead, it is traditionally inadvisable at this time to undergo surgery to the face for beauty enhancement, the breast, ovaries, veins, or female genitalia. This is especially so if natal Venus is in hard aspect or quincunx to Ascendant, Sun or Moon, or if positioned in the 6th, 8th, or 12th houses. This book's focus is not on houses and Saturn's beams can manifest regardless of house. However, he produces more evil potential for health issues specifically in these houses!

Test for potentially lowered levels of copper, blood sugar, thymus gland activity, white blood cells, semen or female hormones.

Herbal Note: For symptoms of low estrogen, the professional herbalist may consider Wild Yam, Red Clover, Sarsaparilla and other estrogenic herbs. Some sexual hormone supporting foods are figs, sunflower seeds, pumpkin seeds, and Saw Palmetto Berries. Do not self-treat.

Transit Saturn Conjunct Natal Mars

Frustrating or cooling to male libido, erectile dysfunction, overtaxes adrenals and testosterone, energy affected, lowers testosterone (but sometimes the reverse), reduces sperm count, influences male hormonal shifts in the lifespan, both puberty and "manopause" (also see *Transit Saturn Conjunct Natal Venus*). Anemia, iron or B12 deficiency, atrophy.

Inclines to disciplined exercise (gym rat's aspect), and abandonment of bad habits (gives willpower). Tightens muscle tone, dries and hardens muscles. Reduces excretion of toxins, which can accrue, and cause rheumatic ailments and skin disease. Constipating, prevents or blocks sweating; slows metabolism burn-rate. Dehydrating. (See discussion: *When Cold and Dry Precipitates Hot Conditions*, under *Saturn's General Action*, beginning of this chapter.)

Field Note: There was one case of Saturn conjunct both Mars and the South Lunar Node within 1° in late Aries, with birth time unknown. The interview was by phone. "Is there something wrong with your brain or eye?" queried the astrologer.

"Oh yes" was the reply. "I was badly cross-eyed in one eye until the age of 14, when they operated. For the next fifty years, I've been unable to see much out of this eye because the brain had become dependent on the good eye."

Positive: Strengthening to muscles, blood building, provides added discipline to energy use, dieting, exercise routines, hard work, and useful work. Reduces excess libido and resultant consequence, more inclined to "safe sex" if any; steadies wild swings of testosterone, iron or adrenalin; toughens sissies (Saturn's opinion). Good for controlling anger, but can produce extreme frustration leading to anger outbursts.

Surgical and Medical Tips: Unless the responsible physician feels it is necessary to move ahead, it is traditionally inadvisable to undergo surgery to muscles, adrenal gland, male genitalia, ears or nose when Saturn transits over natal Mars, especially if in hard aspect or quincunx to Ascendant, Sun or Moon, or if positioned in the 6th, 8th, or 12th houses.

Should symptoms suggest, test for lower iron, hemoglobin, adrenalin, cortisol, testosterone. Check for cell changes or obstruction in or around the prostate gland or testes.

Herbal Note: The professional herbalist may consider male support herbs, such as Saw Palmetto, Sunflower and Pumpkin seeds, and Figs. Iron rich herbs and blood builders may be helpful, such as Nettles, soaked Raisins, and Beets.

Should frozen peristalsis occur at this time, use warming demulcent laxatives, never drying! Flaxseed tea is a good example. Solomon's Seal Root is Matthew Wood's specific for drying ligaments and tendons. Mullein, Boneset and Solomon Seal are excellent for bone injury. Muscle strains respond well to Wintergreen, Rosemary, Peppermint, Camphor, Myrrh, and Cayenne. Muscle wasting counteractive: Nettles. Do not self-treat.

Transit Saturn Conjunct Natal Jupiter

Saturn is opposite in action to all planets. Jupiter governs excess; transit Saturn reigns him in. This transit greatly reduces flexibility of arteries and veins. Hardens or dehydrates the liver, slows its ability to filter toxins; slows production of bile, reduces its ability to break down and repackage foods; may reduce liver's mineral storage (or conversely bring an excess). If someone has suffered from hepatitis or alcoholism, this transit warns of impending problems unless reversed.

Possibly some influence on the blood (the rulerships of the many blood constituents is not yet well understood by traditional medical astrology). Indicated in atrophy, emaciation, lack of necessary oils, reduces or plugs oil glands, breaks down cartilage (or reverse), dries synovial fluids. Can indicate pituitary hormone insufficiency, producing growth and maturation problems, decreased lactation, growth retardation. Psychologically, removes hope and good cheer, but also reigns in euphoria, megalomania, mania, compulsive gambling and other excessive Jupiterian mental states.

Positively, this aspect can assist weight loss, and supports tumor reduction, but this is NOT true for the **natal** conjunction of Saturn and Jupiter. If suffering from tumor growth related to the natal position of Jupiter, Saturn's approach could signal either shrinkage, or negatively, a pending malignancy, depending on the chart. Controls surplus body fluids.

Reduces blood cholesterol (or, conversely, further hardens the arteries; see text above), reduces excess eating and drinking, reduces edema, and can correct liver and blood problems with disciplined approach and nutrition, controls mental excesses and profligacy.

May indicate an increased need for choline or B6, Chromium,

Biotin and is a watch-aspect for diabetic or hypoglycemic tendencies *(Nauman)*. She has a wonderful section on this aspect in natal charts in her book. *(See end of Chapter 1, Additional Texts.)*

Surgical and Medical Tips: Unless the responsible physician feels it necessary to move ahead, it is traditionally inadvisable to undergo surgery to the liver, pituitary gland, arteries, or fat when Saturn transits over natal Jupiter, especially if in hard aspect or quincunx to Ascendant, Sun or Moon, or if positioned in the 6th, 8th, or 12th houses. Should symptoms present, consider a possible blocking or condensing of bile or fats in the liver, gallbladder or blood vessels. In cases of sclerotic liver, do all you can to reverse his influence.

Herbal Note: The professional herbalist may consider warming cholagogues and hepatics, such as Gentian, and Burdock. Do not self-treat.

Transit Saturn Conjunct Natal Saturn

The first Saturn Return" occurs at about age 29 to 30. The skeleton, teeth and brain complete growth and youth ends (with some gender variation). At this time, the innate chronic potentials of natal Saturn may begin to manifest.

Take note and adjust the diet and lifestyle to prevent future consequences. In Saturn we reap as we sow. One tastes the fruits of self-care, or lack thereof, at the second Saturn Return, approximately age 59 to 60. Still, the body is resilient, and many are fortunate enough to turn around the mess they have created.

Surgical Tips: Unless the responsible physician feels it necessary to move ahead, it is traditionally inadvisable to undergo voluntary surgery to the bones, teeth, nails or skin at the Saturn Return, or to any body region governed by the sign Saturn tenants. This is especially so if Saturn is in hard aspect or quincunx to Ascendant, Sun or Moon, or if positioned in the 6th, 8th, or 12th houses.

Transit Saturn Conjunct Natal Uranus

Saturn can block neural transmission or electrical signals. If his transit corresponds with neurological or hormonal extremes, it can suggest a vitamin or mineral deficiency! This transit over Uranus also warns those with seizure disorders to be diligent. Saturn conjunct Uranus either steadies hormonal extremes or brings them on!

Positive: Saturn can also cure! Reduces spasm, tremor, and seizure (if caused by long term nutritive deficiency). If one has gone through a protracted period of hormonal or mental extremes, Saturn can offer a steadying hand.

Uranus (with Aquarius) rules electricity and table salt (sodium) is the mineral so necessary for electrical conduction. This transit can ground and regulate strange electrical issues.

Surgical Tips: Unclear. Unless the responsible physician feels it is necessary to move ahead, it may be ill-advised to undergo surgery to the nerves or spinal cord, especially if Saturn is in hard aspect or quincunx to Ascendant, Sun or Moon, or if positioned in the 6th, 8th, or 12th houses.

Should stricture, extreme "stuck" cramp, frozen limbs or paralysis present, consider an obstruction to the flow of electrical current through either the muscles or nerves.

Herbal Note: In rare cases, the professional herbalist may consider the anti-paralytic herbs. Where warm antispasmodics are suggested, Lobelia and Mistletoe are noted traditional favorites. Moist, demulcent warmth is best for this transit. Do not self-treat.

Transit Saturn Conjunct Natal Neptune

This long-term transit profoundly impacts the psyche and can precipitate chronic depression. Other possible manifestations include: slowed lymphatic drainage, insomnia, lead poisoning, mysterious poisoning, blood cell changes, sepsis, carbon monoxide poisoning (especially in Aquarius), leaky valves or gut.

Neptune has everything to do with substance abuse and the secrecy around it. When transit Saturn arrives at natal Neptune, it is definitely time to stop drinking or drugging. If not, the addiction lurches into the danger zone. Mixing drugs and alcohol (or drugs, drink and boating) is far more risky than usual.

Positive: This aspect encourages a correct diagnosis for those long term puzzling symptoms. This period of time can reveal an existing nutritional deficiency, strengthen weakness, plug pranic leaks, block psychic vulnerability, reduce irrationality, and mature an individual by breaking "rose colored glasses." This transit can provide the discipline or structure for halting addictions of all kinds.

Surgical Tips: Unclear. Unless the responsible physician feels it is necessary to move ahead, it may be inadvisable to undergo surgery or commence chemotherapy when Saturn transits over natal Neptune, especially if also in hard aspect or quincunx to Ascendant, Sun or Moon, or if positioned in the 6th, 8th, or 12th house. If surgery must take place, work with the doctor to preestablish tolerance to the selected anesthetics.

Herbal Note: For prolapse, the professional herbalist may consider astringents, such as Oak, Yellow Dock, Horsetail, and Rutin. For depression or opioid/alcohol withdrawal: Saint John's Wort, Rose Hips, lymphatic cleansers, tonic and sedative nervines, etc. Do not self-treat.

Transit Saturn Conjunct Natal Pluto

Saturn is one of the two "Chronocrats," or keepers of time (Jupiter being the other). Natal Pluto indicates, in part, one's past life karma (as does natal Saturn and the natal South Node).

Transit Saturn's arrival to natal Pluto can signal the onset of disease of karmic or ancestral origin. This combination is also associated with poisoning, radiation, sepsis, gangrene, venom, or cellular changes. The sign of natal Pluto is important.

One's internal powers of healing can manifest at this time to produce miraculous healing, cures and remissions. This transit could be useful for diagnosing and killing long term parasitic infestations including Lyme's disease and STDs. Potentially effective for medically directed cellular cleansing and heavy metal removal.

Note: We do not yet know enough about Pluto to truly designate his full medical properties. To date astrologers have not yet observed him through the entire zodiac.

Surgical Tips: Unclear. Unless the responsible physician feels it is necessary to move ahead, it may be inadvisable at this time to undergo radiation treatment, hormonal treatments, chemotherapy, gender reassignment, organ transplant or any drastic voluntary surgery. This would be especially the case if this conjunction is in hard aspect or quincunx to Ascendant, Sun or Moon, or if positioned in the 6th, 8th, or 12th house.

Transit Saturn Conjunct Natal North Node

When Saturn transits the natal North Node, one receives a surfeit of Saturn's cold, cosmic Violet Ray. This stimulates increased cold, stiffness and mineral delivery in the body parts governed by the sign of the natal North Node, and the sign it inhabits. Possible ramifications include: stiffness, rheumatic pains, cold, trapped fluids or toxins, impactions, plugged ducts, gravel and stones, bone spurs, dryness, arthritis, drying bowel (especially in Virgo or Scorpio), skin disease, strain from overwork, and, in Fire signs, arterial inflexibility.

Field Note: A client suffered lupus, affecting mostly her hands. Her fingers had become so stiff as to feel as though they had turned to stone. She had natal Saturn in Gemini conjunct the North Node in the birth chart's 3rd house.

Let's work this out: Saturn's ray is cold, dry and tense. Being natally in Gemini, she would receive an extra dose of this Saturnian energy in the Gemini body zone. The third sign, Gemini, rules the hands, and the 3rd house echoes this attribution.

Positive: This is perhaps the best aspect for increasing bone density and overall strength!

Surgical and Medical Tips: Impaction and sepsis prone. Excellent for grafts, bone setting and dental replacement, provided that other aspects agree and natal Saturn is fortified.

Cellular changes can occur rapidly under this aspect. Therefore, test all suspicious moles, freckles or lumps without delay. Don't ignore constipation.

Herbal Note: Saturn hordes toxins when passing over the natal North Node. If symptoms suggest, this is a time to assist the bodily excretory systems related most to the North Node's natal sign. Increase fluids and assist circulation. This transit can be drying.

A professional herbalist may use warming alteratives, hepatics and stone-dissolving herbs as necessary, such as Parsley, Gravel Root, Olive oil, Oregon Grape Root, Burdock Root, Black Walnut. Warming bile moving herbs: Chamomile, Bayberry, Flaxseed Tea, Agrimony, Yarrow, Butternut, Burdock, et al. Cayenne and Ginger may be useful should this transit coincide with internal stasis or cold. Do not self-treat.

Conversely, there are few more optimum times for curing atrophy or reversing osteoporosis!

Field Note: One client was born with a tight natal Saturn-North Node conjunction in Aries, the sign of the head, also conjoined with the natal Moon in Aries. Their dispositor (ruler of Aries), is Mars. With the Sun and Mercury, Mars was natally posited in Taurus, the sign of the ears. If unrelieved, this all suggested an inordinate level of pressure occurring somewhere within his head region (Astrological Body Zones 1 and 2).

I inquired as to how this might have manifested in his life. He relayed that he had suffered from multiple ear infections since childhood, and was currently struggling with glaucoma (this last, I guessed). Additionally, he had twice perforated an eardrum during flus, and if fact, was now so suffering. The list went on.

A physician could do great good by working out how to offload this building pressure within the head region.

Transit Saturn Conjunct Natal South Node

Saturn's cold, drying forces and his cold cosmic Violet Ray are on the chart's exit point. This is a troublemaker because it "hatches" the inherent problems associated with the South Node. Genetically inherited disease may manifest in the predisposed, because both Nodes are associated with genetic disease.

Check aspects to natal Saturn. Should natal Saturn be weak, and/or aspects to natal Saturn stressful, this conjunction can signal an escalation of osteoporosis.

Field Note 1: Multiple times, I've observed this transit exactly coinciding with a surprise diagnosis of osteoporosis or osteopenia.

A reliable repetition of performance increases confidence in any aspect! So, the last two times I noted this transit currently active, I made inquiries. Sure enough, osteopenia had been detected.

Field Note 2: Should this transit be approaching, and the native has a related illness, this same energy can be used to turn it around! Here is a revealing tale. One friend had a muscle atrophy disease of unknown origin, steadily declining. However, one year hence, transit Saturn would conjoin South Node simultaneous to the South Node's transit of Saturn! This is a "doubling."

Acknowledging the approaching transit, this individual worked hard to find the cause and reverse symptoms. The arrival of Saturn to the natal South Node instead now indicated a correction of the weakness. And, it did! Saturn rewards those who work with him.

Positive: Saturn's arrive at the natal South Node will bring one's physical weaknesses to light. This is the perfect time to identify and strengthen your weakness, because Saturn is pointing them out! I've witnessed many a difficult case turn themselves around at this time.

Surgical and Medical Tips: Unless the responsible physician feels it necessary to move ahead, surgery of any kind is not advisable at this time, nor until transit Saturn is well past the natal South Node, and not going to retrograde back over it. If surgery is necessary, refer to *Astrology & Your Vital Force, Chapter 18.*

However, stones, gravel, arthritis and cataracts can be more readily dissolved away at this time!

Herbal Note: This is tricky. First, one must figure out what weakness or genetic issue the natal South Node indicates, and in what body part. Saturn's arrival here will either identify and fix the issue or, if ignored, move the native headlong into it (it seems there is a choice at this time). Theoretically, in cases of malnourishment caused maladies, the professional herbalist may prescribe mineral rich nutrient herbs, such as Nettles, Oat Straw, Alfalfa, Fenugreek, and Seaweed. Do not attempt to self-treat.

Transit Saturn Conjunct Natal Ascendant

First, be certain the Ascendant degree is really true. Saturn produces drying and astringent effects to the physical body during this aspect for good or ill, most especially to the regions governed by the Ascendant's sign. Effects last for the duration of Saturn's transit through the Ascendant sign, though are more pronounced within 3° of the true Ascendant degree.

For some natives, this aspect is "just what the doctor ordered," strengthening to bones, and consciously improving to diet and habits., However, should Saturn limit circulation and oxygen, one can see excessive slimming, asthenia, malnourishment and wasting. For older persons, Saturn's arrival to the Ascendant can signal the commencement of old age.

SATURN'S SQUARE
Health Potentials for Predisposed Nativities
The square does not always manifest as health concerns or benefits.

Saturn's transiting squares are generally not as strong as conjunctions. However, they will slow the function of any natal planets involved, especially within a 3° orb. This effect is even more pronounced when transit Saturn is retrograde and backing up to square the natal planet.

For example, the natal Moon is at 3° Sagittarius, and transit Saturn is retrograde in Virgo moving from 4° to 3°. Visualize a truck with a heavy load of stones backing up!

The signs involved in the transit-natal square are very important. See *Chapter 3: Aspect Mechanics.* Simplistically, transit Saturn slows the natal planet from the sign he is transiting. The natal planet and its sign receive Saturn's influence!

An example would be a transit of Saturn in Gemini squaring the natal Moon in Virgo. One of the upper digestion organs (Virgo), or stomach, breast or mucosa (Moon) would be dried and slowed by transit Saturn. The origin sign (Gemini) would suggest the inhibition of function originates in a Gemini body region, such as nerves, mental tension, lungs, hands, and arms.

See *Herbal Notes* and *Surgical Notes* for *Saturn's Conjunctions* earlier in this chapter. **Saturn's squares do not always express themselves as medical issues.**

Transit Saturn Square Natal Sun: Inhibits the vital force, heart, brain, and sometimes vision. This square may indicate an increased need for magnesium, iodine, oil soluble vitamins.

Transit Saturn Square Natal Moon: Dries mucous membranes, chills stomach, reduces digestive fluids, reduces absorption of nutrients and calcium. This square reduces female hormones, fertility and breast milk, and hardens the uterus. Cataract building may signal a need for potassium, B2 or silver.

Transit Saturn Square Natal Mercury: Slows nerves, inhibits hearing or speech, and indicates potential neural malnutrition.

Transit Saturn Square Natal Venus: Inhibits libido, copper absorption, and female hormones; shrinks breasts, hardens ovaries, impairs kidney function, traps or reduces thick white fluids, tumor building.

Transit Saturn Square Natal Mars: Inhibits libido, reduces male hormones, sperm count and virility, may indicate a significant change in iron, adrenalin or testosterone levels. For some natives, this aspect can strengthen bones and muscles, typically through hard work. Restricts or directs energy and exercise in a disciplined manner.

This transit may affect hearing or smell. It slows motor nerves, signals potential muscular-skeletal issues such as rheumatism or arthritis, and may signal a tendency to lactic acid or uric acid retention and resultant skin issues. Drying to muscles, ligaments, tendons. The signs tell you where! (See discussion: *When Cold and Dry Precipitates Hot Conditions,* under *Saturn's General Action,* beginning of this chapter.) May suggest a B12 deficiency.

Transit Saturn Square Natal Jupiter: Slows liver function, may weaken cartilage, inhibit the pituitary. Deficient fats or cholesterol, good for weight management. May indicate an increased need for choline or B6, Chromium, Biotin and is a watch-aspect for diabetic or hypoglycemic tendencies (*Nauman* –on this aspect in natal charts in her book; see end of *Chapter 1, Additional Texts.*)

Transit Saturn Square Natal Saturn: This signals one of Saturn's the four "seven year" pivot points of his 29 years cycle through the twelve signs. The bodily structure undergoes change.

Transit Saturn Square Natal Uranus: This aspect may inhibit the little known electrical forces of the body for good or ill.

Transit Saturn Square Natal Neptune: Inhibits sleep, yet disciplining to addictions.

Transit Saturn Square Natal Pluto: Unclear to this author.

Transit Saturn Square the Lunar Nodes: This aspect does not necessarily manifest physically. However, if natal Saturn is simultaneously under stress, this aspect doubles it. Transit Saturn is "in the bends" *(see page 46).*

SATURN'S OPPOSITION
Health Potentials for Predisposed Nativities
The square does not always manifest as health concerns or benefits.

The following is a helpful formula for discerning the meaning of Saturn's opposition by sign polarity.

Formula for Interpretation of Saturn's Opposition
Transit Saturn is cooling, slowing, and drying in _____ *(give sign of transit Saturn and body parts ruled).* This then influences _____ *(name planet opposed)* and its bodily functions _____*(describe),* in those bodily regions ruled by the sign of the natal planet _____ *(give sign and body parts).* Thus, the entire sign polarity is emphasized. Now check the function of this polarity (figures in *Chapter 3).*

The opposition of transit Saturn works like the conjunction, but not as strong. Additionally, as with other oppositions, Saturn pulls upon the vital force of the natal planet opposed, which is weakening because it pulls from the opposite side of the ecliptic.

The opposition of transit Saturn also cools, dries and slows the planet opposed. Those effects come from the opposite sign, not the same sign, as with a conjunction. It is essential when examining the opposition to note the houses and signs in the polarity concerned. See *Chapter 3: Aspect Mechanics.*

Transit Saturn Opposes Natal Sun

Here, the vital force is at lowest ebb, (second only to the South Node's passage over the natal Sun), as Saturn pulls at the Sun from the opposite side of the ecliptic plane.

This opposition from Saturn inhibits the vital force, heart, brain, and sometimes vision. Frail persons require extra care at this time. Licensed Health practitioners should consider the methods at their disposal for refueling the internal life battery. It is supremely important to sufficiently convalesce if ill at this time. May indicate an increased need for magnesium, iodine, or oil soluble vitamins.

Transit Saturn Opposes Natal Moon

All things governed by the Moon are at low tide. This opposition from Saturn dries mucous membranes, chills stomach and diminishes digestive acids and mucous secretion. It reduces female hormones, fertility and breast milk; hardens uterus and can be cataract building. Poor absorption, especially of calcium. In the age appropriate, may signal menopause. May signal a need for potassium, or silver.

If occurring in an infant's chart, don't leave them, even for a week; as a lifelong abandonment imprint occurs. However, this transit can separate mother and child for any number of perfectly involuntary reasons.

Transit Saturn Opposes Natal Mercury

All Mercury-ruled functions are weighted down. This transit slows the nerves, and can signal neural malnutrition, inhibiting to thinking, hearing, speech or hand acuity. Blocks and dries the upper respiratory tract. This transit is dangerous for those suffering COPD, TB, etc. (See *Herbal Note* in *Transit Saturn Conjunct Natal Mercury*.) This is serious in infants and geriatrics.

Transit Saturn Opposes Natal Venus

Inhibits libido and blocks affection, copper absorption, and female hormones, (lowers hormones); shrinks breasts, hardens ovaries. Tumor building, impairs kidney function, traps or reduces thick white fluids. May thin the hair or correspond with balding. An important aspect for diabetics (influences blood sugar). This aspect can temporarily halt one's sex life.

Transit Saturn Opposes Natal Mars

Energy is at a lower ebb. Inhibits or frustrates libido, reduces male hormones, sperm count, and virility. Can temporarily halt one' sex life, drinking or athletic escapades. Misbehavior of all kinds is confronted or stopped. This is the transit of "consequences". Restricts available energy, and makes the native more aware of a wiser, more conscious use of their energy, body and time.

Positively, directs disciplined exercise or recovery through a partner, program or physician. Shrinks or conversely, builds muscle mass, depending on age, nutritive absorption and other factors. Other possible impacts include: affects to hearing or smell, slowing of motor nerves, muscular-skeletal issues, atrophy, rheumatic, and lactic acid or uric acid retention with resultant skin issues.

Drying to muscles, ligaments, tendons. The zodiac signs tell you where! May indicate need for increased iron, adrenalin, testosterone, or B6. (See discussion: *When Cold and Dry Precipitates Hot Conditions,* under *Saturn's General Action,* beginning of this chapter.)

Field Note: A long-term, incorrigible alcoholic finally succeeded in sobriety when transit Saturn-in-Capricorn exactly opposed his natal Mars-in-Cancer, positioned in his Ascendant (Cancer rising). Assistance arrived in the form of a solid program inclusive of a medication that reduces brain induced craving.

Transit Saturn Opposes Natal Jupiter

Slowed liver function (dangerous if suffering from liver disease), deficient fats or cholesterol, supportive of weight management, weakened cartilage, inhibits pituitary. This transit can signal that "it's finally time" to remove that growth, stop overeating, quit eating junk food, etc. Here are two interesting examples.

Field Note 1: One friend born with Jupiter (growth) natally ascending in the sign Cancer, suffered a decades long, large benign lipoma, happily growing within Cancer's body region, both internally and externally. As transit Saturn arrived to oppose his natal Jupiter, both he and the doctors concluded that it was high time for its removal.

Field Note 2: One lady born with Jupiter in Cancer, the sign of the stomach, had a legendary appetite for years, the subject of jest amongst her friends and relatives. In her sixties, precisely as transit Saturn opposed her natal Jupiter from drying Capricorn, a temporary stomach issue abruptly halted this pattern.

Transit Saturn Opposes Natal Saturn

One of the four essential "seven year" pivot points of Saturn, in his 29 year cycle through the twelve signs. The bodily structure undergoes change.

Transit Saturn Opposes Natal Uranus

Uncertain. May inhibit the electrical forces or centers of the body for good or ill.

Stronger than the square, and more serious. Antispasmodic herbs may be required. Read for the conjunction and for the reverse aspect: Uranus conjunct Saturn. Do not self-treat.

Transit Saturn Opposes Natal Neptune

Inhibits sleep, disciplining to addictions. Suddenly, one can take an honest look at oneself and one's visions. Sometimes a diagnosis is finally achieved after months or years of enduring a mysterious complaint (this is similar for the transit conjunction).

Transit Saturn Opposes Natal Pluto
Unclear to this author.

SATURN'S QUINCUNX
Health Potentials for Predisposed Nativities
Transits do not always manifest as health concerns

An entire book could be written on health-related quincunxes! Essentially, a quincunx by Saturn means that its needful, strengthening and mineralizing rays are not reaching the planet he quincunxes, if occurring either natally or by transit. Doctors rarely can figure out the cause of consequent complaints!

Quincunxes have a secret or puzzling quality, striking from left field. The hidden cause of a mysterious health complaint is so often revealed by the quincunx of transit (or natal) Saturn, Mars, or any large planet, plus the bodily organs of the sign it inhabits. The two signs involved in any quincunx will be central to your interpretation.

The reader may note that some of the effects of Saturn's quincunxes are similar as to those listed for Saturn's conjunctions, squares and oppositions. However the mechanics behind Saturn's quincunx is distinctively that of deprivation.

The quincunxed natal planet is deprived of minerals, strength and bone building forces. Saturn also governs long term timing of bodily functions as in puberty, menopause, etc. Theoretically, it can't receive the rays of Saturn, so strong for Saturn's conjunction! Saturn's quincunx indicates a disconnection with his beams, that when ignored can produce atrophy of an organ or structural wearing of bodily regions, as shown by the planets and signs quincunxed. See *Chapter 4, Quincunx!*

As we see, symptoms for excess and deficient Saturn can be similar, but for different reasons. For example: A deprivation of minerals (Saturn deficient) can wear down bone and cartilage, causing arthritis. On the other hand, an excess of mineral deposits (excess Saturn) can settle in joints, promoting painful inflammation and arthritis!

Transit Saturn Quincunx Natal Sun

Here, the vital force. doesn't receive the building, nutritive rays of Saturn. Possible atrophy of heart muscle, weakening brain integrity, cataracts or weakening vision. Inhibits the vital force.

An unwise time for hospital release! The vital force. may be endangered for the frail elderly, provided other transit testimonies agree. May indicate an increased need for magnesium, iodine, oil soluble vitamins.

Transit Saturn Quincunx Natal Moon

All things governed by the Moon may not receive appropriate minerals. Poor absorption, especially of calcium! Dries mucous membrane, chills stomach and reduces digestive fluids. May signal a need for potassium or silver.

Reduces female hormones, fertility, and breast milk, hardens uterus. The lymph and blood may distribute minerals poorly, resulting in "pockets" of stuck toxins or minerals. This can create cataracts, cancer, bone spurs and a host of hardening pockets, while the rest of the body goes undernourished!

Transit Saturn Quincunx Natal Mercury

Mercury ruled functions may become malnourished. This can result, over time, in the neural malfunction, neural malnutrition, inhibited hearing or speech, "shattered nerves," etc. If unattended, this deprivation can bring on any number of diseases associated with malnourished nerves or genetic predisposition.

Transit Saturn Quincunx Natal Venus

Venus functions are deprived of Saturn's building ray, and therefore, possible copper deficiency and reduced female hormones. Also, can build tumors, impair kidney function, shrink breasts, or hardens ovaries.

Transit Saturn Quincunx Natal Mars

May suggest a lack of minerals available to muscles, atrophy, low libido, reduced male hormones, sperm count, and virility; restricts or shrinks muscle tissue, may block hearing or smell, slows motor nerves, musculoskeletal issues, mysterious rheumatic complaints.

This aspect may signal a tendency to lactic acid or uric acid retention (and resultant skin issues), slowed peristalsis, slowed or blocked catharsis of toxins from orifices, hernia prone, drying to muscles, ligaments, tendons.

Saturn's blood clotting factor may not work well at this time, producing nonstop bleeds. This is a dangerous transit for some types of surgery. The signs tell you where any or all the above may be active! May indicate need for increased iron, adrenalin or testosterone, or B6. Timing mechanisms related to adrenal hormones and male hormones may be offset.

Herbal Note: Nettles are advised for muscle atrophy *(M. Wood).*

Field Note: A person suffered for years with "an impossible to diagnose" muscle-wasting disease. The native had natal Saturn (minerals) in Scorpio, quincunx natal Mars (muscles) in Aries. Here the effect played out upon the muscles (Mars), rather than through the sign Aries (Head). This person was healed with mineral-rich herbs and predigested amino acids, which counteracted the mineral deficiency from the quincunx.

Transit Saturn Quincunx Natal Jupiter

The regulatory action of Saturn is not reaching Jupiter (liver). This can presage undiagnosed liver, cholesterol or blood issues. Slowed liver function (dangerous if suffering from liver disease), deficient or out-of-control fats or blood cholesterol, unexplained weight gain or loss (usually gain), weakened cartilage, growth problems, puberty oddities (Saturn's regulatory action upon the pituitary can be off).

Field Note 1: One lady was born on an exact quincunx of natal Saturn in Libra to natal Jupiter in Aquarius. Here we see a disconnection of Jupiter's growth principle from Saturn's opposing astringent function. Her top half was quite fat and buxom whilst her lower half was extremely lean, with no female-style buttocks apparent.

Field Note 2: I have noted Saturn and Jupiter to be quincunx by sign in approximately 75% of my cases with an unexpected diagnosis of weak cartilage being ground away by bone in the knee, hip, or foot, and also in cases of severe osteoporosis. Somehow the cushioning function (Jupiter) is not integral (Saturn). Or perhaps the bone itself (Saturn) is undernourished (Jupiter), or too hard and dry (Jupiter is warm, moistening and oily).

Field Note 3: I recall a client who had a natal Saturn-in-Aries (Aries rules the eyes), exactly quincunx her natal Jupiter in Virgo (liver). I volunteered that she "may have a slow liver function with consequential obstruction, or poor circulation (toxic buildup) in the region of the upper head, brain or eye."

She explained that she had survived cancer of the outer eyeball. Continuing, she added that a recent scan showed a benign "hard spot" on her liver.

Transit Saturn Quincunx Natal Saturn

When transit Saturn is quincunx its natal position by sign, the emphasis of this period is in a sign very unlike that of natal Saturn. This may cause deficiency to one of the two signs involved! The imbalances indicated by this quincunx could, hopefully temporary, express through the skeletal system and connective tissue.

Transit Saturn Quincunx Natal Uranus

Saturn regulates and balances. Without Saturn's grounding ray, spasticity may result, or all manner of extremes depending on the signs involved. Possibly associated with onset of neurological diseases. Salts and electrolytes may not be blocked from their appropriate electrical functions.

Transit Saturn Quincunx Natal Neptune

The impacts are unclear to the author. This aspect may indicate a secret heavy metal poisoning or impeded lymphatic flow. There may be a leaking or leeching of an essential nutrient (Saturn), supporting a natal weakness (Neptune). Be alert for secret bone loss. Mineral and bone loss is especially relevant at this time for users of opioids, alcohol or chemical meds (Neptune).

The ability to sleep deeply may be impeded from a very earthly cause, i.e., a lumpy mattress, cold feet, or nightly parental duties. This aspect is annoying to dreamy types, and may be experienced as unwanted earthly duties.

Look carefully under the rug when this transit quincunx is within a 1° orb. Something toxic may be building up in the lymphatic system or blood stream unnoticed. Be alert for blood cell changes, deficient white cells, etc. Neptune governs viruses, and the arrival of a transit quincunx from Saturn may signal a period of quietly sinking immune resistance.

Transit Saturn Quincunx Natal Pluto

The effects are not clear to this author. In rare cases this could suggests a hidden or rare cancer, necrosis, bacterial infection, poisoning or potentially mortal disease process setting in, either unnoticed or confounding to the physicians. The secret source will be the sign and house position of transit Saturn, (read as "cold, slow, restricted flow"); whereas the area affected could include the sign (and possibly house) position of natal Pluto.

SATURN'S SEXTILES & TRINES
Health Potentials for Predisposed Nativities
Transits do not always manifest as health concerns or benefits.

This is a book of pathologies and has limited space. So, we are not dedicating all sections to these traditionally "positive" aspects except in the case of Sun and Jupiter where these are extremely relevant health aspects.

All Saturn aspects translate his cold light and vibratory frequency to any natal planet. The sextile (60°), and trine (120°) are considered "positive" by Western astrologers, rarely bringing issues. However, in the East, Saturn's forward sextile is considered as strong and as potentially difficult as his hard aspects.

That being said, sextiles are rarely as forceful as hard aspects in practice. Saturn's transit sextile offers a steadying influence to any planet.

Chapter 15
URANUS
Extremes and Imbalance

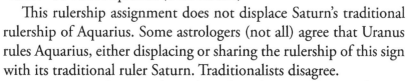

Properties, Rulerships and Actions
Rules: Co-rules Aquarius (with Saturn)

This rulership assignment does not displace Saturn's traditional rulership of Aquarius. Some astrologers (not all) agree that Uranus rules Aquarius, either displacing or sharing the rulership of this sign with its traditional ruler Saturn. Traditionalists disagree.

Uranus was discovered in the relatively recent year of 1781 and therefore its dignities and debilities are speculative. Rulership indicates a strong resonance with a sign. Also, the planet in transit carries with it, wherever it goes, the influence of the house of a horoscope governed by its home sign.

When discovered, Uranus was in the sign Gemini with his personal North Node. This is a "jazzy" sign (statistically, the greatest total number of famous jazz musicians in my "Who's Who in Jazz" study were born in Gemini or Aquarius. Gemini also governs the peripheral nerves, and Uranus rules electricity. Nerves are electrical transmitters!

It therefore surprises me that the erratic, and famously improvisational Gemini is not considered a candidate for Uranus' exaltation. If rulership and exaltation are based on natural affinity, it should be. The currently popular assignments are:

Exalted: Scorpio

Detriment: Leo

Fall: Taurus (This seems apt. Taurus grounds electricity, therefore reducing the impact of this highly electrical planet.)

Metal: Uranium *(Urquart)*

Minerals: Zinc *(M. Uyldert)*. Salt is traditionally assigned to Saturn. However, Saturn is grounding to electricity. Uranus holds the greatest influence over electricity of perhaps any planet. Is salt really ruled by Uranus?

Vitamins: Unknown.

Gem & Cosmic Ray: Not established

Astronomers have established that Uranus has a reversed magnetic field and is the only planet rotating on its side, askew, and spinning in the reverse direction of its fellow planets. Astrologers have noted that Uranus significantly influences electrical current: its surges, reversals and outages.

My experience has been that this eccentric planet brings "undiagnosable" conditions and unpredictable results, agreeing perfectly with what astrologers had already found out about Uranus' action in other areas of life.

Body Rulership & Organ Affinities: The great prophet and medical psychic Edgar Cayce states that Uranus governs the thyroid gland. He is unique in this viewpoint, but my casework lends some truth to this idea. Many cases of severe thyroid disfunction show an angular or highly afflicted Uranus, especially near 0° of a fixed sign.

General Action: Electrical. The great medical psychic Edgar Cayce stated that Uranus rules extremes. This extremism is so often observable in those born with Uranus exactly rising. Uranus also produces structural twists, torsion, dislocations and disorder to structure, such as scoliosis or tilted uterus.

Uranus throws any function off-center, producing imbalance, reversals and extremes. He tends to reverse magnetic fields, suddenly. Uranus' problems are often weird and baffling. Symptoms appear and disappear suddenly, seemingly out of nowhere, mystifying the doctors.

Spasm: Extreme, shocking, paralytic, productive of cramps and seizures, sudden release or relief, electrical arrhythmia or malfunction. The location of spasm is found in the sign he tenants natally or is currently transiting through. Uranus also upsets hormonal balances.

The great physician-medical astrologer, William Davidson, associated Uranus with spasm. Davidson specified that Uranus-caused spasm can occur in any organ, vessel or bodily region.

Uranus stimulates and amps up any region he natally tenants or transits through. However, the manner of stimulation is different than that of fellow stimulant Mars. Whereas Mars' influence is hot and constant, Uranus is rather like cold ice or an electrical current switched on and off.

Compensation: The iconic Dr. William Davidson taught a unique slant on Uranus not heard much elsewhere. He said that this planet produced not just spasm, but compensation.

The problem was that he provided no examples to illustrate his meaning. My *Webster's Dictionary* says: "Compensation: 1. To make up for; counterbalance. 2. To make payment to; recompense." This describes Venus!

However, Uranus always shows where in the chart we have something exceptional, genius, unique, or just plain weird. Uranus also acts as an electrical stimulant. For health problems that are suspected as being due to electromagnetic fields, look to Uranus and Neptune.

Perhaps an exceptionally good function of one body zone or organ would indeed compensate for poor function elsewhere. In my files is one case of natal Uranus in Aquarius exactly opposed to Saturn in Leo, in the Ascendant (rising). This man lived for years on only 17% of heart function (Leo). His circulation (Aquarius) was excellent! Of course, for Uranus to create compensation, it would need to be well-placed and aspected. His was.

Positive: Uranus awakens! Uranus liberates! Uranus can produce a smooth and well-regulated flow of electrical current through the heart, brain and body.

A long-term or puzzling complaint can vanish suddenly, without explanation! Experimental method trials work out. Electrical healing methods can be supported. The Uranus' transit can be amicably utilized to assist the awakening of long dead nerves and reestablish current. Deafness, blindness, paralysis can inexplicably reverse at the time of Uranus' transit passage over the natal planet signifying the problem. *(See Field Note for Uranus Conjunct Natal Saturn.)*

Negative: Surprise! Out of the sheer blue descends an inexplicable medical concern, such as a sports injury that occurs while sitting on the couch. Arrhythmias, spasms, reversal of electrical current, wild hormonal swings, seizures, mental extremes, stroke, paralysis, alarming symptoms, hyperthyroid, neural excitement.

Transit Frame & Orb: Uranus spends approximately seven years in each zodiac sign. His transits best show results in tight orb (0-1°) to any natal planet, bringing an off-and-on spasmodic influence to that planet for about a year.

Temperature: The action of Uranus appears to be ice cold, yet stimulating, but in a manner different from Mars. Much depends on Uranus' current sign and element.

In Fire signs, this planet's frequencies can manifest as mania, panic attack, seizure, heart attack, heart arrhythmia and stroke, all seemingly "hot" complaints. However, Uranus' stimulation produces extreme tension, torsion and spasm; not always accompanied by inflammation, (as is more typical to Mars). Therefore, rather than thinking of temperature per se, think "electricity."

General Field Note: Astrologer Clayton Cruce published a fascinating research monograph entitled *Electrical Series Volume 1: Lightning (Solarion Press)*. The book focuses on several birth charts of electrocution victims, both accidental and human induced, with transits for the date of electrocution.

There is no doubt that Uranus is heavily involved in most electrocutions. One of his many intriguing findings replicated my own: Uranus is so often natally angular, or by transit-to-natal on the angles for persons inclined to electrocution. Cruce and I concur that exact trines of Uranus are productive of sudden, excessive surges of electrical current directed to the natal planet so trined! Cruce made many further important and independent discoveries on this topic.

URANUS THROUGH THE ELEMENTS & SIGNS

Applicable to both natal and transit charts, these partial lists of expressed symptoms apply only to predisposed nativities. These conditions are obviously uncommon and require multiple testimonies beyond the presence of Uranus.

Manifestation of symptoms may be enhanced by lifestyle choices, and taking preemptive measures can reduce, remove or prevent potential issues from manifesting. It is impossible to list all potential manifestations.

Uranus in Fire Signs

Aries: Sudden rush of blood to brain vessels (migraine), electrical brainstorms, epilepsy, seizure, sudden trauma to the head, aneurysm, violent rages, mania, strange eye problems, detached retina, sudden release of excessive testosterone or adrenalin, uncoordinated vision.

Leo: Disturbance to the electrical rhythm of heart (arrhythmia), heart flutter, spasm or anomalies in heart vessels or valves, aneurysm alert, increases body heat, spasm in gallbladder, fits of anger, twisted wrist (with Gemini), scoliosis (natal), back spasms, spinal subluxations, spinal nerve sheath anomaly.

Sagittarius: Excess surges of arterial circulation, excitement of sciatic nerve, hard-to-diagnose diseases of spinal nerves, leg spasms, hip and thigh spasm, extreme muscular tension, religious mania, tremor, epilepsy, excited mental states, ADHD (natal), strokes, electrocution, and paralysis.

Uranus in Earth Signs

Uranus, being electrical, is better grounded in Earth signs. This may lessen the impact of his transit in Earth signs. Conversely, he can upset the normal stability creating functions of these signs.

Taurus: Thyroid disturbances, hearing disorders, tinnitus, misalignment of axis bone or cervical vertebrae, dental oddities, irregular growth of teeth, spasm of vocal cord or larynx, spasm of upper esophagus, choking, vocal oddities, jaw misalignment, bruxism, weird food cravings.

Virgo: Abdominal hernia, duodenal or intestinal spasm, twisted intestine, hard-to-diagnose intestinal issues, spasm in transverse colon, pancreatic or duodenal disturbance, extremes of liver action, immune system peculiarities, splenic malfunction.

Capricorn: Gallbladder spasm (also in Leo), sudden jaundice, sudden skin changes, pituitary disturbance or extremes (see Cancer, Pisces), "trick knee," sudden onset osteoporosis, bone changes, odd bone or nail problems, stomach spasm (reflex to Cancer), changes of appetite.

Uranus in Air Signs

Gemini: Spasm in lungs or bronchial tubes, asthma, whooping cough, frozen shoulder, dislocated shoulder, arm or hand spasm; sprained or twisted arms, hands or fingers; attention disturbances, mental disconnection, mental extremes, stuttering, speech disturbance, disturbance of sensory nerves or afferent nerves, sleep apnea, paralysis; twisted tubes, such as fallopian tubes and ureters.

Libra: Renal spasm, lumbar spasm, hormonal imbalance, adrenal extremes, gender identity change or issues, reversal of sex attraction, social "gender benders," hard to diagnose issues of the urinary tract, ovarian peculiarities, sodium-potassium imbalances, acid-alkaline imbalances, kidney anomalies.

Aquarius: Lower leg spasm, "charlie horses," lower leg thrombosis, venous spasm, twisted ankle, electrical malfunction to heart (reflex to Leo). Inexplicable actions or diseases of spinal nerves, all manner of undiagnosable problems (due to the body's little-understood electrical system); odd mental states, sudden bolts of psychic information, sudden lack of oxygen, sleep apnea, paralysis, weird circulatory disturbances, disturbed imaginative faculty.

Uranus in Water Signs

Cancer: Stomach spasm, lower lung spasm, breast size irregularities, extreme cyclic changes of breast size, pituitary extremes, emotional extremes, emotional attachment disorders, brain fluid or chemistry extremes. Appetite extremes, explosive vomiting, bulimia, anorexia, orthorexia, eating disorders, paranoia, brain tumor (rare).

Scorpio: Excess sexual activity, peculiar sexual obsessions, size extremes of sex organs or ureters, tilted uterus, uterine or bladder spasm, colitis; spasms of the colon, rectum and anus; sudden impotence or frigidity, sudden nose bleed, bed-wetting, enuresis, excess sweating, hernia, prolapsed rectum or vagina, colorectal twists, explosive diarrhea.

Pisces: Uranus behaves slightly similar to Jupiter in this sign. Pisces lacks boundaries, so Uranus' proclivity for extremes knows no bounds in this sign! Pisces is also a bit sloppy, so Uranus can signal a disorganization of overall glandular coordination, the province of this sign.

Inexplicable blood cholesterol extremes, spasm of lymphatic vessels, lymphatic pressure, engorged lymph nodes, glandular extremes and pituitary disturbance, dwarfism and gigantism, large feet, sudden collapse of arch, sudden weight gain or loss, mega-obesity, fluidic collection, phlegmatic; upsets normal sleep rhythms, sleep extremes, insomnia and excess sleep, weird or disturbing dreams, enlightening dreams.

Blows open psychic doors for good or ill, sudden onset of psychic problems or mental illness; those who experiment with psycho-tropics, psychedelics, channeling or magic under this transit tempt shocking results.

URANUS' TRANSIT OF NATAL PLANETS

Applicable to both natal and transit charts, these partial lists of expressed symptoms apply only to predisposed nativities. These conditions are obviously uncommon and require multiple testimonies beyond the presence of Uranus.

Manifestation of symptoms may be enhanced by lifestyle choices, and taking preemptive measures can reduce, remove or prevent potential issues from manifesting. It is not possible to list all potential expressions.

URANUS' CONJUNCTIONS
Health Potentials for Predisposed Nativities
Transits do not always manifest as health concerns or benefits.

Transit Uranus Conjunct Natal Sun

This transit stimulates the vital force, especially in Fire and Air signs. Strongly influences the electrical centers in the heart or brain, for good or ill. Arterial circulation increases, warms, dilates. This may warn of high blood pressure, especially in Fire signs. Migraine, aneurism, or stroke. The human battery amps up or down. Can bring miraculous cures! Potentially, can awaken dull brain centers.

In some cases, the brain and/or heart receives an excess of electritrical magnetic frequency (EMF). This can be productive of brain tumor or change of heart rhythm. Vision may change suddenly, incurring vision anomalies.

Surgical Tip: This transit can bring unpredictable results for heart, brain, spinal cord and eyes. Transit Jupiter or Saturn can assist with an exact trine or sextile. Consult the responsible physician for surgical timing.

Transit Uranus Conjunct Natal Moon

This transit strongly influences the uterus, female hormones stomach, emotions, brain chemistry and mind. Uterine contractions, stomach spasms, emotional extremes, sudden fear, panic attack, breast changes or growth, gynecomastia (male breast tissue growth). This transit may increase peristalsis in the colon, or stimulate sudden emptying of the bladder. May affect autonomic functions, such as breathing, sleep, or heart rhythm. Dietary extremes.

Field Note: Freak emotional winds strike suddenly! My files host several cases of persons who whimsically abandoned home and family, or relocated cross-country during a Uranus conjunction or square of natal Moon within an orb of 3°.

One senior client panicked and committed suicide on this exact conjunction in Sagittarius, following an incident of family distress. Of course, in these cases, their natal Moons were predisposed to extremes in the first place.

Surgical and Medical Tips: This transit suggests unpredictable results for stomach, breast, brain, eye and uterine surgery. It may be advisable now for pregnant women to avoid air flight and take every precaution to avoid shock, vibration and strong EMF fields. Jupiter can help mitigate with an exact trine or sextile.

Psychiatric patients should be watched closely for sudden emotional swings and decisions. A poor time for diet extremes. Hormonal treatments may have extreme or unwanted impact. Consult the responsible physician for surgical timing.

Transit Uranus Conjunct Natal Mercury

This transit is often decisively disturbing to both a native's mental state and neural transmission. Excites nerves and quickens transmission. Gifts the minds for those of fertile imagination!

This transit can also cause inexplicable paralysis through a sudden nerve blockage or spasm. Some people experience neural pains during the exact conjunction. Conversely, deadened nerves can reawaken! Common experiences are headache, earache, eyestrain, or neuritis in the body parts assigned to natal Mercury and its sign placement.

In rare cases, this indicates "bald spots" in the spinal sheath and the onset of muscular sclerosis. Conversely, experience may prove that this transit could reawaken neural current in paralysis cases!

Surgical and Medical Tips:: Unpredictable results for surgery to all nerves or nerve plexus, ear, brain, arms, hands, fingers, and speech centers of brain. Jupiter can assist with an exact trine or sextile. The brain and nerves require protective fats, especially now. This is no time for a low fat diet! Consult the responsible surgeon for surgical timing.

Herbal Notes: Professional herbalists will find that the nutritive nervines are quite helpful. Nettles, Oat Straw, Red Clover, Alfalfa, Dulce and Kelp are excellent sources of neural-grounding minerals. Favorite sedative nervines include St. John's Wort (for neuralgia), Blue Vervain, Scullcap, Lemon Balm (mild) and Lavender. Edgar Cayce states that Passion Flower is a specific for epilepsy and provides details for its precise preparation. (See *Edgar Cayce Encyclopedia of Healing,* by Reba Anne Karp.) Do not self-treat.

Transit Uranus Conjunct Natal Venus

This transit produces an estrogen-progesterone imbalance in women. However, men are also influenced by hormonal changes and consequential sexual effects. Typically, romantic attractions shift suddenly, so never trust that latest infatuation to last. Under this transit, some reverse their gender identity or gender of interest! The libido may suddenly lurch to some extreme. Manifestations include premature menarche (first menstruation), or menopause, menarche, or an unexpected, sudden onset menopause, gynecomastia (male breast tissue growth). These expressions are equally plausible for Uranus-Moon hard aspects.

If Edgar Cayce is correct that Venus governs the thymus gland, we could expect changes there, with effects on the strength of the immune system. The erratic action of Uranus over natal Venus could upset kidney, ovarian, venous and skin functions. If skin changes occur, consider changing estrogen or copper levels as potential causes!

Surgical Tip: Unpredictable results for surgery to kidneys, veins, ovaries, female genitalia, and skin, cosmetic surgery or gender reassignment. This is the most radical time for voluntary cosmetic surgery. Some may be overcome with a sudden passion for cosmetic improvements. Others, for gender transformation. However, results are unpredictable and thus inadvisable when transit Uranus is within at least 3° of natal Venus. Jupiter can assist with an exact trine or sextile. Consult the responsible physician for surgical timing.

Transit Uranus Conjunct Natal Mars

Uranus transit stimulates Mars, a planet that needs calming! This transit signifies energy and libido surges, in spurts, and then you crash. Adrenal burnout and exhaustion are seen in many cases.

This aspect stimulates the hyperactive and temper-prone, especially in Fire and Air signs. Insomnia is typical of this transit *(See Field Note)*. The motor nerves of the brain (ruled by Mars) are strained. This can produce all manner of neuromuscular issues in those prone, such as jerking, extreme neuromuscular tension, spasm, torsion. Spastic colon (Scorpio).

Uranus' transit of natal Mars produces extremes (up or down) in either gender of male hormones and/or adrenalin. Menopausal women may experience extreme hot flashes, while males can experience performance issues (positive or negative). Some males experience sudden impotence or premature ejaculation.

There may be changes to the red blood cells. Iron may swing up or down. This aspect can produce unexpected and extreme expulsion of blood or wastes: hemorrhage, spurting of arteries, vomiting, catharsis, diarrhea, ejaculation, sweating or urination, sudden nose bleeds.

Anaphylaxis is linked to this aspect, especially for Fire signs. Be vigilant to insect bites, bee stings, and plant toxins. Raises blood pressure, suddenly (especially in Fire signs).

This transit is accident-prone. Avoid playing with wild animals, fire, explosives and firearms. Take great care with mechanical equipment, driving, and electricity. Uranus-Mars contacts are typical in electrocution cases (Cruce), both accidental and human induced.

A sudden increase or decrease in Mars' hot cosmic Yellow Ray affects the blood and liver, bile. This can cause high blood pressure, aneurism, stroke and various blood cell or liver issues. There may be an alarming increase/decrease in sperm count, iron, testosterone, male hormones, adrenalin, salt, electrolytes, red blood cells, muscle mass, and available energy.

Those with mania, anger control issues and bipolar disorders need to be on high alert. People experience bouts of emotional and muscular tension. Muscle strains and spasms are common. Hyperthyroid, especially in Sagittarius.

As discussed above, this transit produces an erratic and extreme effect on energy. Some folks feel euphoric because of a spike in their muscular energy and libido! Many drink heavily and carouse (now described as "high risk behaviors"). However, self-induced liver, brain and arterial damage can ensue.

Conversely, energy can surge downward because this aspect can exhaust the adrenals! We then witness a cycle of high energy, insomnia and extreme behaviors followed by fatigue and exhaustion. Indeed, insomnia is a typical manifestation of this transit.

Field Note: A friend was notorious for her profound childhood slumber, prompting her brother to invite his friends to come observe this phenomenon. However, at forty-nine she became suddenly plagued with insomnia.

At onset, transit Uranus was exactly conjunct her natal Mars-in-Aquarius at her natal Midheaven. The Midheaven-Nadir axis acts as a "planetary door" for incoming rays. I've noticed that the Midheaven-Nadir axis appears to influence the spine from top of head to coccyx. And important for her case of insomnia, Aquarius and Sagittarius co-rule the spinal nerves.

The Uranus transit of my friend's natal Mars and Midheaven suggested a reception of excessive electrical current entering her muscular system and spinal cord. This current would enervate her general muscular system and adrenals (Mars), and spinal nerves (Aquarius), thus producing insomnia. The sign of Aquarius would indicate the physical zone of reception for this Uranus-Mars conjunction (calves and ankles).

First, I suggested various interventions to electrically "ground" the bed itself. We had to be ingenious, utilizing various opaque stones and copper wire. Then we ensured the bed was not aligned North-South. The North-South axis of the horoscope align with the North-South directional line in the bedroom, the precise direction where transit Uranus was currently positioned. The South Point is always the Midheaven (MC) and the North Point always the Nadir.

We worked with her personal Mars "receiving zone" in Aquarius (the ankle), to calm the electrical current produced by transiting Uranus. Also, we worked to reduce current arriving through the South point, across the North-South/Midheaven-Nadir axis.

More muscular exercise before bed was also suggested. Because the Mars-ruled muscular system and motor centers of brain may be implicated, we researched sleeping herbs to specifically relax the motor nerves, spinal nerves and muscles. She was to avoid wearing the hot end of the color spectrum: red and yellow.

Within days, her distressing several-month bout with insomnia perfectly resolved.

Surgical and Medical Tips: Reactions move fast! Therefore, take any hint of anaphylaxis seriously! Treat heatstroke, snow blindness, head injuries with exceptional urgency. Expect some temporary disturbance in those prone to male sexual or urinary disfunction. A red-alert for those with adrenal, blood or iron disorders, hyper-activity, bipolar, or mania.

Unpredictable results extend to blood donors, blood transfusions, and surgery in general, especially for male genitals, hormonal treatments, electrical treatments of all kinds, nose, muscles, and gelding animals. Jupiter can assist with an exact trine or sextile. Consult the responsible physician for surgical timing.

Herbal Note: Licensed practitioners can select those anti-spasmodics and muscle relaxants most directed to the muscular system, such as Valerian, Kava Kava, Lobelia (vagus nerve), Wood Betony, Ginger. (For a huge, hyper-specific selection, see the *Earthwise Herbal Repertory* by Matthew Wood.) Magnets and musical tone therapy work well to redirect electrical surges and outages. Do not self-treat.

Transit Uranus Conjunct Natal Jupiter

This long-term aspect is unclear. Pituitary action may be disturbed, resulting in hormonally induced extremes, such as hirsutism (excessive body hair), growth extremes, breast swelling. Liver function may be extreme or imbalanced, affecting digestion, flatulence, blood constituents, cholesterol, and the like. Liver and gallbladder spasm. This combination produces and encourages extremes related to the bodily regions ruled by sign of natal Jupiter.

Surgical and Medical Tips: Unclear. May have unpredictable effects on liver surgery or treatment. Also, miracle prone! Consult the responsible physician for surgical timing.

Transit Uranus Conjunct Natal Saturn

We see two opposite potentials. First, Uranus can awaken a benumbed limb or sense *(see Field Note)*. Or this transit can suddenly release (Uranus) the shackles of a physical karma (Saturn)!

Secondly, Uranus' transit of Saturn can royally upset balances because Saturn is the balance-wheel of the planets. Glandular function is awry, circadian rhythms are thrown off kilter, or the heart rhythm is disturbed. For the age-appropriate candidate, this transit so often signals a disturbingly sudden onset of puberty, menopause, hirsuitness, etc. Sudden bone growth, growth spurts or, conversely, calcium dumping.

Field Note: An elderly client was born with a tight conjunction of Saturn, Mars and South Node in Aries, the primary sign-ruler of the eyes. All his life he suffered from one eye that couldn't adequately transmit images to his brain. At age 78, Uranus' long transit over his natal Saturn-Mars-South Node in Aries corresponded with his blind eye "waking up" and a return of vision!

Transit Uranus Conjunct Natal Uranus

The author cannot comment on exactly how this transit manifests because it occurs at approximately age 84, well beyond the age of the vast majority of her clients.

Transit Uranus Conjunct Natal Neptune

Physical or psychological weaknesses attributed to natal Neptune could either be brought to the fore, or reversed! A sudden psychic awakening could occur, or there could be sudden leaks or toxicity (for example, a breast implant leaks toxins). Look to the bodily regions ruled by natal Neptune.

Surgical and Medical Tips: Hypothetically, one should be careful of unpredictable effects from anesthesia or toxic implants. Possibilities for sudden drug overdoses, sudden release from addictions, sudden diagnoses or revelation of a mysterious complaint. Consult the responsible physician for surgical timing.

Transit Uranus Conjunct Natal Pluto

Drastic results of many kinds are possible when in close orb; examples: surgical accidents, bacterial outbreak, gangrene, and accidental perforation of bowel during colonoscopy. Potential onset of genetic disease.

Transit Uranus Conjunct Natal North Node

Uranus' transit of the North Node signifies sudden surges of electrical energy entering one's field. The bodily region signified by the sign of the natal North Node suggests where this surge enters. This can produce a sudden or even alarming excitement to the organs ruled by the natal planet or sign. For instance, in Aries, it could signify electrical brain storms. Because this aspect induces extremes, it is dangerous for epileptics or those suffering mania, schizophrenia, or bipolar disorders.

When in close orb, Uranus delivers so much electrical charge that it may also affect the signs it squares and opposes! Be careful around electricity and lightning! This transit has potential to awaken impaired nerves.

Surgical and Medical Tips: Treatments related to the natal sign of the North Node may produce exaggerated responses. For example, should this transit occur as one undergoes electromagnetic therapy, then "less is more." This transit could signal the commencement of radical therapies using vibration, oscillation or electricity. Be wary of hormonal injections; results may be strange, indeed.

Transit Uranus Conjunct Natal South Node

Uranus' transit of the natal South Node can awaken sleeping genetic issues or bring latent psychological issues to the forefront. Past-life memories are stimulated. Electrically related diseases may ensue for predisposed nativities. This is a significant aspect and often mentally unsettling.

Avoid drugs, channeling spirits, playing with kundalini, or anything else that might suddenly open psychic boundaries. The natal sign of this conjunction is extremely important in the assessment of psychological or physical effects.

Surgical and Medical Tips: This is an all-around unpredictable time. Electrical malfunctions may occur either within the body or in necessary medical equipment; exercise caution around electricity!

Be wary of therapies using oscillation, vibration or electricity. Because this aspect induces extremes, it is dangerous for those with seizure complaints, mania, schizophrenia, or bipolar disorder. Consult the responsible physician for surgical timing.

Transit Uranus Conjunct Natal Ascendant

First, be certain the Ascendant is really true. This long-term aspect stimulates electrical current to the body, for good or ill, most especially to the regions governed by the Ascendant's sign.

Although this book does not include discussion of the houses, the transit of Uranus to the exact Ascendant degree is so powerful that it must be included! In many cases, the arrival of Uranus to this essential life-giving angle signifies an unexpected change (good or bad). The sign indicates the body zone potentially involved and the element suggests the style of the sudden shift. The change, should it occur, is unexpected and cannot be ignored.

Typically, one cannot be certain of birth times and, therefore, of precise Ascendant degrees without performing a rectification. The important medical astrologer Carl Jansky worked in obstetrics wards. He recounts that in almost all cases he attended, the nurses recorded the birth time late by roughly fifteen minutes, after they washed up!

Effects last for the duration of Uranus' transit through the Ascendant sign, though are more pronounced within 1° of the true Ascendant degree.

Field Note: To the week that Uranus arrived at a dear friend's Ascendant in Aries (rules the brain and eyes), she began experiencing bizarre seizures, resulting in the discovery of a glioblastoma (type of brain tumor). Many other brain transits were concurrent.

In this case, the friend was also afflicted by Uranus' quincunx to her natal Sun, plus an eclipse conjunct her Sun, while transit Mars simultaneously opposed her Sun! The Sun is one of the traditional co-rulers of the brain. This is a perfect example of *The Planet In Trouble,* as in *Chapter 5.*

Please be reminded that not everyone experiences negative results from Uranus. Because Uranus is a liberator, a similar aspect could just have easily corresponded to the sudden release of life-long deafness or blindness!

THE URANUS SQUARE
Health Potentials for Predisposed Nativities
Transits do not always manifest as health concerns or benefits.

Uranus' transit squares behave similarly to his conjunctions at perhaps 75% strength, yet strike suddenly with great force! In a sense, one gets used to a long conjunction of Uranus over a natal planet, whereas the square creates an ongoing, palpable friction, when in a tight orb of 1°.

Due to retrogrades and direct motion, Uranus typically revisits a natal planet at least twice, sometimes three times

Refer to the previous text of this chapter for Uranus' conjunctions to each planet. However, there is an important difference. In considering the square aspect (90°) we have the electrical stimulus of Uranus coming from the sign he is transiting and going to the sign of the natal planet he squares. The signs and quadruplicity of the planets involved would seem of paramount importance. (For square types by sign and mode, see *Chapter 3: Aspect Mechanics.*)

If you know the bodily regions ruled by each sign, you can readily use the following formula:

Formula for Interpreting Uranus' Transit Squares

Transit Uranus delivers an unpredictable off/on electric current from the bodily zone of his current position_____ *(give sign and bodily regions ruled)* to the bodily zone of the sign _____ *(give sign and bodily regions ruled)* of the planet he squares and to the bodily functions of the planet he squares _____ *(give bodily functions)*.

Special Note on Transit Uranus Square the Natal Lunar Nodes: This may result in electrical oddities, surges and outages, or activate latent genetic diseases.

THE URANUS OPPOSITION
Health Potentials for Predisposed Nativities
Transits do not always manifest as health concerns or benefits

The transit opposition of Uranus is similar to its conjunction, but with some marked differences:

1) This effect is the same as the conjunction, although its source is the opposite sign. Thus the opposite sign of the natal planet is activated, demanding balance of the principles of the sign polarity.

2) Uranus causes a "wobble" or imbalance to functions of the natal planet he opposes, and the body region of its natal sign. This stems from the bodily region or organs governed by the sign thatUranus passes through. Also, think "electrical current,"

3) The opposition typically brings the Uranian effects from an outside source, such as a person, healer, spouse, or something presenting itself to the native.

4) The opposition produces sudden break-offs or "divorces" to the physical function of the natal planet opposed. This is not a consistent affair, but off/on, much like electric current.

5) The opposition influences the medical function of the polarity. *See Chapter 3* regarding the medical interpretation of polarity.

The houses and signs concerned are essential to note. It is beyond the scope of this text to discuss all sign and polarity combinations.

Here is a formula emphasizing the sign polarity to help use this section. (See *Chapter 3: Aspect Mechanics* for discussion of sign polarity.) Uranus' oppositions do not always manifest themselves as health concerns or benefits.

Formula for Interpreting Uranus' Transit Opposition

Uranus transiting through the sign _____ *(give sign)*, will exert an electrical pull, strange behavior or magnetic current reversal to the natal planet he opposes _____ *(name planet)* and its bodily functions _____ *(describe planets bodily functions)*, in the bodily regions ruled by the sign of the natal planet_____ *(give bodily regions)*. The polarity of these two signs is stimulated. Give the action of this sign polarity _____.

Transit Uranus Opposes Natal Sun

This transit might throw off the heart rhythm or brain chemistry. There can be a break in current. This can be dangerous to life when accompanied by an eclipse conjunct the Sun (within 3°), and adjunct transit stresses.

Transit Uranus Opposes Natal Moon

Hormones, emotions, and brain chemistry may go periodically "out of whack," swinging up and down.

Divorce prone. Note the sign polarity and elements involved. Gives glandular and mood changes.

Transit Uranus Opposes Natal Mercury

This transit confuses the mental focus. Thoughts and mental forces are influenced and irritated by Uranus' oscillating vibration. Exacerbates mania, schizophrenia, epilepsy, and many neurological conditions. Weird, new, radical or extreme ideas are introduced into the life. Sudden epiphanies are possible! Breathing rhythm may be disturbed. Note sign polarity and elements involved.

Transit Uranus Opposes Natal Venus

Sudden changes to female hormones, veins, kidney function, copper levels, libido. Can produce surprising results such as. sudden hair growth or loss, genital changes, breast size change, voice change. Similar to the conjunction, though associated more with external events or relationship shocks and shifts.

Transit Uranus Opposes Natal Mars

Can produce extreme swings of energy and libido. Sperm count or red blood cell count may swing up or down; anemia. Adrenal and iron levels are affected. There may be unusual effects upon the motor nerves or muscles. Strange changes in bone marrow possible. Note the sign polarity and elements involved.

Read the more extensive discussion in the section *Transit Uranus Conjunct Natal Mars.*

Transit Uranus Opposes Natal Jupiter

Unclear to this author. May produce odd imbalances in liver function or blood chemistry. Pituitary function can be disturbed, producing growth extremes, premature or delayed puberty.

Changes possible in blood, blood volume or pressure. It is unclear, but there may be some association with diabetes. Note the sign polarity and elements involved. Sudden weight gain/loss.

Transit Uranus Opposes Natal Saturn

Challenges Saturn's authority from opposite viewpoint. For example, radical treatments may counter the physician's advice. A patient may divorce his/her physician or vice versa!

Mental and/ or physical stability threatened, prone to falls, potential sudden mineral loss influencing bone integrity. General life timing, such as puberty, menarche, and menopause, can be thrown off-kilter. Note the sign polarity and elements involved.

Transit Uranus Opposes Natal Uranus

Unclear to this author. May impact the conduction, flow, or timing of electricity throughout the bodily electrical systems, or specific to one organ. This transit may change, reverse, stop, start or alter the influx of subtle electrical currents into one or more of the chakras. Note the sign polarity and elements involved.

Transit Uranus' Oppositions to Trans-Saturnian Planets

Not enough information available.

THE URANUS QUINCUNX
Health Potentials for Predisposed Nativities
Transits do not always manifest as health concerns

The quincunxed planet, and therefore, its functions, cannot "digest" enough Uranus (electrical stimulus) at this time. All quincunxes are sneaky and hard to diagnose, or they hide in latency. However, they are not mild aspects! In fact, they are "the" primary health aspect.

A quincunx of Uranus signals a possible neural or cellular change brewing secretly, often going unnoticed or ignored. If occurring with additional stressors to the natal planet concerned, the quincunx of Uranus is perilous.

Astrologers, including this author, have much to explore about the medical effects of quincunxes.

Transit Uranus Quincunx Natal Sun

The Sun or brain may either not receive enough electrical current, or is electrically disturbed in a manner difficult to diagnose. In other cases, the brain suddenly receives too much current. The life force is suddenly affected.

I have witnessed sudden death when this quincunx coincided with multiple testimonies in predisposed charts. Not a good time for risky sports, altitude changes, and the like.

Transit Uranus Quincunx Natal Moon

The brain chemistry is affected in ways hard to diagnose (look to the sign of transit Uranus for clues). This quincunx upsets menstrual cycles and most monthly bodily rhythms; can indicate gyneco-mastia (male breast tissue growth) or similar hormonal anomalies.

Strange moods, odd effects to pregnancy. The delivery system for electro-magnetic energies to the whole body is distracted. May suddenly affect emotional health and stability or precipitate an inexplicable onset of mental illness.

This transit can signal the beginning of cellular change due to excess EMF exposure. This is a good time to investigate how one's symptoms are influenced by magnets, magnetic fields, computers, cell phones, WIFI, the neighbor's radio dish, and so forth.

Transit Uranus Quincunx Natal Mercury

The nerves may have some difficulty receiving and/or channel-ing electricity. Synapses are affected. Sensory information may be addled. Tremors and other nerve-related disease may be indicated. There may be problems with neural coordination (e.g. in the hands or speech), including reception interpretation of sensory data.

Breathing may become imbalanced. This aspect can upset mental balances or indicate onset of mental illness. Nerves may be strained. This is a perfect time to research the influence upon one's symptoms of magnets, magnetic fields, computers, cell phones, WIFI, the neighbors radio dish, and the like.

Field Note: A client's onset of epilepsy occurred on this aspect within a 1° orb. Many other transits were congruent, as was the underlying natal tendency. Hypothetically, natal Mercury, (ruling synapses in general, brain nerves, and peripheral nerves) was not able to receive enough electrical current at this time.

Conversely, was the seizure caused by an electrical "zap attack" from Uranus, similar to how Mars attacks from 150°? I wonder if the Uranus quincunx can act that way.

Transit Uranus Quincunx Natal Venus

The ovaries, kidneys and veins may not receive enough electri-cal charge. Strange effects or hard-to-diagnose issues. Kidney hor-mones may release erratically, producing electrolyte imbalance.

Estrogen extremes. This aspect can signal hidden changes in ovarian or kidney cells.

There could be odd sexual feelings or changes of inclination or tastes. If hair is falling, or skin is changing, look for clues to the cause in the sign of transit Uranus.

Transit Uranus Quincunx Natal Mars

Muscles and motor nerves may not receive consistent electrical charge, resulting in spasm, strains, jerking, tremors, and the like. Timing and muscular coordination and contraction may be "off."

Accident-prone and clumsy. Up or down extremes can afflict energy, adrenalin, iron and testosterone. Balancing hormones is essential at this time. Strange sexual effects or lack of performance coordination may ensue, especially for males.

Be careful with electricity. This is a very important transit and may signal the onset of puzzling neuromuscular issues. For clues, study the signs of transit Uranus and natal Mars carefully, and remember the word "electricity." This aspect sometimes revs up the thyroid.

The impact of this quincunx may remain latent for months, striking suddenly when triggered by other transits.

Transit Uranus Quincunx Natal Jupiter

Unclear to this author. May disturb pituitary or liver function. Effects would be entirely hidden, or if not, baffling to doctors. For clues, consider the signs and elements of both planets involved and the signs they tenant. Weight gain/loss. Inexplicable change in blood volume or pressure may occur.

Transit Uranus Quincunx Natal Saturn

This is a prime time to watch for sudden calcium and mineral depletion. Osteopenia or osteoporosis can develop. Sudden instability, "trick knee," falls or spinal subluxations. Teeth may grow in strangely. In children, may signal a sudden halt to normal growth or development, or conversely, an age-inappropriate surge!

Electrical charge is not reaching the bones. Broken bones may set incorrectly. This transit may upset the regulation and timing of bodily processes or larger life cycles, such as premature menopause. The native may experience a nagging feeling of instability, without necessarily knowing the source.

Transit Uranus Quincunx the Natal Trans-Saturnian Planets

Not enough information available.

Transit Uranus Quincunx the Natal Lunar Nodes

Not enough information available. However, almost any planet arriving on the same numeric degree of the natal Lunar Nodes, in any sign, is capable of stirring up health issues of either genetic or karmic origin.

THE URANUS TRINE
Health Potentials for Predisposed Nativities
Transits do not always manifest as health concerns

As explained in the introductory chapters, this book is focused on what are called the "hard aspects." However, it is important to bear in mind that the exact orb trine of Uranus is capable of delivering an unblocked surge of electrical charge to the planet he trines. This is often noted in. cases of electrocution *(Cruce, Hill)*, where Uranus is seen performing as strongly as do his hard aspects and quincunxes!

Be especially alert to Uranus' precise transit trine of Mercury, Mars, Sun, Moon, or Ascendant.

Chapter 16

NEPTUNE
Leaks, Misdiagnosis
Supernatural Influences
Concealment

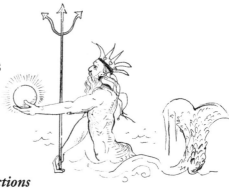

Properties, Rulerships and Actions

Rules: Co-ruler of Pisces (with Jupiter). This rulership was designated by astrological writers of the 20th century and is not accepted by all traditionalists.

The rulership system is an ancient and well-devised system in its own right, and thus, the unnecessary reassignment of planetary rulerships upsets the entire system. The same caveat also pertains to Neptune's remaining dignities and debilities:

Exalted: Cancer

Detriment: Virgo

Fall: Capricorn

Metal: Aluminum *(M. Uyldert)*

Minerals: Unknown

Vitamins: Unknown

Gem & Cosmic Ray: Not established

Substances: Opioids, marijuana, alcohol

Body Rulership & Organ Affinities: Neptune's organ affinities have not been definitively established. The great prophet and medical psychic Edgar Cayce stated that Neptune governs the "leyden" glands. He is unique in this viewpoint. Cornell assigned the spinal fluid to Neptune.

"The arterial stream is supreme but the cerebrospinal fluid is in command." – W. G. Sutherland, DO

Temperature and Moisture Influence: Neptune's 1846 discovery prevents us from sourcing earlier opinions regarding Neptune's temperature effects upon the human organism. Astrologers didn't know he existed.

Modern astrologers rate Neptune as "cold and wet" because of his obvious association with oceans and the cold-moist Water sign Pisces. However, Neptune's actions are decisively relaxative, a quality antithetical to cold per se. Increasing cold acts to mass atoms more closely together, creating tension and shivering in the physical body.

Could Neptune be simultaneously cold and relaxing? Anomalies do exist in nature. For example, herbal stimulants are typically warming, although we do see an exception in the cooling stimulant Peppermint.

Although warmth is stimulating, it can just as easily be relaxing. Energetically speaking, hot-moist has some obviously relaxing effects, responsible for the popularity of hot tubs. Hot water stimulates while simultaneously relaxing the tissues. That being said, I opine that Neptune is warm and moist, because he manifests as magnetic, sleepy, relaxing, receptive, permeable and sexy!

Despite some thinking Neptune cold, there are in truth, few Neptunian maladies that manifest as physically cold. Sleepy, romantic energies are not cold. However, Neptune is draining to the vital force. As we noted in *Chapter 6*, Sol brings the heat of life, our essential vital force. Neptune appears thus to reduce the vital force through excessive laxity. This creates cold through default, quite in reverse of cold Saturn's method.

Saturn is cold because his violet ray is cold. This concentrates atoms, producing tightness in the body. Conversely, Neptune causes cold because he drains away the vital force with diffused laxity, while not himself being cold! Drifting fog gives us the best feeling for Neptune.

Conversely, an argument in favor of cold temperature for

Neptune might be Neptune's association with sleep and coma. We think of dying as cold, and indeed the body grows frigid as life departs. However, frigidity per se is definitely not Neptune's province!

Rather, Neptune is primarily diffusive in nature, signifying permeability of consciousness. Perhaps no planet signifies psychic and/ or physical permeability to the degree of Neptune, save the Moon, in some conditions.

However, Neptune's permeability extends to the astral plane— that plane just above the physical in vibrational density. Neptune's action is strongly involved in coma, psychism, sleep and astral projection. He blurs the boundaries between worlds through diffusion.

I've closely observed scores of folks born with Neptune either exactly rising or exactly conjunct their natal Sun. They are anything but cold! Sometimes remote, yes. Escapist, yes. Sometimes weak-willed and usually highly-sensitive.

Depressed? Oh, yes. But never emotionally cold, and they are so magnetically attractive, every one. Supported by the foregoing arguments, I offer that Neptune's temperature is not consistent, but drifts according to element between warm-moist and tepid-moist. However, Neptune's warmth is sleepy warmth, quite unlike the heat of booming Jupiter or lusty Mars.

General Action: Diffusive, permeating, draining, fatiguing, psychic, anesthetic and sleepy, Neptune veils symptoms and conceals pathogens. He relieves pain, and governs anesthesia. His transit medical influence is primarily weakening, relaxing, sleepy, dreamy, seeping, sagging, fatiguing and draining.

Neptune transits open the psychic doors and can be hypnotic, highly magnetic, sexy, soothing and lazy. He enhances either hedonism or spirituality (all depending upon how one chooses to escape this reality). He confers psychic healing tips and enhances fantasy. This planet works well with vibrational remedies that adjust the astral body such as Bach Flower remedies, homeopathy, music therapy, color.

In the natal chart, Neptune is our proverbial Achilles heel, that irresistible siren of temptation, bliss and escape. Because his influence lowers the veil between the worlds, his transits are essential to note for those suffering mental illnesses involving involuntary clairaudience, clairvoyance, trance or fantasy.

Davidson states that Neptune's position in the natal chart suggests a porousness of the etheric shield, inclined to the leakage of prana (vital force). This explains the vague and fatiguing impact of this planet upon the bodily regions of any sign it tenants, and upon the planets it aspects, either natally or by transit.

Neptune exerts a considerable influence upon memory extremes inclusive of photographic memory, reincarnation memory, forgetfulness and dementia. These extreme effects on memory are noted when Neptune is in a close-orb transit or natal relationship with the natal Sun, Moon, Mercury or Lunar Nodes.

Neptune has a strong association with unconsciousness, "being stoned," and coma.

Neptune conceals things, making diagnosis difficult or faulty. Envision a slowly moving cloaking fog. Neptune rules misdiagnosis!

EMF Field Issues: It is possible that Neptune rules magnetism (along with Venus). Uranus rules electricity. Both Neptune and Uranus are implicated in health problems arising from EMF (computers, cell phones, etc). Neptune contributes to cellular change and cell traveling, apparent in some cancers.

Hidden Entities and Poison: Neptune appears to govern viruses, molds and hidden, sneaky poisons in the air or water. In the natal chart, he can represent a region of lowered guard and greater permeability.

Supernatural Etiologies: Neptune is strongly associated with spirit attachments, ghosts, possession, past-life memories, clairvoyance and clairaudience. Medieval and Renaissance physicians considered "elf-shot" and other fairy-induced illness as legitimate etiologies.

Positive: Deep sleep, relaxed disposition, magnetism and soothing.

Passively sexy. Neptune can bring angelic intervention and miraculous healings. With help from Neptune, psychic information and vibrational remedies can "save the day." Dreams provide healing tips. Davidson and I have both independently noted the strangely lucky quality of Neptune (it's amazing how often he dominates the charts of heirs to fortune, windfall recipients and jackpot winners).

Negative: Absorbs negativity from others or, conversely, drains positive charge from others! Presents as chronic, undiagnosed fatigue; fuzzy mind; disinclination to work or attend to worldly matters; weakness of body and/or mind; depression ("I can't face the world!"); psychic boundary issues.

Transit Frame & Orb: Neptune's transits are most strongly felt within an orb of 0-3°. Neptune can visit and revisit these few degrees for approximately two years (variable). Neptune's "Sidereal period," i.e. one completed revolution through the twelve tropical signs, is 164.79 tropical years. So we do not experience Neptune natal return.

NEPTUNE THROUGH THE ELEMENTS & SIGNS
Health Potentials for Predisposed Nativities
Transits do not always manifest as health concerns or benefits.

Applicable to both natal and transit charts, these partial lists of expressed symptoms apply only to predisposed nativities. These conditions are obviously uncommon and require multiple testimonies beyond the presence of Neptune.

Manifestation of symptoms may be enhanced by lifestyle choices, and taking preemptive measures can reduce, remove or prevent potential issues from manifesting. It is not possible to list all potential expressions.

Neptune in Fire Signs

Aries: Strange eye problems, detached retina, fuzzy vision, glaucoma; astral visions, brain fatigue, fluidic brain, brain tumor; involuntary fantasy, decay of upper teeth or jaw.

Leo: Weakened heart muscle, leaking heart valves, hidden or undiagnosed heart issues, fluidic heart; spinal subluxations, weak back, weak gallbladder action; spinal sheath anomaly.

Sagittarius: Hard to diagnose diseases of spinal nerves; religious mania, euphoria, mystical mental states; weak legs, cellulite on hips or buttocks; alcoholism and drug addiction.

Neptune in Earth Signs

Taurus: Thyroid disturbances, hypothyroid, thymus gland issues bearing on calcium absorption, hearing weakness, deafness, excess ear wax, fluid in ear, misalignment of axis bone or cervical vertebra, dental decay, hidden poison or abscess in teeth causing mysterious illness, bleeding gums, vocal polyps, throat virus, tongue or esophageal cancer (with other testimonies), choking, weak swallowing action, vocal oddities, jaw misalignment, weak neck, weak lower jaw, eating disorders and addictions, malnourishment, heavy metal poisoning.

Virgo: Abdominal hernia; duodenal, liver, pancreatic or intestinal cysts or cellular changes; hard to diagnose intestinal issues; lazy gut, leaky gut, candida (with Venus); mysterious pancreatic, duodenal, liver or intestinal disturbance; worms; peculiar liver action; liver torpor; sluggish portal circulation; inefficient immune system; spleen malfunction; leukemia (rare); poor nutrient absorption or assimilation; bloating and fermentation, dietary extremes ("dying to be healthy"); weak abdominal wall; hernia, intestines floating out of place, blood sugar issues.

Capricorn: Sluggish gallbladder, skin changes or skin cancer, pituitary disturbance or extremes, "trick knee," weak knees, weak bones or cartilage, instability, slippery ligaments or hyper-elastic tendons, osteoporosis, bone changes, nail fungus, moles and warts, stomach issues and nausea (reflex to Cancer), dental caries, receding gums, changes of appetite, heavy metal poisoning, gallbladder malfunction contributing to brain or eye changes (by reflex to Aries).

Neptune in Air Signs

Gemini: Dislocated shoulder, mental disconnection, fuzzy mind, clairvoyance, clairaudience, slurred speech, dumbness, poor coordination, poor hand acuity, mental addictions, media addiction, phone addiction, numbing or confusion of sensory nerves or afferent nerves, lazy in studies, weakening arms or hands, leaking capillaries, dirty CPAP machines, first or second hand smoke, sleep apnea, weak lung action, mysterious spot on lung, tuberculosis.

Libra: Dizziness, vertigo, hormonal imbalance, adrenal tumor, gender identity change or issues, social "gender benders," hard to diagnose issues of the urinary tract, ovarian cysts, enuresis, sodium-potassium imbalances, bed-wetting, alcoholism, sex and love addiction, weak kidneys, low kidney "chi."

Aquarius: Venous insufficiency, varicose veins, blood clots in lower leg, twisted ankle, weak lower legs, electrical malfunction to heart (reflex to Leo), inexplicable actions or disease of spinal nerves, hidden spinal tumors, issues of spinal fluid, odd mental states, psychic reception, lack of oxygen to heart or brain, angina, anemia, leukemia, mysterious blood disorders, blood poisoning, carbon monoxide poisoning, autointoxication, malformed cells, dysthenia, depression sleep apnea, dirty CPAP machine, first or second hand smoke, opium addiction.

Neptune in Water Signs

Cancer: Breast cysts or tumors, pituitary extremes, emotional attachment disorders, unfulfilled parenting issues and longings *("I wasn't nursed," etc.)*, brain fluid or chemistry extremes, eating disorders or addictions, paranoia, excessive weeping, depression, unexplained nausea, dark spot on lower lung, fluidic lower lungs, tuberculosis, weak lung function, leaking breast implants, plastic poisoning, excess hidden estrogens, waterborne parasites, bleeding gums, tooth decay; living above negative *"sha"* water currents *(Feng Shui)*.

Scorpio: Sex addiction, nymphomania, bladder prolapse, uterine prolapse, bladder tumors, secret bleeding, incontinence, cancer, enuresis, excess sweating, hernia, prolapsed rectum or vagina, colorectal cysts or cellular change, colorectal bacterial imbalance, candida, genital fungus, diarrhea, peculiar sexual obsessions, undiagnosed STDs, parasites, oddly-smelling sweat, chronic nasal infection, plastic poisoning, hormone poisoning, dirty water, fecal or urine contamination, vermin caused disease. Influences hearing and thyroid, gut fermentation, gas, living above graveyards, hauntings, hidden oil.

Pisces: Behaves slightly similar to Jupiter in this sign. Pisces lacks boundaries, so Neptune's psychic openness knows no bounds in this sign! Neptune contributes to the Piscean tendency to glandular non-coordination.

Inexplicable blood cholesterol issues, lymphatic toxicity, engorged lymph nodes, glandular extremes and pituitary disturbance, dwarfism and gigantism, large feet, flat feet, mega-obesity, fluidic collection; lazy cecum or upper intestines; phlegmatic and excess sleep, weird or engrossing dreams, enlightening dreams. Psychic doors are open for good or ill, onset of psychic problems or mental illness, spirit possession, problems due to reincarnation-related memory.

Blood chemistry issues, blood toxicity, problems from mixing drugs and alcohol, drug overdoses, STDs. Reflexes to digestive organs and can be associated with cellular changes or strange growths in pancreas, duodenum, liver, and intestine. Plastic poisoning, water pathogens, hormone poisoning, negative *"sha"* water currents *(Feng Shui)*, hauntings.

NEPTUNE'S TRANSIT TO NATAL PLANETS

Applicable to both natal and transit charts, these partial lists of expressed symptoms apply only to predisposed Nativities. These conditions are obviously uncommon and require multiple testimonies beyond the presence of Neptune.

Manifestation of symptoms may be enhanced by one's lifestyle choices, and taking preemptive measures can reduce, remove or prevent potential issues from manifesting. It is not possible to list all potential expressions.

TRANSIT NEPTUNE'S CONJUNCTIONS
Health Potentials for Predisposed Nativities
Transits do not always manifest as health concerns or benefits.

The conjunction is the strongest of Neptune's transit aspects. Therefore, more attention, *Field Notes* and *Herbal Notes* are devoted to this specific aspect.

Transit Neptune Conjunct Natal Sun
This transit considerably attenuates the vital force. The individual may feel sleepy or fatigued. The vital force may be draining away due to some hidden source that should be brought to light. Some gradually wax psychically sensitive under this long transit. Clairvoyance and clairaudience increases.

Other potential manifestations: heart muscle weakens or atrophies, leaky valves, undiagnosed hole in heart, heart virus, fluid on brain, eyesight or eye muscles weaken, low or high blood pressure (depending on condition and physical type), glaucoma, cataracts, vision may blur or decline.

Disinclination to worldly matters, the brain and/or heart may receive an excess of magnetic energy, addictions may develop or increase. Neptune's transit of the Sun can sometimes be productive of brain tumors or sub-oxygenation of heart or brain. Vitamin or mineral deficiencies are common manifestations, as is atrophy due to poor protein assimilation. However, considerable creative genius can manifest at this time.

Medical Tip: Check for hidden viruses, tumors or heart valve issues. Test for nutritional deficiencies. Increase the inflow of the vital force through the element of the natal Sun. Strengthen the heart muscle and check for blood pressure changes. This is a good period to visit your opthalmologist.

Transit Neptune Conjunct Natal Moon
This transit strongly sensitizes the feelings and mind. Manifestations include escapism, mysticism, clairvoyance or clairaudience, vivid dreams, fatigue and extreme sensitivity to vibration and thoughts. Weakens eyesight, cataracts, brain fog, excess sleeping,

thins blood and is addiction prone. This transit is sexy and pleasure seeking. Neptune can signal an ongoing virus or psychic parasite, or being drained or hypnotized by others.

Neptune's transit of the Moon can provoke edemic conditions and increase fluidic buildups in the bodily zone governed by the natal Moon. Symptoms include: fluidic brain, swelling of lymph nodes, breast swelling, ovarian cysts or tumors, endometriosis, menorrhagia, bleeding.

Prolapsed bladder, ongoing stomach virus, lazy stomach or insufficient stomach enzymes, prolapsed uterus or bladder, insufficient lung action, heightened senses (especially hearing), unplanned pregnancy. Increases female receptivity. Neptune influences memory extremes when near the Moon (past-life memory or conversely, present-life dementia).

Mental and emotional confusion are typical, and sleepiness. Danger of drowning, possible association with leukemia, drug addiction (or being involuntarily drugged), strange longings. Musical.

Neptune can induce cellular changes and cyst growth, usually hidden. Strange cloud on lung, insufficient lung action, emphysema, mucus or fluid in lungs. Enhances the love of the sublime.

Surgical and Medical Tips: Check anesthesia for compatibility and dose. Neptune's aspects to the Moon can indicate an inability of the lymphatics and blood to process medications or alcohol quickly. This is a nice time to "get away from it all," sleep and convalesce.

Herbal Note: Lymphatic assistance of the breast and brain tissue may be in order. Dandelion Root is one of the traditional herbs for clearing the breast. Manifold choices exist to treat confusion, "brain fog," and depression (see Wood's *Earthwise Herbal Repertory*). Moonstones and amethyst exacerbate astral porousness. Do not self-treat.

Transit Neptune Conjunct Natal Mercury

This transit behaves similarly to Neptune's conjunction of the Moon. Decisively attenuating to mental states, this aspect slows and "fuzzes" neural transmission, reduces alertness, enhances mental receptivity, opens the imaginative and inspirational faculties, reduces concentration on worldly tasks, enhances fantasy and clairaudience and either dulls or sensitizes hearing (because of strange, relaxing effects on auditory nerves).

This transit can coincide with the onset or worsening of dementia. Vertigo, cysts or fluidic buildup near nerves, bronchial tubes, lungs or in spinal column. Interest in drugs, confused brain chemistry, poor judgment. Musical. May influence hand acuity. Narcolepsy, sleeping or stoned at the wheel, weakened respiration, pneumonia.

Medical Tip: This transit potentizes schizophrenia and similar mental states where the normal boundaries between the physical plane and the astral world are blurred. This is a dangerous time to ingest psychotropics. Stay awake and alert when driving!

Herbal Note: Nutritive nervines and grounding remedies are helpful: Oat Straw, Alfalfa, Parsley, Fenugreek, Sunflower. Respiratory herbs may be useful: Mullein, Osha, Coltsfoot, Inula, Horehound, Sunflower seeds, etc. Choose "cooling" or "warming" by Mercury's element. Traditionally, Peppermint combined with Linden, Elder or Yarrow flowers is used to open and relieve congested bronchial tubules, especially for pneumonia, and those coughs that won't quit. For "brain fog," see earlier *"Herbal Note"* under *"Transit Neptune Conjunct Natal Moon."* Do not self-treat.

Transit Neptune Conjunct Natal Venus

Neptune is "the higher octave of Venus." This is a sexy aspect! Magnetism increases. Seduction prone. Cyst prone. Neptune is sneaky and productive of slow-growing secret cysts or tumors when in relationship with Venus, Jupiter, Saturn or the Moon! Ovarian and kidney cysts are especially related to Venus. Venous insufficiency or prolapse, genital yeast, candida, STDs, prolapsed vagina, sugar extremes (diabetes), sugar addiction, copper excess, excess wine drinking.

If Edgar Cayce is correct that Venus governs the thymus gland, we could expect changes there, with effects on the strength of the immune system, probably weakening.

Field Note: The observations below lend support to both the

Jyotish idea that Venus "rules the thick lymphs," and Cayce's assignment of the thymus gland to Venus. The upshot here is that Venus may have some influence on the immune system and the white blood cells.

Traditionally, the immune system is related to the Virgo-Pisces polarity. Mars (the fighter) must also be involved as is Saturn (the demarcator of boundaries), and Jupiter (the protector).

Two clients with natal Venus exalted in Libra and Leo Ascendants never catch colds or flus, although they have both worked long years in hospitals. Conversely, a third client who is almost always sick has natal Venus in detriment (Virgo), simultaneously conjunct restraining Saturn, in the malefic 12th house. There are many more examples supportive of Venus' role in immune extremes.

Medical Tip: Practice safe sex! Avoid excess sugar and alcohol.

Transit Neptune Conjunct Natal Mars

This aspect is famous for blood poisoning! This includes poisoning by alcohol, food, drugs, carbon monoxide, insecticides, date drugs, venoms and bee stings, etc. (See *Field Notes* for the reverse aspect in *Chapter 12,* section: *Transit Mars Conjunct Natal Neptune.*)

This planet combination is linked to weird, insect-borne diseases and STDs. This transit increases opportunities for being infected with AIDS, Lyme disease, oral herpes, genital herpes, strep, staph, shingles, genital fungus, etc. This transit brings fermentation and putrefaction.

Neptune-Mars also produces wet, itchy rashes: poison oak and sumac, fungus. Neptune's conjunction to Mars can signify changes in blood cells or hemoglobin content. All manner of excess or deficient blood conditions are possible: anemia, leukemia, excess or deficient blood iron, minerals or salts leaching out through urine, electrolyte imbalance, hemophilia, mysterious bleeding, rash.

Fatigue. Mars throws wastes out through all bodily orifices and Neptune relaxes. This can present in any number of ways: excessive nocturnal emissions, excess sweating, diarrhea, excess urination, leaking urine, enuresis, incontinence.

Male performance issues including impotency or, conversely, sexual addiction. Unsafe sex, chronic drug addictions, drug overdose, drowning. ("Don't talk to strange mushrooms." Somebody on the radio actually said that!)

This aspect is weakening to muscle strength and integrity; over time, it may contribute to disorders of the blood cells, including anemia. The immune system is significantly impacted in some cases, especially when long-term, concealed viruses or pathogens are present.

Surgical and Medical Tips: Beware of exceptional reactions to beestings and medications, especially if transit or natal Uranus is also involved. Strictly avoid drug-alcohol combinations, or drug/drink and swimming. Practice safe sex or observe continence.

Herbal Note: Blood and muscle building herbs are helpful at this time. Nettles are good for both anemia and muscle atrophy. Beets, Lentils, Raisins (especially soaked) are helpful sources of natural iron. Consult a licensed medical professional and do not self-treat.

Transit Neptune Conjunct Natal Jupiter

Pituitary action may become disturbed, resulting in hormonally induced extremes such as hirsutism, growth extremes, breast swelling and flatulence. Liver porosity increases, liver function may become extreme or imbalanced, affecting: digestion, blood constituents, cholesterol, alcohol sensitivity, etc. This combination encourages any extremes related to Jupiter and its natal sign position. Lazy liver function. Edema (in Libra, Aquarius, or Water signs).

Surgical and Medical Tips: Unclear. May have unpredictable effects on liver surgery or treatment. Miracle prone too! Alcohol may create greater danger to the liver at this time. There is also an increased tendency to bad reactions from mixing drugs and alcohol.

Transit Neptune Conjunct Natal Saturn

This transit is distinctly weakening to bones, gradually leaching minerals (especially calcium). In rare cases, Neptune-Saturn disturbs calcium metabolism, and potentially promotes cellular change in bodily area ruled by the sign of natal Saturn (or signs in hard aspect or quincunx).

Typical manifestations include osteopenia, osteoporosis, tooth decay, instability (mental or physical), poor focus, elasticizing influence on ligaments and tendons, joints slipping out of alignment, weakening cartilage, atonicity, peculiar skin growths, and mysterious wasting diseases. This aspect differs considerably from its reverse: transit, Saturn conjunct natal Neptune! There can be profound psychological changes.

Herbal Note: Ladies, this is a great time to read Susan Weed's books on menopause! She provides excellent herbal combinations for counteracting age-related calcium leaching and consequent bone loss. Men benefit too! Oat Straw, Nettles, Alfalfa, Dandelion and Red Cover are excellent herbs for bone support. Consult a licensed herbalist and do not self-treat.

Transit Neptune Conjunct Uranus

The effects of this aspect are unclear to this author. Neptune rules magnetism (with Venus), and Uranus governs electricity. Thus, there may be an influence on the body's electromagnetic field or little-known electrical functions within the body. EMF fields may be influencing the body's magnetic field in an adverse manner. This aspect may not be felt in all persons.

Transit Neptune Conjunct Natal Neptune

People do not live long enough to experience their "Neptune Return." It would require a life of nearly 165 years in length.

Neptune Conjunct Natal Pluto

This aspect is unclear to this author and may not be felt in all nativities. Potentially carcinogenic.

This Neptune conjunction could indicate an ongoing misdiagnosis of a chronic Pluto-type ailment (e.g. radiation poisoning, bacterial infection, Lyme disease), because both planets govern poisoning (along with Mars, Saturn, Nodes and certain signs).

This conjunction could testify to the secret leaking of poisons within the body or environment, e.g. breast implants. Neptune may govern plastics, therefore, plastic poisoning should be considered. Neptune-Pluto combinations may be active in hormone therapies, stem cell transplants, organ transplants, and blood transfusions.

Transit Neptune Conjunct Natal South Node

Neptune's transit of the South Node can awaken diseases in remission, genetic issues, or bring latent psychological issues to the front lines. Past life memories are stimulated. This significant, long term aspect is often mentally unsettling. Latent or genetic mental illness can awaken. Avoid drugs, channelling spirits, trying LSD or mushrooms, moving kundalini or anything else that might suddenly open psychic boundaries.

The natal sign of this conjunction is extremely important in the assessment of psychological or physical effects. Consider supernatural etiologies (causes). This aspect lowers resistance to unseen contagious pathogens in general, and is no time to visit hospitals without a mask, share fluids, etc. This transit enhances any innate bodily weaknesses or pranic leaks suggested by the sign and house placement of the Natal South Node.

If, during this transit, an eclipse occurs here, this may produce a significant flushing, leaking or fatiguing incident within the organ or body zone ruled by the sign of the transit South Node.

Generally, Neptune conjunct the South Node, either natally or by transit, alerts to a secret "etheric leak" in the bodily region governed by the sign of the natal South Node. This might express as lassitude, weakness, torpor, decay. Hidden virus is typical. Secret poison is another classic manifestation.

This transit is associated with alcohol or drug danger, faulty prescriptions or dangerous combinations of medication, dementia, foggy thinking, excess sleeping, sleep disorders. One's psychic boundaries are very slack at this time. Avoid playing with spirits or astral entities, or taking psychotropic drugs. Conversely, increase psychic protections and stay grounded!

Drownings are associated with this transit and its reverse (transit

South Node over Natal Neptune). This tendency is strongest for Air and Water signs. It's certainly no time to get drunk and hang out alone in a hot tub. Important bodily functions are hypoactive (slowed), unless the chart is receiving counteractive stimulus.

Medical astrologers do not yet understand all the things Neptune means, and more will be revealed.

This transit has a significant effect on mental states. I've seen the onset of psychiatric conditions with transit Neptune on the natal South Node. Depression is typical. Also, "past life memory" and other reincarnation-related issues. Sometimes one hears voices or sees visions because the normal screen between this world and the astral plane is loosened.

Be careful of secret poisoning or self-poisoning. Relaxing Neptune has a great deal to do with alcohol, marijuana and opiates. To imbibe at this time qualifies astrologically as "self-undoing" through these substances. Mysterious wasting problems can occur. This is no time to dismiss the potential for supernatural influences upon health! The entry of puzzling viruses is very typical of this transit. Those suffering mysterious fatigue at this time should consider overlooked invisible pathogens and/or poisons.

Potential danger is shown from inexpertly provided chemical medicine, or the unconsidered mixing of medications, alcohol, drugs. Toxic water. This conjunction suggests misdiagnosis. If coinciding with same, it is best to obtain several opinions.

Field Note: One client had transit Neptune conjunct his natal South Node simultaneous to a transit of the South Node over his natal Neptune! Because Neptune rules the waves, I advised him not to swim in the ocean. He did so anyway (as clients do), and drowned. Luckily, his wife (who was swimming nearby) rescued his body from the deep and resuscitated him. She was a retired lifeguard.

Surgical and Medical Tips: See previous warnings. If you must undergo anesthesia under this transit, pre-test type and dose, and give extra recovery time. Blood transfusion must be attended with great care because this conjunction heightens risk of contracting HIV.

Avoid hormonal injections because results can be strange indeed. Because of Neptune's fluid-leaking tendencies, removal of tumors must be attended with great care. Obviously, this would be an inadvisable time for breast implants or any introduction into the body of a potentially leaking poison.

Never, never play around with channeling spirits, trance, astral projection or psychotropics while this transit is current!

Medications (especially opiates, anesthesia) can cause strange reactions or addictions. Symptoms range from the onset of an unnoticed pain medication addiction to poisoning by disharmonious anesthesia.

For those pursuing diagnosis: Neptune on the South Node produces a veiling effect, thus it is wise to seek multiple medical opinions. Those with supernaturally induced psychic problems; schizophrenia and/or depression require vigilant support at this time.

Herbal Note: Practitioners might find useful the tonifying, high mineral content herbs good for convalescence: Fenugreek, Seaweeds, Oat Straw, Nettles, and Alfalfa, etc. Vervain is a traditional herb for preventing bad dreams. Avoid Mugwort and other dreaming herbs at this time—it's too much! Juniper Berries and Leaves worn about the neck help close the astral door (hearing voices, etc.). Antiviral herbs might be useful for dragging viruses: Chaparral, Olive Leaf, Oregano. Don't self-treat.

Transit Neptune Conjunct Natal North Node

Neptune's transit of the North Node signifies an influx of Neptune's sleepy, permeating energy into the bodily system. This could manifest in a great number of interesting ways including excess self-medication, drinking binges, sugar addiction, music or media addiction, surfing (Neptune rules the ocean), spirit possession, receiving angelic messages, onset of chronic contagious illness, onset of psychic states, spiritual inspiration, artistic genius, spiritual gifts, and onset of clairvoyance or clairaudience.

Neptune at either Lunar Node can coincide in predisposed persons with the onset of schizophrenia or other mental states presenting astral-physical blurring symptoms. Spirit entities can more readily gain entrance at this time (as with Neptune-South Node). This aspect potentially increases moisture, lubrication and mucous.

This conjunction is a secret cyst and tumor builder, and can signal cellular changes in the bodily region governed by the natal North Node or its opposite sign.

Herbal Note: Licensed practitioners might note that anti-cancer, cyst removing and lymphatic assisting herbs may be useful: Red Clover, Cleavers, Red Root (Ceanothus), Violet, Poke Root, etc. It would seem best to add a warming herb (most lymphatic specifics are cooling). Do not self treat.

Field Note: Several clients reported ongoing puzzling illnesses when Neptune was transiting their natal North Nodes in Aquarius. Doctors were of no use. The first case turned out to be "poisoning through the air," a suggested astrological idea that escaped multiple doctors. Indeed, visiting workmen discovered a secret carbon monoxide leak! Both stories are recounted in *A Wonderbook of True Astrological Case Files.*

Two subsequent clients were independently poisoned under this transit by toxic gases ingested through plastic tubing and hoses they were using for various purposes. Aquarius is the sign of "fixed air," thus indicating poison gas. Aquarius also co-rules the veins (with Venus) and is the general governor of the circulation. Hence, the correlation to hoses!

Surgical and Medical Tips: Neptune's transit of the natal North Node is one testimony of success through vibrational therapies (homeopathy, Bach flower essences, spiritual healing, reiki, gem therapy, color therapy. Potentially positive for hypnotherapy).

Great care should be taken not to over-medicate or mix drugs/ alcohol. Hormonal treatments could be successful or extreme. Because of Neptune's diffusive, fluid-leaking tendency, removal of tumors must be attended with great care.

Transit Neptune Conjunct Natal Ascendant

First, be certain the Ascendant is really true. This long term aspect is profoundly relaxing and/or fatiguing on multiple levels for good or ill, most especially to the regions governed by the Ascendant's sign. Effects last for the duration of Neptune's transit through the Ascendant sign, though are more pronounced within 3° of the true Ascendant degree.

Be prepared to observe strong, impelling spiritual and/or escapist urges befall the native. I recall how one close friend abandoned his real estate office for the woods when this transit arrived! Others just become confused or tired with the world.

Field Note: One client began to experience mysterious symptoms of fatigue as Neptune arrived exactly upon her Ascendant and North Node degree, being together in Aquarius. It so turned out to be carbon monoxide poisoning.

TRANSIT NEPTUNE'S SQUARES
Health Potentials for Predisposed Nativities
Transits do not always manifest as health concerns.

Neptune's squares behave similarly to his conjunctions at perhaps 50 to 75 percent strength. Use the basic text for Neptune's conjunctions to each planet. Strongest at 1°, and will operate as long as the planet continues to visit this degree. In most cases, Neptune's influence is not much felt at orbs larger than 1°.

There is an important difference between Neptune's conjunctions and squares. In considering the square aspect (90°), we have a draining influence of transit Neptune coming from Neptune's current sign to the sign of the natal planet he squares by transit. To determine a square's meaning, the signs and quadruplicity of the planets involved are of paramount importance. (See *Chapter 3, Aspect Mechanics,* for square delineation by sign combination.)

However, if you know the bodily regions governed by the signs, and the planetary functions you can do this yourself with the following formula.

Square Interpretation Formula

Transit Neptune slowly drains and weakens the functions of the natal planet he squares _____

(name that planet, and its specific functions), from the bodily region governed by the sign he currently is transiting _____*(give that sign, and the bodily regions it governs)*.

TRANSIT NEPTUNE'S OPPOSITIONS
Health Potentials for Predisposed Nativities
Transits do not always manifest as health concerns.

Neptune's opposition is quite similar to Neptune's conjunction although there are two marked differences:

1) A weakening effect upon the natal planet is sourced from the bodily region of the opposite sign. The entire sign polarity is strongly involved. *See Chapter 3 for polarity delineation tips.*

2) The source of confusion, misdiagnosis, faulty advice, poisoning (or if positive, angelic intervention) is brought from others outside oneself to the natal planet opposed.

Sign Polarity: The houses and sign polarity concerned are essential to note. It is beyond the scope of this text to discuss all sign and polarity combinations. Here is a formula to help use this section.

Opposition Interpreting Formula for Neptune

Transit Neptune in_____ *(give sign and the bodily region it governs)*, produces a fatigue-inducing drain upon the natal planet he opposes _____ *(name planet)* and its bodily functions_____

(describe). *See the medical implications of polarity in, Chapter 3 Aspect Mechanics.*

Transit Neptune Opposes Natal Sun

Weakens the heart muscle, brain or eyesight. Produces lassitude. Note sign polarity involved.

Herbal Note: Licensed practitioners might find that cardiac tonics herbs and foods are useful. Renaissance physicians fed beef hearts to the weak-hearted, and hung strengthening herbs, or gold above the heart. Turquoise and amber works well in specific cases. Hawthorn berries assist the heart in many ways, including bringing more oxygen to the heart muscle. Do not self-treat. See *Herbal Tips* for *Transit Neptune Conjunct Natal Sun.*

Transit Neptune Opposes Natal Moon

Produces a feeling of malaise, lassitude, insecurity or confusion. Mentally and emotionally confusing. The native may feel profound ennui, boredom or depression. Uncertainty in relationships causes confusion. Optically weakening. Note the sign polarity involved.

Herbal Note: See *Herbal Note* for *Transit Neptune Conjunct Natal Moon,* and directly below, *Transit Neptune Opposite Natal Mercury.*

Transit Neptune Opposes Natal Mercury

This transit attenuates the mental focus and is exacerbating to depression, schizophrenia, epilepsy, addictions and many neurological conditions. Sudden epiphanies are possible. The native feels as though he or she is straining to see through thick fog. It is a difficult time to receive correct information. Medical advice may be in error.

One may experience spirit visitations, visits or voices. Medical misdiagnoses or outright deception are common. Be on high alert for potentially faulty prescriptions and/or medication errors! Hospital paperwork is confused. However, incoming psychic information regarding health may be useful. Note sign polarity involved.

Herbal Note: To treat increasing forgetfulness: Sage, Rosemary Gingko and Periwinkle. Do not self-treat.

Transit Neptune Opposes Natal Mercury

Atonic, relaxing, loosening. Reduces common sense, lowers emotional boundaries and sexual guard. Temptation.

Potentizing to anesthesia, alcohol, opiates. Reduces willpower.

May relax kidney function; suggests hormonal confusion, sexual dreams, psychic-sexual influences or draining .

Transit Neptune Opposes Natal Mars

This aspect produces sudden downward swings in energy or libido. Anemia. Strange changes in bone marrow or cells is possible. Sperm count may swing up or down. This is a notable combination for blood poisoning, alcohol poisoning, drug overdose and drowning. Avoid water sports.

If someone is bleeding, it is difficult to stop it. Temptations and tempters of many kinds appear, typically negative. This transit is notable when occurring when Mars is strongest life, the teenage years and twenties. Safe sex is a must. Note delineation for sign polarity involved *(Chapter 3)*.

Beware of a misdiagnosis of Mars-related conditions. A first rate warning to avoid contagious diseases and STDs caught from fluid or blood exchange. Fermentation, and all manner of weird, disharmonious chemical blendings (internal).

Surgical Tip: This aspect warns of inattentiveness on the part of the surgeon or mistakes with anesthesia. Danger of contagion or infection through blood transfusions or sloppy hospital hygiene. Check for changes in testosterone, adrenalin, cortisol, red blood cells or iron levels.

Herbal Note: Licensed medical practitioners might find Nettles and water-soaked Black Raisins useful should blood iron levels lower. Support and tonify Mars' functions (adrenal gland, iron, testosterone, white and red blood cells, muscles). Sesame tahini is traditionally believed to assist the integrity of the blood cells. Do not self-treat.

Transit Neptune Opposes Natal Jupiter

Unclear to this author. Because Jupiter rules growth and neither planet respects boundaries, we suggest all manner of dribbling, "out of control" conditions.

Strange things may be going on in the blood-stream, hormones or liver that the doctors cannot readily define. The liver may become sloppy, imprecise.

Psychologically, this opposition could suggest drug or medication induced grandiosity, euphoria, prophesying, religious mania, especially with Mars involvement, or similar over-expanded mental states. Note sign polarity involved.

Herbal Note: Warming hepatic herbs are useful for Neptune-Jupiter symptoms of damp, cold, liver torpor: e.g. Sage, Bayberry, et al. It is difficult to find warming hepatics, so one might consider a mixture of cooling hepatics (Gentian, Agrimony, Centaury) with the inclusion a warming stimulant. Sesame Tahini has been traditionally used to assist the integrity of the blood cells. Do not self-treat.

Transit Neptune Opposes Natal Saturn

Neptune's opposition quietly challenges Saturn's stability with confusion. Poisoning from outside sources, e.g. air pollution or the water supply. Heavy metal or plastic poisons can leak into the body, especially Saturn-ruled lead. If, under this aspect you suspect that heavy metals are leaking from dental fillings, etc., you might be right!

Saturn can signify the medical profession. This transit baffles physicians, making diagnosis faulty or difficult. Conversely, physicians may be unreliable at this time.

This aspect weakens bone integrity and behaves similarly as the conjunction, though less strong.

Herbal Note: See *Transit Neptune Conjunct Natal Saturn.*

Transit Neptune Opposes Natal Uranus

Neptune (confusion, veiling) stands opposite to electricity and electrical current reversal (Uranus). Because Neptune governs magnetism (with Venus), and Uranus rules electricity, this transit could manifest as peculiar changes in the body's electrical current, or EMF related problems (excess screen use, et al.).

Transit Neptune Opposes Natal Pluto

Neptune and Pluto both govern poisoning, so Neptune-Pluto contacts could signify dangerous hidden poison, mold, bacteria or viruses. This transit may correspond with psychedelic experimentation with LSD, mushrooms, Peyote, etc. Blood transfusions and needles are more prone to contamination. This transit is similar to the conjunction, although not as strong. Sepsis. (Read: *Transit Neptune Opposes Natal Mars.*)

Transit Neptune Opposes South Lunar Node

This means that Neptune will be conjunct the natal North Node! Read for Neptune conjunct North Node. The Nodes are always opposite.

TRANSIT NEPTUNE'S QUINCUNX
Health Potentials for Predisposed Nativities
Transits do not always manifest as health concerns.

The functions of the quincunxed natal planet are secretly influenced by a hidden poison, virus, chemical, mildew or magnetic or supernatural problem. The wonderful thing about Neptune's quincunxes is that you immediately know that there is a probable poison, virus, ghost or parasite at work! However, if not caught, it will go undiagnosed, quietly weakening the patient for years. Where relevant, consider the possibility at this time of supernatural etiology. Do you live above an old grave?

Neptune's quincunx can also signal a slow weakening or atrophy in either the body zone governed by the sign it currently passes through, and/or those of the natal planet and sign that transit Neptune is currently quincunxing.

All quincunxes are sneaky and hard to diagnose. A quincunx of Neptune can signal a possible cellular change brewing secretly, often going undiagnosed or ignored. Neptune is associated with some kinds of metastasizing tumors and cancers (with the help of Saturn, Jupiter, Nodes, or Pluto).

The quincunx of Neptune is best observed with an orb of 1°. This planet will revisit this degree, hanging around for months.

Transit Neptune Quincunx Natal Sun

The vitality is drained from an unknown source. Search for a hidden virus, mildew chemical, poison, or depressed or ill person. Consider supernatural etiology (ghost, psychic draining, etc.) The heart may be weakened by a concealed parasite, virus, mold, alcohol, drug or poison. Leaking or weakened valves are typical. Fluidic conditions can weaken the heart or brain. Eyesight may weaken. Use orb of no more than 1°.

Herbal Note: If relevant, this is a good time to fortify the heart muscle, and valves with heart tonifying herbs: Hawthorne, Stone Root, et al. Do not self-treat.

Transit Neptune Quincunx Natal Moon

The brain chemistry is affected in ways hard to diagnose. Neptune rules fluids, drugs and opiates. One may feel uneasy without knowing why. A medication may be slowly disturbing normal brain or lymphatic function. Check for hidden poisoning, memory lapses, fluidic leaks, valve leakage, hidden water on brain or paranoia without known cause. If suffering infertility at this time, look to Neptune for hidden clues.

This transit can signal the onset of hidden cysts or tumors anywhere in the body, but classic to brain, uterus, breasts, stomach or lung. Use orb of no more than 1°.

Herbal Note: Assist the lymphatic filtration of the brain: Periwinkle, Ginkgo, Betony, (brain); Sage, Rosemary (memory); and breasts: Dandelion Root, Poke Root, Red Clover (breasts). These last are also excellent for assisting the general lymphatics, as is Mullein: Do not self-treat.

Transit Neptune Quincunx Natal Mercury

The nerves may have some difficulty receiving and/or interpreting incoming data. Synapses are effected. Sensory information may be addled. Neural coordination problems, clumsy hands or slurred speech. Breathing may weaken, depriving the body of oxygen.

This aspect can cause mental lapses or the onset of dementia. Inappropriate sleeping or trance states. Nerve enervation may be reduced in the body region governed by the sign of natal Mercury, producing strange effects. Lymphatic clearance of chemicals is slowed. Be very careful with medication and dosage!

A perfect time to research the influence upon one's symptoms of magnets, magnetic fields, computers, cell phones, WIFI, the neighbor's radio dish, and the like. May indicate the onset of neurological decline.

This is the type of transit where the doctor keeps telling you that you have no problem, but you know that you do! In this case, look to transit Neptune's sign position for clues, noting the body parts that sign rules.

Herbal Note: See *Transit Neptune Conjunct Natal Mercury*.

Transit Neptune Quincunx Natal Venus

Strange effects, unsuspected poisoning or hard to diagnose issues of ovary, kidneys or veins. This aspect can signal hidden changes in ovarian or kidney cells. Potentials increase for odd sexual fantasies or changes of sexual inclinations. Supernatural-sexual problems, e.g. entity inspired dreams or ghostly visitation. Secret admirers, wanted or otherwise. Peeping Toms.

Attempts to secretly influence the object of affection (the native) through magic or hypnosis. If hair is falling out or skin is changing, look for clues in the sign of transit Neptune.

A pleasant experiment—"Just try it once!"—turns into a serious addiction without being acknowledged as such. Unacknowledged addictions to sugar, wine, sex, fantasy, music or movies.

Transit Neptune Quincunx Natal Mars

Muscles and motor nerves may weaken without known cause. Timing and muscular coordination and contraction may be "off."

Accident prone and clumsy. Blood cell changes. Hidden anemia or bleeding, blood cell integrity affected, possible leukemia (rare).

Strange sexual effects; clandestine affairs and temptations; crossing the tracks in any number of illicit ways without intending to do so; drunken blackouts; excesses, especially for males. Be wary of alcohol and boating, surfing, scuba diving, secret sex and drugs.

This is a very important transit and may signal the onset of puzzling blood deficiency or muscular atrophy issues. Sexually active people can contract an STD without knowing it.

Supernatural-sexual encounters, misuse of music, latent virus, slowly spreading bacteria or virus, sepsis, blood poisoning from unknown source, accidental body fluid transference of contagion (use extreme caution with needles, blood and sperm banks), viral issues that remain latent for months. This transit suggests accidents due to carelessness, drugs, alcohol or sleep-walking.

Because Mars is thought to rule the bone marrow, there could be a mysterious disturbance to marrow production or blood cells. Be very careful with medication and dosage! Immune insufficiency.

Herbal Note: See *Transit Neptune Conjunct Natal Mars.*

Transit Neptune Quincunx Natal Jupiter

May disturb pituitary, pancreatic, liver function, or blood. May indicate hidden tumors or cysts on liver or pituitary (rare). Effects would be baffling to doctors. For clues, consider the signs involved. May produce odd changes in blood chemistry or hormones. May relax the arteries.

This transit can signal plethora of blood and engorgement from hidden cause, fluidic problems, secret hepatitis, undiagnosed virus in liver or blood. The liver may be slowly weakening from an unknown cause, unconscious behavior or alcoholism. Beware smoking "safe" herbs that are secretly laced with chemical field sprays. This is the time when, unknown to us, a poison or plastic is quietly working away at weakening the liver, pituitary or pancreas function. May signal onset of cellular change in liver or pancreas (rare, and requiring multiple planetary testimonies).

Transit Neptune Quincunx Natal Saturn

This is a prime time to watch for an unnoticed calcium and mineral depletion. Osteopenia can develop. Some body part or organ quietly weakens. For some, this transit could indicate a felt instability, vertigo, "trick knee," falls or spinal subluxations.

In children, this transit may signal a sudden halt to normal growth or development, or conversely, an age-inappropriate surge! Teeth may grow in strangely. Broken bones may set incorrectly. Regulation and timing of bodily processes or larger life cycles may be interrupted. This aspect signals a secret weakening of structural integrity. A feeling of insecurity.

Field Note: Three healthy, athletic friends were recently stunned by their unexpected diagnoses of advanced osteoporosis. It is notable that two were men, as this condition is uncommon to males. All were born with natal Neptune in quincunx to natal Saturn by sign.

Transit Neptune Quincunx Natal Uranus

Mysterious disturbances to electrical rhythm. May influence the thyroid gland. Consider the signs involved of both transit Neptune and natal Uranus.

Transit Neptune Quincunx Natal Pluto

Neptune and Pluto both signify parasites and poisons (of different types). Therefore, this aspect can signal hidden parasites, sepsis or blood poisoning. This aspect warns of unsuspected contagion or underestimated issues that may kill, if ignored—e.g. that unseen tick or spider bite that later endangers the life; toxic shock from a tampon (toxic shock syndrome), unrecognized bubonic plague, the fever after the salad bar, etc.

Never lightly regard a minor bite, fever or strange symptom under a close-orb quincunx of transit Neptune to natal Pluto! Dispose of bodily fluids with great care, and avoid dead animals or fish. This aspect could warn of contagion through organ, skin or blood transplant/transfusion. Gangrene. Avoid traditionally dangerous foods (e.g. old fish). Strongest within an orb of 1°.

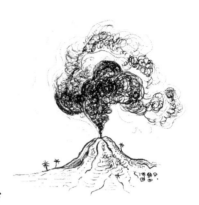

Chapter 17
PLUTO
Temperature Extremes

Properties, Rulerships and Actions

There are two fundamental considerations to keep in mind when looking at the impact that transit Pluto has on the health of the native. First, astrologers, current to this writing, are still getting acquainted with Pluto, as he was discovered in 1930. With an orbital period of 248 years, astrologers have only been able to observe Pluto in half the signs. Therefore, it is wise to approach interpreting the influence of Pluto with humility and a spirit of discovery.

The second important thing to consider is that most people will not experience the effects of a Pluto transit. This may be due to its incredible distance from the Earth (averaging 40 times the distance of the Earth from the Sun) combined with its diminutive size—it would take 22 Plutos to match the mass of tiny Mercury, and 7,000 Plutos to match Neptune. Additionally, Pluto's orbit roams far afield of the ecliptic plane, the geocentric pathway of the "original" Ptolemaic planets of ancient astrology.

The great American prophet and medical psychic, Edgar Cayce, stated that Pluto did not influence all persons, but was gradually gaining in impact since the time of its discovery in 1930. My observations have confirmed this. However, when this tiny lightweight exactly conjoins by transit a natal planet within a tight orb of 1°, its influence so often outweighs all other current transits! (See the special note on this below in the *"Transit Orb"* section.)

This phenomenon was first discovered and imparted to me by Arthur Young, the significant physicist who solved the flight dynamics of the Bell Helicopter. Alerted, I've watched Pluto's exact transit conjunctions of natal planets for decades, and can whole-heartedly corroborate Young's finding.

Consensus Rulership: Scorpio (co-rules with Mars)

However, Mars' traditional rulership of Scorpio is not displaced just because Pluto was discovered, and modern astrologers assigned this celestial body to Scorpio. The best case for Pluto's assignation to Scorpio was presented by researcher Fritz Brunhuber in his book *Pluto*, 1934, republished in English by the A.F.A. Inc. in 1966.

Exalted: Pluto is thought to be exalted in Leo.

However, there are good arguments for Taurus, now assigned to its detriment because this sign is opposite Scorpio.

Detriment: Taurus (debatable)

Fall: Aquarius

Metal: Possibly Plutonium *(M. Urquart)* and Radium *(Brunhuber)*

Minerals: Radium, as an alkaline Earth metal.

Brunhuber suggests this correlation for contemplation and further research. Plutonium, an actinide metal. Sulphur *(unique to Davidson)*. Brunhuber suggests obsidian.

Vitamins: Unknown

Cosmic Ray and Gem: Unknown.

This author suggests infrared. However, infrared is already assigned to the Lunar South Node in the Jyotish tradition. Why cannot both vibrate infrared?

Body Rulerships: Unknown.

May rule some aspect of the DNA molecule. Almost everything we know about the DNA and genetic codes has come to light shortly after the discovery of Pluto. He may have some association with the lymphatic system, blood cells or marrow (an educated guess). Research needs to be directed to these topics. Brunhuber suggests Pluto as the ruler of the pineal gland, an honor the great medical psychic Edgar Cayce gave to Mercury. Brunhuber also suggests that Pluto influences a seat of vital force found at the "nape" of the neck (presumably, the medulla).

General Action: Pluto is a tiny, mustard colored celestial body, at the far reaches of the Solar system. Although frequently compared in influence to Mars, we note significant differences!

Pluto's symptoms run chronic whereas Mar's maladies are acute. For instance, Mars brings the beesting with potential for anaphylaxis, whereas the flesh-eating spider bite that goes septic is more akin to Pluto!

Pluto's deeply ingrained diseases can go latent for years (such as syphilis or Lyme disease), surfacing when awakened by transits or other factors. Or, they behave like HIV, slowly morphing into new forms and deadly. Sepsis leading to gangrene would be a prime example of an unchecked transit Pluto influence hard at work.

Pluto researcher Brunhuber mentions Pluto's penchant for "rays," and their many healing uses. The introduction of radiation and chemotherapy for cancer treatment have occurred since Pluto's discovery in 1930. Initially, these intense therapies destroy healthy cells in order to kill the cancerous cells while they are at it. This is a perfect Plutonian logic, as Pluto shows no mercy.

Pluto may possibly govern stem cell, marrow and organ part transplants, gender reassignment and all manner of tampering about with DNA, including Frankenfood (i.e. genetically modified).

AIDS was discovered in 1981 coincident with Pluto's entrance into Scorpio in 1983, the very sign which implicates body fluid exchanges. The Scorpio period inducted the plague gone wild, and a defined etiology.

Neptune conceals, and Pluto reveals. Pluto's deep heat boils up long-hidden issues to the surface. One often sees the reappearance of a long-lost parent or discovery of a sunken ship under Pluto's exact transit.

His actions work deep down at the cellular level and are drastic, invading, and septic. Pluto may signal physical invasions of pathogenic bacteria, or the onset of plagues. Pluto's exact-orb transit is often witnessed in amputation, transfusion and introduction of drastic life saving measures.

Gangrene is certainly related to Saturn, the Nodes, and Pluto.

Radiation poisoning may belong to this planet. Pluto is probably involved in many kinds of cellular change, including cancer.

The desire for synthetic hormone therapies or steroid use may be related to an exact transit of Pluto to natal Venus or Mars. These therapies have gained speed after Pluto's discovery.

It is important to mention that the great medical psychic Edgar Cayce stated that not all people were influenced by Pluto, and that its influence was growing stronger since its discovery in 1930.

Positive: Pluto can give supernatural strength and courage, an indomitable will, remarkable healing ability, surgical genius.

This planet could be associated with all manner of new medical treatments, especially those involving body part transplants, DNA, radiation, lasers, and gender reassignment. Miraculous healing and intervention: "Nobody understands how his malignant tumors simply vanished!"

Negative: Sepsis, malignancy, chronic hidden maladies, plagues, destruction to cells, sociopathic coldness, mortal danger.

Field Notes: Tradition notes that any planet rising at birth will stamp itself upon the physiognomy and character *(see my book "The Astrological Body Types")*. The below entertaining observations offer priceless instruction into the nature of Pluto's true influence.

Five of my close friends were born with Pluto exactly rising (with four in Leo and one in Virgo). For starters, all five have Herculean muscular strength. Two possess supernatural powers in this regard.

All five are emotional extremists. This varies from Uranus' mental extremes. They all possess the curious trait of banishing a family member, spouse or friend forever, for trivial transgressions, without either sentimentality or remorse. Truly, Pluto is the higher octave of angry Mars. Mars forgets and forgives, but never Pluto!

Four of them chose intensely physical occupations in the healing arts: Rolfer, Physical Therapist, and Hospice Manager, and a Massage Therapist who had first considered a career as an ambulance technician. The fifth also became involved in the healing arts. All five achieved mastery of their respective medical fields.

Curiously, all five ladies enjoy being in the deep woods alone, four having lived fearlessly for years in that state (Pluto is the farthest out planet). Brunhuber's research supports this trait for Pluto in the 1st house: "...Always full of riddles and secrets, an inaccessible person with whom it is almost impossible to maintain a friendship...," and, "If Pluto is near the Ascendant, they have enormous power to force their way through life...."

All five evince immense courage in the face of their own death, or surgery, or that of others, appearing to find these events interesting instead of scary. All five are extremely fit and body conscious. "I'd rather be dead than fat," said one, who proceeded to kill herself with an extreme diet. Here are a few examples to illustrate these points:

The first was a slight woman in her late forties, born with Pluto exactly rising in Virgo. I looked on in disbelief as she plucked up a large, obstinate pig named Pablo, and threw him into the back of her truck with no more aplomb than had he been a dachshund. While working as a lighthouse keeper, the strapping young men of her crew would call for her whenever they needed to lift something really heavy!

A second woman I knew was born with Pluto exactly rising in Leo. One day she encountered an injured wild bobcat, huddling in her yard. He allowed her to place him in a cage without fuss. At the vet's, he morphed into a spitting nightmare.

A third natal Pluto-rising-in Leo case leapt from her car one night, futilely attempting to resuscitate a deceased car crash victim, still lying in the intersection. She appeared emotionally unfazed by this stunning event, recounted to me only minutes later with no more excitement than had she just raked up the leaves.

The similarity of their unusual characteristics, when bundled, are truly astonishing. Pluto's influence when closely ascending at birth appears productive of Olympian strength and courage, indomitability, interest in death and danger, profound healing talent, the proclivity for long periods of solitude (while being perfectly sociable in company), and emotional extremism ranging from unselfish heroism to sociopathic coldness. My cases second many of Brunhuber's findings. However, I am cherry-picking his quotes. Those interested in more character detail for Pluto in all positions should read Brunhuber's seminal work, *Pluto*.

Transit Orb: The brilliant physicist Arthur M. Young privately imparted to me that his personal astrological research revealed that Pluto possessed almost no transit influence except when found within a tight 0-1° orb of a natal planet, at which time its influence on the life would overpower that of all other current transits! My cases have shown Young's rule to be exactly right.

Although transit Pluto has a tiny orb, the aspects it makes are felt long-term. Pluto is the slowest planet. Its transit moves back and forth over a natal planet several times for two to three years, slowly going in and out of orb.

Pluto's station is extremely strong, doubling his impact for 1-3 days. In general, a stationing malefic is pathologically "worse." Thus, we can deduce that Pluto will be more dangerous when it stations within 1° of any natal planet, most especially a "personal planet" (Venus, Mercury, Mars), a "light" (Sun, Moon), or a Lunar Node.

Temperature and Moisture Levels: Extreme cold (Buryl Payne Ph.D.) and extreme heat on a deep cellular level, not surface fever. I have observed that the "Plutonian" person either simmers hot beneath the surface or glows ice cold!

This opinion is supported by Brunhuber, who suggested that Pluto was both Fiery and Watery at the same time. However, Fire and Water either conflict with one another or cancel each other out. Thus, more work is necessary to settle the question of moisture attribution.

The late significant physicist Buryl Payne, Ph.D. statistically observed Pluto's role in large storms. He determined that Pluto was influential in producing extreme cold on Earth. Payne's work provides our first useful proof of Pluto's role in temperature. Davidson errs toward intense heat: "In Pluto's aspects you want antipyreticness; you want anything that will lessen the temperature and the internal feverish tendency." *("Pluto," Davidson, pg 134.)*

PLUTO THROUGH THE ELEMENTS & SIGNS
Health Potentials for Predisposed Nativities
Transits do not always manifest as health concerns or benefits.

Applicable to both natal and transit charts, these partial lists of expressed symptoms apply only to predisposed nativities and with multiple testimonies. Even then, as discussed previously, most people will not feel the effects of transit Pluto.

Manifestation of symptoms may be enhanced by lifestyle choices, and taking preemptive measures can reduce, remove or prevent potential issues from manifesting. It is not possible to list all potential expressions.

Pluto was discovered in 1930 when it was transiting Cancer. Since its orbital period is 248 years, astrologers have not yet had the opportunity to study his influence in every sign, and even then, during only one transit of the sign.

At the time of this writing, Pluto has made it half way around the ecliptic to Capricorn. Therefore, the descriptions provided below will be necessarily based on limited observation and on theory. We have much study to do on the effects of Pluto. The following ideas are not well researched and therefore, hypothetical.

Pluto in Fire Signs
Aries: In exceptionally rare cases, Pluto in this sign may potentize cellular changes in the brain or eyes, or bizarre genetic diseases within the Aries body zone of possible karmic origins.

Leo: In exceptionally rare cases, Pluto in Leo may potentize cellular changes in the sheath of the spinal cord, heart, thoracic spine or present bizarre genetic diseases of possible karmic origin within the Leo zone.

Sagittarius: In very rare cases, Pluto may potentize cellular changes in the spinal cord, neural coordination, voluntary nervous system, muscular system, coccyx, hips, femurs, thighs. In exceptional circumstances, this transit (or natal placement) could suggest bizarre or unprecedented genetic diseases of possible karmic origin in these same regions (such as neuromuscular diseases). Hyperactivity, panic.

Pluto in Earth Signs

Taurus: In very rare cases, Pluto in Taurus may potentize cellular change in the throat, ears, teeth, lower jaw, neck, cervical vertebra, tongue, saliva glands, tonsils, upper esophagus, lips, mouth, vocal cords, larynx, thyroid, parathyroid, thymus. In exceptional circumstances, this transit (or natal placement) could suggest bizarre or unprecedented genetic diseases of possible karmic origin in these same regions.

Virgo: In very rare cases, Pluto in Virgo may potentize cellular changes in the pancreas, spleen, appendix, duodenum, liver, upper intestine, transverse colon. In exceptional circumstances, this transit (or natal placement) could suggest bizarre or unprecedented genetic diseases of possible karmic origin in these same regions. If symptoms present, this transit may signal a parasite infestation of the upper digestive organs. Pluto in Virgo may also suggest autoimmune diseases of the intestines.

Capricorn: In very rare cases, Pluto in Capricorn may potentize cellular changes in the skin, bones, knees, ligaments, tendons, (or areas ruled by opposite sign Cancer). In exceptional circumstance, this transit (or natal placement) may suggest bizarre or unprecedented genetic diseases of possible karmic origin in these same regions.

Pluto in Air Signs

Gemini: In very rare cases, Pluto in Gemini may potentize cellular changes in the lungs, nerves, shoulders, hands, capillaries, bodily tubes, coordination, or speech. In exceptional circumstances, this transit (or natal placement) could suggest bizarre or unprecedented genetic diseases of possible karmic origin in these same regions.

Libra: In very rare cases, Pluto in Libra may potentize cellular changes in the kidneys, adrenals, ovaries or testes. In exceptional circumstances, this transit (or natal placement) could suggest bizarre or unprecedented genetic diseases of possible karmic origin in these same regions, or influence kidney filtration.

Aquarius: In very rare cases, Pluto in Aquarius may potentize cellular changes in the veins, blood, spinal cord, cones of eyes, lower leg, ankle, blood cells. In exceptional circumstances, this transit (or natal placement) could suggest bizarre or unprecedented genetic diseases of possible karmic origin in these same regions.

Pluto in Water Signs

Cancer: In very rare cases, Pluto in Cancer may potentize cellular changes in the breasts, stomach, pituitary gland, lower lung, mucous membrane, uterus, thoracic duct, meninges, membranes of lungs or heart. In exceptional circumstances, this transit (or natal placement) could suggest bizarre or unprecedented genetic diseases of possible karmic origin in these same regions. Paranoia caused by past life memory-recall is common for those sensitive to Pluto's rays.

Scorpio: In very rare cases, Pluto in Scorpio warns of cellular changes in the bladder, genitals, colon, pelvis, rectum, anus, sweat glands, nose, or excretory system. In exceptional circumstances, this transit (or natal placement) could suggest bizarre or unprecedented genetic diseases of possible karmic origin in these same regions. Parasites and STDs are common for this sign position for those sensitive to Pluto's rays.

Pisces: In rare cases, Pluto in Pisces may potentize cellular changes in the lymphatic system, cellular matrix, or feet. In exceptional circumstances, this transit (or natal placement) could suggest bizarre or unprecedented genetic diseases of possible karmic origin in these same regions.

Spirit possession is of concern with this transit for those weak, selfless persons who psychically place themselves in harms way. Pluto in Pisces can correspond with past life memory-recall problems, pathological fear, psychic parasites and sexual-psychic control.

PLUTO'S TRANSIT OF NATAL PLANETS
Health Potentials for Predisposed Nativities

Transits do not always manifest as health concerns or benefits.

Applicable to both natal and transit charts, these partial lists of expressed symptoms apply only to predisposed nativities and with multiple testimonies. Even then, as discussed previously, most people will not feel the effects of transit Pluto.

Manifestation of symptoms may be enhanced by lifestyle choices, and taking preemptive measures can reduce, remove or prevent potential issues from manifesting. It is not possible to list all potential manifestations.

The descriptions provided below will be necessarily brief because astrologers have not yet observed Pluto complete one round of signs, being about half way through at the time of this writing. Nobody is expert on Pluto's effects. All statements below are based on limited observation and theory. We will review in detail only the conjunction aspect, because it is the most likely to be felt.

PLUTO'S CONJUNCTIONS

Transit Pluto Conjunct Natal Sun

Deeply energizing. Those who know how to use Pluto's energy could revitalize their battery with vital force. This long-term aspect is potent within a 1° orb. Effects are more typically psychological and spiritual. In rare cases, there may be a threat of death should the natal Sun receive exceptional additional transit stress.

In rare cases, this transit may potentize cellular changes in the brain, eye or heart (or to one's father or husband). In exceptional circumstances, this transit (or natal placement) could suggest the onset of bizarre or unprecedented genetic diseases of possible karmic origin.

Transit Pluto Conjunct Natal Moon

This long-term aspect is potent within a 1° orb. Effects are more typically psychological and spiritual. In rare cases, there may be a threat of death should the natal Moon receive exceptional transit stress. In rare cases, this transit may potentize cellular changes in the brain, eye, stomach, breast, uterus, mucous membrane, lung, meninges, membranes of heart or lung.

In exceptional circumstances, this transit (or natal placement) could suggest the onset of bizarre or unprecedented genetic diseases of possible karmic origin in these same regions. Female hormones could undergo significant change over a long period. This transit's influence often tends to relate more to one's mother or wife than to oneself.

This is an excellent period to obtain assistance to overcome addictions (before they overcome you).

Transit Pluto Conjunct Natal Mercury

This period is excellent for students of medicine, chemistry, surgery, anatomy, diagnosis, homeopathy, medical astrology. Diagnostic abilities are greatly enhanced. The mental force and mentation are intensified. This transit is highly productive for geniuses, but dangerous for some mental states. Latent viruses or bacteria hiding in nervous system may awaken. Effects are more typically psychological and spiritual. This long-term aspect is potent within a 1° orb.

In exceptionally rare cases, this aspect may potentize cellular changes in the brain or nerves, or ears. Speech may be affected. In exceptional circumstances, this transit (or natal placement) could suggest the onset of bizarre or unprecedented genetic diseases of possible karmic origin in these same regions, or within the sign of natal Mercury.

Transit Pluto Conjunct Natal Venus

This long-term transit is potent within a 1° orb. Effects are typically psychological and spiritual. In exceptionally rare cases, this aspect may potentize cellular changes in the ovaries, kidneys, lips, breasts, veins, female genitalia, and possibly skin. In exceptional circumstances, this transit (or natal placement) could suggest the onset of bizarre or unprecedented genetic diseases of possible karmic origin in these same regions. Significant changes to sexual hormones and libido are typical with long term effects.

Although, most will experience no effects, this transit may correspond to notable health changes, life threatening illness, or death in the lives of female friends of relatives.

Field Note: In the years when Pluto exactly crossed the Venus of one case study, this individual lost to death two ex-spouses plus fifteen additional close friends, family and acquaintances. Obviously, this was an extreme manifestation of Pluto's "death and rebirth" principal and not the expected outcome for most charts!

Transit Pluto Conjunct Natal Mars

This conjunction can intensify sexual instincts and desires. The entire panoply of survival instincts is amplified. And yet, this transit offers the native an opportunity for spiritual decision in regards to these urges. Pluto-Mars can act to enhance the spiritual will power necessary to conquer chronic disease "I'm not a statistic!". One witnesses this same quality in Scorpio natives (recall the famous double Scorpio spoon-bender Uri Geller.)

This long-term aspect is potent within an orb of 1°. Significant and long-term changes can occur with the male hormones. The adrenal gland is stressed.

Together, these planets signal bacterial invasion of an especially dangerous species. In rare cases: frostbite, gangrene, amputation.

Pluto can be both a killer and a radical life-saver when joined with Mars! If under exceptional stress with collaborating testimonies, there is a threat of accident or surgery. Can provides courage, determination, fearlessness and toughness. Excellent for overcoming dangerous illness with the power of will, belief and thought.

Davidson links these two planets in concert with terrible, intense inflammation, deep seated. Brunhubner says this combination gives fermentation and putrefaction.

In exceptionally rare cases, Pluto's transit may potentize cellular changes in the nose, male genitals, prostate, genitourinary system, adrenals, red blood cells, muscles, or process of bodily excretion, sweat, or could suggest bizarre or unprecedented genetic diseases of possible karmic origin in these same regions.

Surgical and Medical Tips: Beware of exceptional reactions to beestings and medications. This transit can enhance the adrenal and immune responses, aka anaphylaxis.

Transit Pluto Conjunct Natal Jupiter

This long-term transit is potent within a 1° orb. Effects are typically manifest psychologically and spiritually. In exceptionally rare cases, this transit may potentize cellular changes in the pituitary, liver or arteries. In obscure cases, Pluto's transit can suggest bizarre or unprecedented genetic diseases of possible karmic origin in these same regions or in the sign of natal Jupiter.

If positive, this aspect brings heightened energy and spiritual faith are available now for heroically overcoming serious issues. This transit can produce both religious manias and great healing miracles of faith.

Transit Pluto Conjunct Natal Saturn

This long-term transit is potent within a 1° orb. Effects are typically manifest psychologically and spiritually. In exceptionally rare cases, this transit may potentize cellular changes in the bones, skin, tendons, ligaments, nerves, hearing. In obscure cases, Pluto's transit (or natal placement) may suggest bizarre or unprecedented genetic diseases of possible karmic origin in these same regions. If felt by the native, this is a life changing aspect, sometimes positive (the surgery relieves the karma).

This transit heralds in an ideal time to purge out toxic metal, lead or mineral accretions in the body parts ruled by natal Saturn's sign.

Transit Pluto Conjunct Natal Uranus

This long-term transit is potent within a 1° orb. Effects are typically manifest psychologically and spiritually. For some, it may exert a significant effect on the little-known electrical system of the human body and/or the distribution of finer energies moving into and through the chakras.

In rare cases, suggests bizarre or unprecedented genetic diseases of possible karmic origin in these same regions.

Transit Pluto Conjunct Natal Neptune

This long-term transit is potent within a 1° orb. Effects are typically manifest psychologically and spiritually. In rare cases, this aspect may potentize cellular changes in the lymph, or in the bodily regions governed by the sign of natal Neptune. In obscure cases, this transit may suggest bizarre or unprecedented genetic diseases of possible karmic origin in these same regions.

Spirit possession is a concern for weak and predisposed individuals. Dementia or Alzheimer's may be a consideration. Those whom are addicted to alcohol or opioids are entering a danger zone where overdose is more likely. This is a time for exceptional caution with anesthesia, medication, venoms, poisons, gas. Heightened vigilance is called for regarding the psychic influences entering one's mind, including from the media.

Transit Pluto Conjunct Natal Pluto

This transit, or "Pluto Return," will not occur within a person's lifetime because Pluto's orbital period is 248 years.

Transit Pluto Conjunct Natal North Node

Recall that Pluto rules temperature extremes. Pluto's transit of the North Node signifies an influx into the bodily system of either deep, slow, stimulating heat, or, conversely, intense cold.

Astral temperature extremes could manifest in a great number of interesting ways over a long period of time, either in general or specific to the bodily region ruled by the sign of natal North Node. These changes could include tissue inflammation, sepsis, hyperoxidation, cellular change, metabolism changes, cancer, hormonal or DNA changes. This long-term transit is important within a 1° orb. Effects are typically psychological and spiritual. If relevant, consider supernatural etiology.

In rare cases, this transit could be a precursor to genetic, rare or unprecedented disease. Because the North Node is the prime entry point for celestial energy, this transit provides an enhanced opportunity for bacterial or parasite invasion and STDs. Obviously, this is no time to visit a plague zone.

In some cases, Pluto's arrival at the North Node would signal the arrival of a life-saving new therapy, such as a stem cell transplant or new type of laser. Pluto appears to be associated with all manner of fluid transfusions or organ transplants, including cadaver grafts, fecal transplants, etc.

Surgical and Medical Tips: Pluto's transit of the North Node signals a surfeit and enhancement of Pluto's incoming rays, dangerously potentizing effects of chemo, hormone and radiation therapy. Doses should be carefully monitored at this time!

Herbal Note: This may be a perfect time for deep, powerful cleansing of the lymph, blood, cells. The pink-magenta-colored blood cleansing herbs come to mind: Poke Root, Red Root, Beets, Grapes, Seaweeds, and Red Clover. Sanicle is excellent for clearing morbid secretions. Do not self-treat.

Transit Pluto Conjunct Natal South Node

This long-term transit is important within a 1° orb. Effects are typically psychological and spiritual, and most people will experience no effects. Pluto at the South Node warns of "danger from Pluto." Those with drug addictions move into a danger zone.

This is perhaps the most dangerous time for channeling spirits, taking psychotropic herbs or psychedelics, or any activity that loosens the psychic boundaries.

This transit can awaken mental illness and psychiatric problems (especially depression, addictions, and paranoia). The old memories leak from the deep unconscious to the upper level of the subconscious, thus influencing the conscious mind. Spontaneous past-life recall may occur for those so open. The transit may suggest the entry of dangerous parasites, bacteria, STDs or even nefarious astral entities (similar to Pluto conjunct North Node).

Conversely, Pluto's transit of the South Node could assist a powerful cleansing release of toxins, evil cells, and the like. The pores open. This transit is profoundly diuretic, diaphoretic, and cathartic. If relevant, consider supernatural etiology.

At this time, the native faces a spiritual choice. He or she can summon their spiritual willpower to overcome their weaknesses and fears. If not, the fears and bad habits may overcome them! Pluto, Mars and Saturn all produce this same effect at the South Node, albeit the type of choice is different in each case.

Herbal Note: Potent herbs may be an "undoing" at this time. Step carefully, and watch doses. Be alert for copious or dangerous secretions, internal bleeding, and parasites. Do not self treat.

Surgical and Medical Tips: Hypothetically, this is a dangerous time for hormonal therapy, lasers, chemotherapy, radiation, blood transfusions, organ or marrow transplants, fecal transplants and the like. The effects may not go as planned or produce unexpectedly intense side effects. However, the treating physician remains the authority on the necessity and timing of these treatments. Psychiatric patients must be watched closely.

Transit Pluto Conjunct Natal Ascendant

This long-term aspect can be important within a 1° orb. Effects are typically psychological and spiritual. The problem is that the exact degree of the Ascendant is rarely known with certainty (who stood by with an atomic clock at your first breath for the purpose of an accurate birth chart?). Therefore, it is difficult to anticipate the timing of potential effects, making only approximate time frames possible. However, if someone experiences relevant "Plutonian" symptoms as Pluto hovers near their assumed Ascendant degree, then they can use that information in the analysis of causes and potential interventions.

In very rare cases with more planetary testimonies, this transit can mark the onset of a dangerous illness or potential death (I have witnessed this). However, most people need not worry!

Speaking of Ascendants, Pluto's exact quincunx to a known Ascendant degree could suggest a sneaky parasite or poison issue, coming from the bodily zone ruled by the sign of transit Pluto as affecting the bodily zone governed by the natal Ascendant. *(See the discussion of quincunxes below).*

PLUTO'S SQUARES
Health Potentials for Predisposed Nativities
Transits do not always manifest as health concerns.

Use at 0-1°. If physically effective, this aspect would be far less strong then the conjunction. This is a very long term transit, with results best understood on hindsight. *(See Chapter 3 for delineation of squares by sign combination.)* Here is a helpful formula. Not all transits express themselves as medical issues.

Square Interpreting Formula for Pluto
Transit Pluto slowly and deeply "boils," inflames, intensifies, purifies (or conversely putrefies) the functions of the natal planet he squares
_____ *(name that planet, and its specific functions)*; from the bodily regions governed by the sign he currently is transiting _____
(give that sign, and the bodily regions it governs).

PLUTO'S OPPOSITIONS
Transits do not always express themselves as medical issues.

Use at 0-1°. If physically effective, this aspect will be. less strong then the conjunction. This is a long term aspect, with effects best understood on hindsight. See *"Chapter 3: Aspect Mechanics"* for delineation of oppositions by sign polarity. Here is a helpful formula.

Opposition Interpreting Formula for Pluto
Transit Pluto in _____ *(give sign and body parts ruled)*, confronts, and then demands regeneration and conscious awareness regarding the meaning of the natal planet he opposes _____
(name that planet); and bodily parts and functions ruled by that planet_____, in the bodily regions ruled by sign of this natal planet _____ *(give the sign and its body parts).*

The nature of this pull, if effective, will be Plutonian, i.e. huge impact, permanent. Manifestations are usually psychological, and only sometimes physical. The entire sign polarity is involved.

PLUTO'S QUINCUNX
Health Potentials for Predisposed Nativities
Transits do not always manifest as health concerns.

Pluto's exact transit quincunx to any natal planet could be useful in understanding odd symptoms arising as related to the function of the quincunxed natal planet. The astrologer can approach the analysis in this way:

Pluto would represent one of the following items: toxins, cellular change, genetic issues, STDs, parasites or bacteria that are concealed somewhere in the bodily region or organs governed by the sign of the currently transiting Pluto. Transits do not always express themselves as medical issues.

Quincunx Interpreting Formula for Pluto

First, list the sign that Pluto is transiting through _____.
Now, list the bodily regions governed by that sign_____.
"Something dangerous" may be lurking somewhere within these bodily regions. This is then seen as influencing the natal planet that Pluto quincunxes,_____*(name that planet)* and one or more of its associated organs and functions_____*(name those organs and functions)*. The sign of this natal planet, and the body regions associated with this sign are also involve. Name those bodily regions

_____.

Maintaining Prudence
Planetary aspects do not always manifest as health concerns or benefits.

Applicable to both natal and transit charts, the partial lists of expressed symptoms in each section apply only to predisposed nativities. These conditions are obviously uncommon and require multiple testimonies beyond the presence of any one celestial body.

Manifestation of symptoms may be enhanced by lifestyle choices, and taking preemptive measures can reduce, remove or prevent potential issues from manifesting.

This material is published for informational purposes only. It is not intended to be a substitute for professional medical advice and should not be relied on as health or personal advice.

EPILOGUE

Cornell's Dream

H. L. Cornell, M.D., the legendary physician who left us the seminal classic *Encyclopedia of Medical Astrology*, fostered a dream shared by many. In his Foreword, he writes:

"...It is my plan to make a World Lecture Tour, and speak before the various Healing Centers and Schools in the U.S.A. and other Nations, and to make an effort to have the various Faculties make Medical Astrology one of the required studies for their students who are aspiring to be Healers..."

"Cornell's Dream," has almost come true with a twist. Although our medical schools, on policy, remain staunchly opposed to Medical Astrology, many members of our exploding alternative healing community are indeed studying and utilizing this ancient science! I've personally taught this subject, both singly and in groups, to a wide array of herbalists, RNs, chiropractors, osteopaths, naturopaths, psychologists, midwives, hypnotherapists and acupuncturists. Occasional clinical physicians also use this system, but keep quiet about it, fearful of rebuke from on high. I've known several personally.

Instead of considering long-established cosmic principles, the current conventional medical community has gone in another direction to correct this lack of what we might call "time awareness" in modern Western medicine. After all, it's common knowledge among the nurses that medical events, psychosis, and hemorrhage increase at full Moon! (Why then, is this fact ignored when booking delicate surgeries?)

Chrono Medicine is a newly recognized field, exploring the impact of biological rhythms, and clock time, upon the commencement of medication. It is puzzling that Medical Astrology, with two thousand years of empirically based "time wisdom," isn't yet invited to this party.

It is obvious that modern Western Medicine has made colossal strides in most aspects of medicine. We all owe a great debt to its courageous practitioners and intrepid researchers. Personally, I would not be here without it, and most of us would be dead by forty without the gifts of hygiene, germ theory, and surgical innovation. However, it is in the knowledge of the unseen patterns *behind* disease, and of the influence of planetary frequencies upon physical bodies, (both imprinted at birth, and current), that this paradigm falls woefully short. And, despite this shortfall, it remains unspoken policy to refuse the substantial insight provided from Medical Astrology!

This mental recalcitrance recalls the great American folk singer Pete Seeger's ode to a stubborn World War II sergeant:

"... We were knee deep in the Big Muddy, but the big fool said to push on...."

It is my dream that the tentative partnership between Medical Astrology and the new sciences, once briefly conflated in the Renaissance, will return for another round. Together, "cosmos-biology" and modern medicine would produce a new, superior medicine, blending chemical-molecular awareness with an acceptance of the astral light frequencies behind apparent physical form, time influences, individuality, and imbalance. A new medicine would be achieved, and thus too, a new Astrology.

Mystical dance, which yonder starry sphere
Of planets and of fixed in all her wheels
Resembles nearest; mazes intricate,
Eccentric, intervolved, yet regular,
Then most, when most irregular they seem;
And in their motions harmony divine,
So smooths her charming tones that God's own ear Listens
delighted.
– Extracted from Milton's Paradise Lost, Book 5, 620-27

BIBLIOGRAPHY
AND SUGGESTED READING

Bhattacharjee, Shivaji, *Astrological Healing Gems*, Passage Press, Salt Lake City, UT, 1990.

Beckman, Howard, *Vibrational Healing with Gems*, Balaji Publishing House, Pecor, NM; Gyan Publishing House, New Delhi, 2000.

Bhattacharya, A. K. and Ramchandra, D. N. *The Science of Cosmic Ray Therapy or Teletherapy*, Firma KLM Private LTD, Calcutta, 1976.

Bhattacharyya Benoytosh, M.A., Ph.D., revised and enlarged by A. K. Bhattacharya, *Gem Therapy*, Firma KLM Private LTD., Calcutta, India 1992.

Brown, Richard, S. G.I.A., *Ancient Astrological Gemstones & Talismans*, A.G.T. Co. Ltd., Publishers, Bangkok, Thailand, 1995.

Blagrave, Joseph, *Blagrave's Astrological Practice of Physick*, London, 1671, edited by David R. Roell, Astrological Classics, 2010.

Cayce, Edgar: *See "Winston"*

Cornell, H.L. M.D., L.L.D., *The Encyclopaedia of Medical Astrology*, Llewellyn Publications and Samuel Weiser, Woodbury, MN, 1972.

Cramer, M.s., Diane, *How to Give an Astrological Health Reading,* The American Federation of Astrologers, Inc., 2005.

Davidson, William, *Davidson's Medical Lectures,* edited by Vivia Jayne, The Astrological Bureau, Monroe, NY, 1979.

Davison, Alison, Metal Power, *The Soul Life of the Planets*, Borderland Sciences Research Foundation, Garberville, CA,1991.

Grey, W. E., *Know Your Magnetic Field*, Christopher Publishing House, Boston, MA, 1947.

Heindel, Max, *Astro-Diagnosis, A Guide to Healing*, 11th edition The Rosicrucian Fellowship, Oceanside, CA, 1928.

Jain, Manik Chand, *The Occult Power of Gems*, Ranjan Publications, New Delhi, India, 1988.

Jansky, Robert Carl, *Modern Medical Astrology*, AstroAnalytics Publications, Van Nuys, CA, 1978.

Johari, Harish, *The Healing Power of Gemstones in Tantra*, Ayurveda, Astrology Destiny Books, Rochester, VT, 1988.

Kapoor, Dr. Gouri Shanker, *Gems & Astrology*, Ranjan Publications, New Delhi, India, 1985.

Kollerstrom, Nick, *The Metal Planet Relationship*, Borderland Sciences Research Foundation, Garberville, CA, 1993.

Light, Phyllis, *Southern Folk Medicine*, North Atlantic Books, 2018.

Millard, Margaret, *Case Notes of a Medical Astrologer*, Red Wheel, Weiser, Boston, MA, 1980.

Montgomery, Ruth, *Born to Heal: The Amazing True Story of Mr. A. and the Astonishing Art of Healing with Life Energies*, Montgomery, AL, 1973.

Nauman, Eileen, *Medical Astrology*, DHM, Blue Turtle Publishing, Cottonwood, AZ, 1982.

Payne, Buryl, Ph.D., "Apparatus For Detecting Emanations From The Planets," The Journal of Borderlands Research Sciences, Vol. XLVI, No. 6, Nov-Dec 1990, pp 7-11.

Popham, Sajah, *Evolutionary Herbalism*, North Atlantic Books, California, 2019.

Ridder-Patrick, Jane, *A Handbook of Medical Astrology*, Penguin Books, London, NY, 1990.

Saha, N. N. Stellar, *Healing: Cure and Control of Diseases Through Gems*, Sagar Publications, New Delhi, 1976.

Simmonite, W. J., *The Arcana of Astrology*, North Hollywood: Symbols & Signs, 1977.

Tansley, David V., D.C., *Radionics & the Subtle Anatomy of Man*, Health Sciences Press, Bradford, Devon, Holsworthy, England, 1972.

Starck, Marcia, *Healing with Astrology*, Crossing Press, 1997.

Tarnas, Richard, *The Passion of the Western Mind*, Ballantine Books Edition, 1993, by arrangement with Harmony Books, a division of Crown Publishers, Inc, NY.

Uyldert, M., *Metal Magic: The Esoteric Properties and Uses of Metals*, Turnstone Press Limited, UK, 1980.

Westlake, Aubrey T., M.D., *The Pattern of Health*, Shambhalla, Berkeley and London, 1973.

Winston, Shirley Rabb, *Music as the Bridge*, based on the Edgar Cayce Readings, A.R.E. Press, Virginia Beach, VA, 1972.

Wood, Matthew, *The Practice of Traditional Herbalism*, North Atlantic Books, Berkeley, CA, 2004.

Wood, Matthew, Francis Bonaldo, and Phyllis Light, *Traditional Western Herbalism and Pulse Evaluation*, Lulu Publishing, 2004.

Wood, Matthew, with David Ryan, *The Earthwise Herbal Repertory*, North Atlantic Books, Berkeley, CA, 2017.

Yogananda, Paramahansa, *The Bhagavad Gita, Royal Science of God-Realization*, verse 29 p. 634, Self-Realization Fellowship, Los Angeles, CA, 1996.

Young, Arthur M., *The Geometry of Meaning*, A Merloyd Lawrence Book, Delacorte Press, 1976; and *The Reflexive Universe*, Robert Briggs Associates, Mill Valley, CA, 1976.

More Works by the Author

Books by Judith Hill

The Astrological Body Types, revised and expanded, Stellium Press, 1997.

An illustrated compendium of zodiac sign, planet, element and mode types, includes vast commentary and vocational attributions. Includes fascinating appendixes, including the research of Mars position in redheaded populations, medical nodes.

Medical Astrology: A Guide to Planetary Pathology, Stellium Press, 2005.

Complete A-Z guide. Medical information for Sun, Moon, planets and Lunar Nodes in all signs. Beginning to advanced material and rare topics (surgery, death, medical nodes). Includes one of the most thorough works on safe surgery timing. A "Dave's Top Ten" book by genre.

Astrology & Your Vital Force: Healing with Cosmic Rays and DNA Resonance, Stellium Press, Portland, OR, 2017.

The Sun's Master Cycle, William Gray's healing method, Sun Water for healing use, corroborative research of Buryl Payne, Ph. D, and others. Jyotish gem prescription methods and discussion of styles; zodiac-color theory and use; malefic houses and how to remediate; Moon-planet conjunctions for medicinal use; much more.

Medical Astrology for Health Practitioners, Stellium Press, Portland, OR, 2019.

The Layman's Prequel to Medical Astrology: A Guide to Planetary Pathology. Provides immediately useful method for health practitioners and beginners. "Let's Get Started!"

The Lunar Nodes: Your Key To Excellent Chart Interpretation,
Stellium Press, 2010.

> Includes "The Medical Nodes." Also: South and North Node in houses, signs; transit Nodes to natal planets; transit planets to natal nodes, thorough comparison of Eastern and Western traditions.
>
> A "Dave's Top Ten" book by genre.

Eclipses and You: How to Align with Life's Hidden Tides,
Stellium Press, 2013.

> Includes significant medical sections for eclipses in each sign.

Vocational Astrology: A Complete Handbook of Western Astrological Career Selection and Guidance Techniques,
A. F. A. Inc., 1999.

> Winner of the Paul R. Grell "Best Book Award" for A. F.A., Inc. publications, 1999; A "Dave's Top Ten" book.

A Wonderbook of True Astrological Case Files,
(co-authored with A. Gehrz), Stellium Press, 2012.

The Part of Fortune in Astrology, Stellium Press, 1998.

Astroseismology: Earthquakes and Astrology, Stellium Press, 2000 (research compendium).

The Mars-Redhead Files, Stellium Press, 2000 (research compendium).

Mrs. Winkler's Cure, (by Judith Hill as Julia Holly), Stellium Press, Portland, Oregon, 2010.

> Non-violent fairy tales for the modern age.
> For ages 7-100.

Self-Study Courses for the Independent Student

MEDICAL ASTROLOGY 101
12 Module Course for the Independent Student
Available at: JudithHillAstrology.com
Optional: Final Exam and Certificate of Passage.
See: JudithHillAstrology.com

MEDICAL ASTROLOGY ADVANCED
Available Fall 2019

WEBINAR CLASS
"Astrological Medicine and Renaissance Herbalism"
with Matthew Wood and Judith Hill.
Available at:
The Matthew Wood Institute of Herbal Medicine.
See: JudithHillAstrology.com

Articles by Judith Hill

Judith Hill & Mark W. Polit, "Correlation of Earthquakes with Planetary Placement: The Regional Factor," NCGR Journal, 5 (1), 1987.

Judith A. Hill & Jacalyn Thompson, "The Mars–Redhead Link," NCGR Journal, Winter 88-89 (first published by: Above & Below, Canada; Linguace Astrale (Italy); AA Journal (Great Britain); FAA Journal (Australia).

"The Mars Redhead Link II: Mars Distribution Patterns in Redhead Populations," Borderlands Research Sciences Foundation Journal, Vol. L1, No. 1 (part one) and Vol. L1, No 2 (part 2).

"Commentary on the John Addey Redhead Data," NCGR Journal, Winter 88-89 "Redheads and Mars," The Mountain Astrologer, May 1996

"The Regional Factor in Planetary-Seismic Correlation," Borderlands Research Sciences Foundation Journal, Vol. L1,Number 3, 1995 (reprint courtesy of American Astrology).

"American Redhead's Project Replication," *Correlation*, Volume 13, No 2, Winter 94-95.

"Octaves of Time," *Borderlands Research Journal*, Vol. L1, Number 4, Fourth Quarter, 1995.

"Gemstones, Antidotes for Planetary Weaknesses," *ISIS Journal*, 1994.

"Medical Astrology," *Borderlands Research Journal*, Vol. L11, Number 1, First Quarter, 1996.

"Astrological Heredity," *Borderlands Research Journal*, 1996.

"The Electional and Horary Branches," *Sufism, IAS*, Vol. 1, No 2.

"Astrology: A Philosophy of Time and Space," *Sufism, IAS*, Vol. 1, No 1.

"Natal Astrology," *Sufism, IAS*, Vol. 1, No 3.

"An Overview of Medical Astrology," *Sufism, IAS*, Vol. 1, No 4.

"Predictive Astrology in Theory and Practice," *Sufism, IAS*, Vol. 11, No 1.

"Esoteric Astrology," *Sufism, IAS*, Vol. 11, No 2, 3.

"Mundane Astrology," *Sufism, IAS*, Vol. 11, No 4.

"Vocational Astrology," *Sufism, IAS*, part 1 and 2, Vol. 111, No 1, 2.

"Astro-Psychology," *Sufism, IAS*, Vol. 111, No 3, 4.

"The Planetary Time Clocks," *Sufism, IAS*,
    Vol. 4, No 1, 2, 3, 4.

"Astrophysiognomy," *Sufism, IAS*, Vol. 4, No 1, 2.

"Spiritual Signposts in the Birth Map," *Sufism, IAS*,
    Vol. V, No 2, 3.

"The Philosophical Questions Most Frequently Asked of the
    Astrologer," *Sufism, IAS*, Vol. 5, No 4, Vol. 6, No 1, 2.

"Music and the Ear of the Beholder,"*Sufism, IAS*, 1999.

"The Astrology of Diabetes," *Dell Horoscope*, October 2003.

"A Life Time of Astrology," published interview with
    Judith Hill, by Tony Howard, *The Mountain Astrologer*,
    Nov-Dec, 2010.

"Great Earthquakes of Northeastern Honshu (1900-2011):
    A Planetary Portrait," *The Mountain Astrologer*, 2011.

"The Astrology of Depression," *Skyscript*, 2017.

"The Lost Secrets of Renaissance Medicine," *ANS*,
    (Astrological News Service) 2017.

Judith Hill is a second-generation, and lifetime consulting astrologer, having performed over 9,000 readings to date. She is also an astrological researcher, teacher, publisher and award-winning author of thirteen books. These include her medically relevant titles:
> *Medical Astrology: Your Guide to Planetary Pathology;*
> *Astrology & Your Vital Force: Healing with Cosmic Rays*
>   *and DNA Resonance;*
> *Medical Astrology for Health Practitioners*
and the classic, *The Astrological Body Types.*

Some of her writings have been translated into Russian, Vietnamese, Italian, Lettish and Arabic.

Hill is a Chartered Herbalist with *The Dominion Herbal College.* Judith Hill and Matthew Wood created the Webinar course "Astrological Medicine and Renaissance Herbalism" through *The Matthew Wood Institute of Herbalism*, produced by Tara Baklund.

Judith created the course "Medical Astrology 101" for the independent student and later introduced traditional Western medical astrology to students in Szechuan, China (2017-18).

Hill conceived and co-produced the first exclusively medically oriented astrology conferences in Portland, Oregon:

> "Medical Astrology Day," (with OAA board members, M. Neuner and S. Scott) and obtained sponsorship from AFAN (1992); and "Medical Astrology Day," with the assistance of D. Tramposh (2008).

She later created and produced the annual *Renaissance Medicine Conference©* in Portland, Oregon, pioneering the conflation of medical astrology and herbal-alchemical conferences in the USA.

One of Judith's contributions to medical astrology is her original documentation of the comprehensive medical and physical implications of the Lunar Nodes through both their natal and transit conjunctions to each planet and sign; and also by detailing the medical impact of eclipses through each zodiac sign and in aspect to planets.

Judith served as the Educational Director for the San Francisco Chapter of *The National Council of Geocosmic Research*. She worked for ten years in the statistical study of astrology, receiving an unsolicited research grant from The Institute for the Study of Consciousness; and produced two widely acclaimed research compendiums: "The Mars-Redhead Files" with Jacalyn Thompson, and "Astro-Seismology" with Mark Polit.

As a pioneer in astro-seismology and astro-genetics, she founded *The Redhead Research Project*; Stellium Press ("for stellar minds"), and San Francisco's first "NCGR Research Day" in the late 1980s. Near this time she briefly worked as an astrological research project assistant for the renowned physicist Arthur Young in Berkeley, California, and assisted KCBS radio's Editorial Director Joan Margalith with her pioneering *Infinity* radio show.

As a "road tested" astrologer, Hill successfully matched five charts to five biographies in a 1989 NCGR-sponsored skeptic's challenge, and successfully predicted (and pre-published) the magnitude, general time and location of California's famous "Loma Prieta" earthquake.

Her breakthrough astrogenetic research was featured on television's syndicated program, *Strange Universe*.

Additionally, she segregated and documented the impact of eclipses according to their nodal polarity (North vs. South Node eclipses, for both Solar and Lunar eclipses); and published possibly the first eclipse calendar for astrological use, inclusive of stated nodal polarity. Hill also documented the potential physical and health effects of most transits in her pioneering work *Medical Astrology in Action: the Transits of Health* (2019).

In the 1980's, Hill authored what may be the first serious column on real astrology outside of the popular press, entitled "Astrology, a Philosophy of "Time and Space" for *Sufism Magazine*.

Judith has lectured widely for multiple conferences, groups, podcasts, radio and television shows both inside, and outside of the astrological world. A biographical interview with Judith by noted producer and astrologer Tony Howard was featured in the December, 2010 issue of *The Mountain Astrologer Magazine.*

In her spare time, she is a professional musician and vocalist in multiple genres, producer, sculptor, teacher, tree advocate, illustrator, "roadside anthropologist," and Jewish heritage historian.

JudithHillAstrology.com

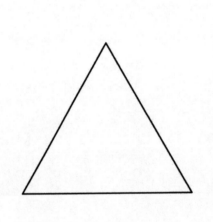

CPSIA information can be obtained
at www.ICGtesting.com
Printed in the USA
LVHW040420290220
648578LV00018B/222

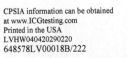